Perioperative Hemodynamic Monitoring and Goal Directed Therapy: From Theory to Practice

Perioperative Hemodynamic Monitoring and Goal Directed Therapy: From Theory to Practice

Edited by

Maxime Cannesson
Professor of Anesthesiology and Perioperative Care,
University of California Irvine, Irvine, CA, USA

and

Rupert Pearse
Professor of Intensive Care Medicine, Queen Mary,
University of London;
Consultant in Intensive Care Medicine,
Barts and The London NHS Trust, London, UK

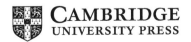

CAMBRIDGE
UNIVERSITY PRESS

University Printing House, Cambridge CB2 8BS, United Kingdom

One Liberty Plaza, 20th Floor, New York, NY 10006, USA

477 Williamstown Road, Port Melbourne, VIC 3207, Australia

314-321, 3rd Floor, Plot 3, Splendor Forum, Jasola District Centre, New Delhi-110025, India

79 Anson Road, #06-04/06, Singapore 079906

Cambridge University Press is part of the University of Cambridge.

It furthers the University's mission by disseminating knowledge in the pursuit of education, learning and research at the highest international levels of excellence.

www.cambridge.org
Information on this title: www.cambridge.org/9781107048171

First published 2014
Reprinted 2015

A catalogue record for this publication is available from the British Library

Library of Congress Cataloging in Publication data
Perioperative hemodynamic monitoring and goal directed therapy : from theory to practice / edited by Maxime Cannesson and Rupert Pearse.
    p. ; cm.
Includes bibliographical references and index.
ISBN 978-1-107-04817-1 (Hardback : alk. paper)
I. Cannesson, Maxime, editor. II. Pearse, Rupert, editor.
[DNLM: 1. Hemodynamics. 2. Monitoring, Physiologic–methods. 3. Perioperative Care. WG 106]
RC670.5.H45
616.1´0754–dc23   2014006286

ISBN 978-1-107-04817-1 Hardback

....

Contents

List of contributors   vii
Foreword – Emanuel P. Rivers   xi
Abbreviations list   xiii

Section 1 – Surgery and Critical Care: Epidemiology and Public Health Approach

1 **Patient outcome following major surgery**   1
Elisa Kam and Rupert Pearse

2 **Statistical methods in hemodynamic research**   8
Yannick Le Manach and Gary Colins

3 **New trends in perioperative medicine**   14
Gautam Kumar, David Walker, and Michael Mythen

4 **The surgical home: a paradigm shift toward perioperative practice**   24
Shermeen B. Vakharia, Zeev N. Kain, and Leslie M. Garson

Section 2 – Cardiovascular Physiology Applied to the Perioperative and Critical Care Settings

5 **Overview of the circulation**   29
Michael R. Pinsky

6 **Cardiac function and myocardial perfusion**   39
Jason H. Chua, Rudolph Nguyen, and Aman Mahajan

7 **Blood pressure regulation**   47
Sheldon Magder

8 **Microcirculation and mitochondrial dysfunction**   56
Daniel De Backer and Diego Orbegozo Cortes

9 **Hemoglobin function and patient blood management**   62
Aryeh Shander, Faraz Syed, and Mazyar Javidroozi

10 **A rational approach to fluid and volume management**   74
Daniel Chappell and Matthias Jacob

11 **Vasopressors and inotropes**   85
Robert H. Thiele and James M. Isbell

12 **Cardiovascular physiology applied to critical care and anesthesia**   95
Nils Siegenthaler and Karim Bendjelid

Section 3 – Hemodynamic Monitoring in the Perioperative Environment

13 **Integrative approach for hemodynamic monitoring**   107
Christoph K. Hofer, Steffen Rex, and Michael T. Ganter

14 **Evaluation of a cardiac output monitor**   120
Lester A. H. Critchley

15 **Invasive hemodynamic monitoring systems**   132
Paul E. Marik

16 **Semi-invasive and non-invasive hemodynamic monitoring systems**   146
Cédric Carrié, Mathieu Sèrié, and Matthieu Biais

17 **Mean systemic pressure monitoring**   157
Michael R. Pinsky

18 **Fluid responsiveness assessment**   163
Xavier Monnet and Jean-Louis Teboul

19 **Non-invasive and continuous arterial pressure monitoring** 171
Berthold Bein and Christoph Ilies

20 **Monitoring the microcirculation** 180
Daniel De Backer and Katia Donadello

21 **ScvO$_2$ monitoring** 186
Alice Carter and Rupert Pearse

Section 4 – Goal Directed Hemodynamic Optimization

22 **Goal directed therapy in the intensive care and emergency settings: what is the evidence?** 191
Joseph Meltzer

23 **Goal directed therapy in the perioperative setting: what is the evidence?** 197
Eric Edison and Andrew Rhodes

24 **Endpoints of goal directed therapy in the OR and in the ICU** 203
Nathan H. Waldron, Timothy E. Miller, and Tong J. Gan

25 **What is a fluid challenge and how to perform it?** 213
Maurizio Cecconi and Hollman D. Aya

26 **The relationship between anesthesia, hemodynamics and outcome** 224
Tom Abbott and Gareth L. Ackland

27 **Goal directed fluid and hemodynamic therapy in cardiac surgical patients** 231
Byron D. Fergerson and Gerard R. Manecke Jr.

28 **Goal directed therapy and hemodynamic optimization in the critical care setting: practical applications and benefits** 237
Trung Vu, Davinder Ramsingh, William Wilson, and Maxime Cannesson

29 **Goal directed therapy at the bedside: the nurse perspective** 246
Elizabeth J. Bridges and Debra R. Metter

30 **A nurse anesthetist perspective: does perioperative goal directed fluid management yield better patient outcomes compared to the traditional method?** 255
Ann B. Singleton

31 **How to implement GDT in an institution and at the national level** 262
Timothy E. Miller and Michael Mythen

32 **Decision support and closed-loop systems for hemodynamic optimization and fluid management** 267
Joseph Rinehart

Index 275

Contributors

Tom Abbott, MA, BM, BCh
The Royal London Hospital, Barts Health NHS Trust, London, UK

Gareth L. Ackland, PhD, FRCA, FFICM
Department of Medicine, University College London, and Department of Anaesthesia, University College Hospital NHS Trust, London, UK

Hollman D. Aya
Department of Intensive Care, St George's Healthcare NHS Trust and St George's University of London, London, UK

Berthold Bein, MD, PhD, MA, DEAA
Department of Anesthesiology and Intensive Care Medicine, University Hospital Schleswig-Holstein, Campus Kiel, Kiel, Germany

Karim Bendjelid, MD, PhD
Intensive Care Service, Geneva University Hospitals, Faculty of Medicine, University of Geneva, and Geneva Hemodynamic Research Group, Geneva, Switzerland

Matthieu Biais, MD, PhD
Bordeaux University Hospital, Emergency Department, Pellegrin Hospital, Bordeaux, and University Bordeaux Segalen, Bordeaux, France

Elizabeth J. Bridges, PhD, RN, CCNS, FCCM, FAAN
University of Washington School of Nursing and University of Washington Medical Center, Seattle, WA, USA

Maxime Cannesson, MD, PhD
Department of Anesthesia and Perioperative Care, University of California Irvine, Irvine, CA, USA

Cédric Carrié, MD
Bordeaux University Hospital, Emergency Department, Pellegrin Hospital, Bordeaux, and University Bordeaux Segalen, Bordeaux, France

Alice Carter, MRCP, FRCA
Department of Intensive Care Medicine, Royal London Hospital, London, UK

Maurizio Cecconi, FRCA, FICM, MD (UK)
Department of Intensive Care, St George's Healthcare NHS Trust and St George's University of London, London, UK

Daniel Chappell, MD
Department of Anaesthesiology, University Hospital Munich, Munich, Germany

Jason H. Chua, MD
Department of Anesthesiology and Perioperative Medicine, David Geffen School of Medicine at UCLA, Los Angeles, CA, USA

Gary Colins, PhD
Centre for Statistics in Medicine, Botnar Research Centre, University of Oxford, Oxford, UK

Diego Orbegozo Cortes, MD
Department of Intensive Care, Erasme University Hospital, Université Libre de Bruxelles (ULB), Belgium

Lester A. H. Critchley, MD, FFARCSI, FHKAM
Department of Anaesthesia and Intensive Care, The Chinese University of Hong Kong, Prince of Wales Hospital, Shatin, New Territories, Hong Kong, SAR

Daniel De Backer, MD, PhD
Department of Intensive Care, Erasme University
Hospital, Université Libre de Bruxelles (ULB), Belgium

Katia Donadello, MD
Department of Intensive Care, Erasme University
Hospital, Université Libre de Bruxelles (ULB), Belgium

Eric Edison
Department of Intensive Care Medicine, St George's
Healthcare NHS Trust and St George's University of
London, London, UK

Byron D. Fergerson, MD
Department of Anesthesiology, University of
California San Diego School of Medicine, San Diego,
CA, USA

Tong J. Gan, MD, MHS, FRCA
Department of Anesthesiology, Duke University,
Durham, NC, USA

Michael T. Ganter
Institute of Anesthesiology and Pain Medicine,
Kantonsspital Winterthur, Switzerland

Leslie M. Garson, MD, MIHM
Department of Anesthesiology and Perioperative
Care, University of California Irvine, Irvine, CA, USA

Christoph K. Hofer
Institute of Anesthesiology and Intensive Care Medicine,
Triemli City Hospital Zurich, Zurich, Switzerland

Christoph Ilies, MD, DESA
Department of Anesthesiology and Intensive Care
Medicine, Herz- und Gefäßklinik, Bad Neustadt/
Saale, Germany

James M. Isbell, MD, MSci
Department of Surgery and Co-Director, Thoracic
and Cardiovascular Critical Care, School of Medicine,
University of Virginia, Charlottesville, VA, USA

Matthias Jacob, MD
Department of Anaesthesiology, University Hospital
Munich, Munich, Germany

Mazyar Javidroozi, MD, PhD
Department of Anesthesiology, Critical Care and
Hyperbaric Medicine, Englewood Hospital and
Medical Center, Englewood, NJ, USA

Zeev N. Kain, MD, MBA
Department of Anesthesiology and Perioperative
Care, University of California Irvine, Irvine, CA, USA

Elisa Kam
Adult Critical Care Unit, Royal London Hospital,
London, UK

Gautam Kumar, MBChB, FRCA
University College London, London, UK

Yannick Le Manach, MD, PhD
Departments of Anesthesia & Clinical Epidemiology
and Biostatistics, Michael DeGroote School of
Medicine, Faculty of Health Sciences, McMaster
University, and Population Health Research Institute,
Perioperative Medicine and Surgical Research Unit,
Hamilton, Ontario, Canada

Sheldon Magder
Department of Critical Care, McGill University
Health Centre, Montreal, Quebec, Canada

Aman Mahajan, MD, PhD
Department of Anesthesiology and Perioperative
Medicine, David Geffen School of Medicine at UCLA,
Los Angeles, CA, USA

Gerard R. Manecke Jr., MD
Department of Anesthesiology, University of
California San Diego School of Medicine, San Diego,
CA, USA

Paul E. Marik, MD, FCCM, FCCP
Division of Pulmonary and Critical Care Medicine,
Eastern Virginia Medical School, Norfolk, VA,
USA

Joseph Meltzer, MD
Cardiothoracic Intensive Care Unit and
Department of Anesthesiology and Perioperative
Medicine, UCLA School of Medicine, Los Angeles,
CA, USA

Debra R. Metter, MN, RN, CCRN, CCNS
Trauma and Critical Care Clinical Nurse Specialist,
Harborview Medical Center, Seattle, WA, USA

Timothy E. Miller, MBChB, FRCA
Department of Anesthesiology, Duke University
Medical Center, Durham, NC, USA

Xavier Monnet, MD, PhD
AP-HP, Hôpitaux Universitaires Paris-Sud, Hôpital
de Bicêtre, Service de Réanimation Médicale,
Le Kremlin-Bicêtre, France

Michael Mythen, MBBS, FRCA, MD
Department of Anaestheis and Surgical
Outcomes Research Centre (SOuRCe), UCL/UCLH
National Institute of Health Research Biomedical
Research Centre, University College London,
London, UK

Rudolph Nguyen, MD
Department of Anesthesiology and Perioperative
Medicine, David Geffen School of Medicine at UCLA,
Los Angeles, CA, USA

Rupert Pearse
Department of Intensive Care Medicine, Queen Mary,
University of London, and Barts and the London
NHS Trust, London, UK

Michael R. Pinsky, MD, CM, Dr hc
Department of Critical Care Medicine, University of
Pittsburgh, Pittsburgh, PA, USA

Davinder Ramsingh, MD
Department of Anesthesia and Perioperative Care,
University of California Irvine, Irvine, CA, USA

Steffen Rex
Department of Anesthesiology, University Hospitals
Leuven, and Department of Cardiovascular Sciences,
KU Leuven, Leuven, Belgium

Andrew Rhodes
Department of Intensive Care Medicine, St George's
Healthcare NHS Trust and St George's University of
London, London, UK

Joseph Rinehart, MD
Department of Anesthesia and Perioperative Care,
University of California Irvine, Irvine,
CA, USA

Mathieu Sèrié, MD
Bordeaux University Hospital, Emergency
Department, Pellegrin Hospital, Bordeaux,
and University Bordeaux Segalen, Bordeaux,
France

Aryeh Shander, MD
Department of Anesthesiology, Critical Care and
Hyperbaric Medicine, Englewood Hospital and
Medical Center, Englewood, NJ, USA

Nils Siegenthaler, MD
Intensive Care Service, Geneva University Hospitals,
Faculty of Medicine, University of Geneva, and
Geneva Hemodynamic Research Group, Geneva,
Switzerland

Ann B. Singleton, CRNA, DNAP
Department of Anesthesia and Perioperative Care,
UCI Medical Center, Orange, CA, USA

Faraz Syed, MD
Department of Anesthesiology, Critical Care and
Hyperbaric Medicine, Englewood Hospital and
Medical Center, Englewood, NJ, USA

Jean-Louis Teboul, MD, PhD
Université Paris-Sud, Faculté de Médecine Paris-Sud,
EA4533, Le Kremlin-Bicêtre, France

Robert H. Thiele, MD
Departments of Anesthesiology and Biomedical
Engineering, Divisions of Cardiac, Thoracic, and
Critical Care Anesthesia, and Director, Technology in
Anesthesia & Critical Care Group, School of
Medicine, University of Virginia, Charlottesville,
VA, USA

Shermeen B. Vakharia, MD, MBA
Department of Anesthesiology and Perioperative
Care, University of California Irvine, Irvine, CA, USA

Trung Vu, MD
Department of Anesthesia and Perioperative Care,
University of California Irvine, Irvine, CA, USA

Nathan H. Waldron, MD
Department of Anesthesiology, Duke University,
Durham, NC, USA

David Walker, BM (Hons), FRCP, FRCA, FFICM
University College London, London, UK

William Wilson, MD
Department of Anesthesia and Perioperative Care,
University of California Irvine, Irvine, CA, USA

Foreword

Perioperative hemodynamic monitoring and goal directed therapy: after 80 years, a therapy that is ready for prime time

Albert Einstein quoted that "Intellectuals solve problems, geniuses prevent them." This is the essence and intent of perioperative hemodynamic monitoring and goal directed therapy (PHM-GDT). This book establishes the scope of the problem, the physiology, the instruments, and the tools necessary. Without goals and endpoints, these tools become continued sources of controversy. Including them makes this book comprehensive in all respects.

George Washington Carver quoted that "excellence is performing common things in uncommon places." Thus, recognizing and treating the patient at the most proximal phase of the insult or even before only makes sense. When GDT was applied to severe sepsis and septic shock before hospital admission, not only were morbidity and mortality reduced but also health care resource consumption. It worked because the average wait time for an intensive care unit (ICU) admission to the emergency department (ED) was over 5 hours.[1] Whether in the ED, general practice floor, operating or recovery room and intensive care unit interventions, GDT has been shown to improve outcomes by robust confirmatory outcome evidence. Lastly, the most important component of realizing the success of PHM-GDT is the human element which includes the collaboration of clinicians and the organization framework in each clinical setting. In this modern era of health care practice, applications of decision support and closed-loop systems to optimize care are even more relevant.

Otto Weininger once quoted that "Among the notable things about fire is that it also requires oxygen to burn; exactly like its enemy, life. Thereby are life and flames so often compared." Oxygen is the primary substrate for cellular respiration (internal combustion), which is fundamental for human life. In its absence, tissue hypoxia leads to inflammation, cellular dysfunction, organ failure, and certain death. In the absence of systemic oxygen consumption, there can be no life. Thus, restoration of global tissue normoxia is one of the most important therapeutic interventions to prevent this pathologic cascade. We have known for over 80 years that physiologic insults increase systemic oxygen consumption and demands creating an oxygen debt.[2,3] While treating this seems so intuitive and physiologically sound, like hand washing, its adoption has been a long time coming nonetheless.

George Bernard Shaw once quoted "Beware of false knowledge; it is more dangerous than ignorance" and Bob Edwards "A little learning is a dangerous thing, but a lot of ignorance is just as bad." All one has to do is to look at the history of the pulmonary artery catheter. How can instruments improve outcomes without understanding the physiology and individualizing patient care in a goal directed fashion? In this book one would find that a comprehensive goal directed provision of adequate oxygenation to the tissues is through a manipulation of preload, afterload, arterial oxygen content, contractility, and cardiac output in order to optimize delivery. The metabolic feedback confirming that oxygen delivery is adequate uses metabolic indicators (i.e., lactate, base deficit, pH, SvO2), which signify that the microcirculation and tissue beds are no longer in distress. Whether the tools are a pulmonary artery catheter or a non-invasive device, the concept is the same and must be tailored to each patient as "one size or endpoint does not fit all."

Ernest Hemingway once quoted that "Critics are men who watch a battle from a high place, then come down and shoot the survivors. . . ." While the concept of ensuring the adequacy of cellular respiration is so fundamental and intuitive, where is the controversy and why has it taken over 80 years to make it part of our everyday practice? While the merits of GDT has been repeatedly shown in the literature, criticism remained a refuge for some over the years. Robert Louis Stevenson quoted "Saints are sinners who kept on going" and Alexis Carrel once quoted "Life leaps like a geyser for those who drill through the rock of inertia." This characterizes the many investigators who overcame the doubt and criticism. These investigators, including the late Dr. David Bennett (February 21, 2012),[4] one of the international founding fathers of critical care medicine and original investigators of PHM-GDT would be proud of this comprehensive book.[5–9] After 80 years, PHM-GDT is ready for prime time.

Emanuel P. Rivers, MD, MPH
Department of Surgery and Emergency Medicine
Henry Ford Hospital, Detroit, Michigan

Clinical Professor, Wayne State University
Detroit, Michigan
Institute of Medicine, National Academies
48202, USA

References

1. Rivers E, Nguyen B, Havstad S, et al. Early goal-directed therapy in the treatment of severe sepsis and septic shock. *N Engl J Med* 2001;**345(19)**:1368–77.

2. Cuthbertson DP. Observations on the disturbance of metabolism produced by injury to the limbs. *Q J Med* 1932;**25**:233–46.

3. Cuthbertson DP. Post-shock metabolic response. *Lancet* 1942; i:433–47.

4. Watts G. Ephraim David Bennett. *Lancet* 2012;**379(9823)**:1294.

5. Boyd O, Grounds RM. Our study 20 years on: a randomized clinical trial of the effect of deliberate perioperative increase of oxygen delivery on mortality in high-risk surgical patients. *Intens Care Med* 2013;**39(12)**:2107–14.

6. Boyd O, Grounds RM, Bennett ED. A randomized clinical trial of the effect of deliberate perioperative increase of oxygen delivery on mortality in high-risk surgical patients. *JAMA* 1993;**270 (22)**:2699–707.

7. Pearse R, Dawson D, Fawcett J, et al. Early goal-directed therapy after major surgery reduces complications and duration of hospital stay. A randomised, controlled trial [ISRCTN38797445]. *Crit Care* 2005;**9(6)**:R687–93.

8. Rhodes A, Cecconi M, Hamilton M, et al. Goal-directed therapy in high-risk surgical patients: a 15-year follow-up study. *Intens Care Med* 2010;**36(8)**:1327–32.

9. Bennett ED. Goal-directed therapy is successful – in the right patients. *Crit Care Med* 2002;**30 (8)**:1909–10.

Abbreviations list

AAMI	Association for the Advancement of Medical Instrumentation		**cvBGA**	central venous blood gas analysis
aBGA	arterial blood gas analysis		**CVC**	central venous catheter
AC	adenylate cyclase		**CvO₂**	venous blood oxygen content
ACC/AHA	American College of Cardiology/American Heart Association		**CVP**	central venous pressure
			DBP	diastolic blood pressure
ACLS	acute cardiac life support		**delta-POP**	respiratory variations in the pulse oxymeter plethysmographic waveform amplitude
ACS	American College of Surgeons			
ACS-NSQIP	American College of Surgeons National Surgical Quality Improvement		**DO₂**	oxygen delivery
			DO₂I	oxygen delivery index
ACTH	adrenocorticotropic hormone		**EBM**	evidence-based medicine
ADH	antidiuretic hormone		**ECG**	electrocardiography
AF	atrial fibrillation		*ED*	*emergency department*
AKI	acute kidney injury		*ED*	*esophageal Doppler*
ALI	acute lung injury		**EDM**	esophageal Doppler monitoring
ANP	atrial natriuretic peptide		**EDV**	end-diastolic volume
ANZASM	Australian and New Zealand Audit of Surgical Mortality		**EEG**	electroencephalography
			EEO	end-expiratory occlusion
APACHE	Acute Physiology and Chronic Health Evaluation		**EF**	ejection fraction
			ELWI	extra-lung water index
αAR	α-adrenergic receptor		**EMR**	electromagnetic radiation/ electronic medical record
APRV	airway pressure release ventilation			
ARDS	acute respiratory distress syndrome		**EO₂**	oxygen extraction from blood
ASA	American Society of Anesthesiologists		**ER**	enhanced recovery
ASA-PSS	American Society of Anesthesiologists' Physical Status Score		**ERAS**	Enhanced Recovery After Surgery
			ESA	European Society of Anaesthesiology
AUC	area under the curve		**ESAs**	erythropoiesis-stimulating agents
AV	atrioventricular		**ESC**	European Society of Cardiology
AVP	arginine vasopressin		**ESL**	endothelial surface layer
βAR	β-adrenergic receptor		**ESPVR**	end-systolic pressure–volume relationship
BIS	Bispectral Index		**ESV**	end-systolic volume
CABG	coronary artery bypass grafting		**Et**	time-varying elastance
cAMP	cyclic AMP		**ETAC**	end-tidal anesthetic concentration
CaO₂	arterial oxygen content		**EuroSCORE**	European System for Cardiac Operative Risk Evaluation
CCO	continuous cardiac output			
CDSS	clinical decision support systems		**EVLW**	extravascular lung water
CEDV	continuous end-diastolic volume		**FDA**	Food and Drug Administration (of the USA)
CI	cardiac index			
CL	closed-loop		**FEAST**	fluid expansion as supportive therapy
CNAP	Continuous Non-invasive Arterial Pressure Monitor		**FTc**	corrected flow time
			FVP	femoral venous pressure
CO	cardiac output		**GEDV**	global end-diastolic volume
COMT	o-methyl-transferase		**GDT**	goal directed therapy
CPB	cardiopulmonary bypass		**HAA**	hospital acquired anemia
CPET	cardiopulmonary exercise testing		**Hb**	hemoglobin
CQUIN	Commissioning for Quality and Innovation		**HES**	hydroxyethyl starch
			HIFs	hypoxic inducible factors
CRP	C-reactive protein		**HR**	heart rate
CSP	carotid sinus pressure		**hs CRP**	high-sensitivity C-reactive protein

IAP	invasive arterial pressure
IBP	invasive arterial blood pressure
ICC	interclass correlation coefficient
ICU	intensive care unit
IOH	intraoperative hypotension
IR	interventional radiology
ITBV	intrathoracic blood volume
ITBVI	intrathoracic blood volume index
ITP	inosine (5'-) triphosphate
ITTV	intrathoracic thermal volume
IVC	inferior vena cava
LOS	length of stay
LV	left ventricular
LVOT	left ventricular outflow tract
LVR	liberal versus restrictive
MAC	mean alveolar concentration
MAP	mean arterial pressure
MET	metabolic equivalent task
MOA	monoamine oxidase
MPI	myocardial performance index
MRI	magnetic resonance imaging
MSFP	mean systemic filling pressure
MVO_2	myocardial O_2
NADH	nicotinamide adenine dinucleotide hydrogenase
NCEPOD	National Enquiry into Patient Outcome and Death
NE	norepinephrine
NELA	National Emergency Laparotomy Audit
NIBP	non-invasive blood pressure
NICE	National Institute for Health and Care Excellence
NICU	neonatal intensive care unit
NIRS	near-infrared spectroscopy
NNT	number needed to treat
NP	natriuretic peptides
NS	normal saline
NSQIP	National Surgical Quality Improvement Program
NT pro-BNP	N-terminal pro-B-type natriuretic peptide
NTAC	National Technology Adoption Centre
OPS	orthogonal polarization spectral (imaging techniques)
OR	odds ratio
$PaCO_2$	arterial oxygen tension
PAC	*Preassessment Clinic*/ pulmonary artery catheter
PACU	postanesthesia care unit
PAH	pulmonary arterial hypertension
PAOP	pulmonary artery occlusion pressure (wedge pressure)
PAP	pulmonary artery pressure
Parm	arm equilibrium pressure
PBM	Patient Blood Management
PCO_2	arterial carbon dioxide tension
PCWP	pulmonary capillary wedge pressure
PE	percentage error
PEEP	positive end-expiratory pressure
PHM-GDT	perioperative hemodynamic monitoring and goal directed therapy
PICC	peripherally inserted central venous catheter
PLR	passive leg raising
Pms	mean systemic pressure
Pmsf	mean systemic filling pressure
Pmsa	mean systemic filling pressure analog
PO_2	oxygen partial pressure
POMS	Postoperative Morbidity Survey
PONV	postoperative nausea and vomiting
ΔPOP	pulse oximetry plethysmographic waveform amplitude
POSSUM	Physiological and Operative Severity Score for the Enumeration of Mortality and Morbidity
PP	pulse pressure
Ppao	pulmonary artery occlusion pressure
PPV	pulse pressure variation
Pra	right atrial pressure
PRAC	Pharmacovigilance Risk Assessment Committee
PRAM	pressure recording analytic method
PSH	Perioperative Surgical Home
PTV	pulmonary thermal volume
PVI	pleth variability index
PVP	*peripheral venous pressure*
PVP	*pulmonary vascular permeability*
PVR	pulmonary vascular resistance
PWTT	pulse wave transit time
Pzf	pressure at zero flow
Q	cardiac output
QIPP	Quality, Productivity and Prevention in Practice
RaFTinG	Rational Fluid Therapy in Germany
RAP	right atrial pressure
RBC	red blood cell
RCRI	Lee Revised Cardiac Risk Index
RCT	randomized controlled trial
ROC	receiver operating characteristic
RRT	renal replacement therapy
RV	right ventricular
Rv	venous resistance
RVR	resistance to venous return
SA	sinoatrial
SAFE	saline versus albumin fluid evaluation
SAH	subarachnoid hemorrhage
SaO_2	arterial oxygen saturation
SASM	Scottish Audit of Surgical Mortality
SBP	systolic blood pressure
$ScvO_2$	central venous blood oxygen content
SDF	sidestream dark field
SDM	shared decision making
$SfvO_2$	femoral venous oxygen saturation
SEE	standard error of the estimate
SIMV	spontaneous intermittent mandatory ventilation
SIRS	systemic inflammatory response syndrome
SO_2	oxygen saturation

sPAP	pulmonary artery systolic pressure	TEG	thromboelastography
SpHb	total Hb	Tn	troponins
SPSP	Scottish Patient Safety Programme	TPTD	transpulmonary thermodilution
SPV	systolic pressure variation	TRACS	transfusion requirements after cardiac surgery
SR	sinus rhythm		
StO$_2$	somatic tissue oxygenation	TRICC	Transfusion Requirements in Critical Care
SvO$_2$	venous O$_2$ saturation		
SV	stroke volume	TTE	transthoracic echocardiography
SVC	superior vena cava	UGI	upper gastrointestinal
SVI	stroke volume index	UOP	urine output
SVR	systemic vascular resistance	VEGF	vascular endothelial growth factor
SVRI	systemic vascular resistance index	VHAs	viscoelastic hemostatic assays
SVrv	right ventricular stroke volume	VO$_2$	oxygen consumption/demand
SVV	stroke volume variation	VR	venous resistance
TBI	traumatic brain injury	VTI	velocity time integral
TEE	transesophageal echocardiography	WMD	weighted mean difference

Chapter

1

Patient outcome following major surgery

Elisa Kam and Rupert Pearse

Introduction

An enormous volume of surgical procedures are performed worldwide each year, particularly in high income nations. While the overall mortality after surgery is relatively low, these figures hide a subpopulation of patients who have much worse outcomes. Given the expansion of the volume of surgery year on year and an increasing tendency to offer surgical treatments to older and high-risk patients, prevention of postoperative deaths has become an important international public health issue. In this chapter, we will review the current knowledge on the mortality and morbidity in patients who undergo surgery, the tools we currently possess to identify the high-risk patient, and the direction of future research.

Surgical outcomes

The need to understand how complications occur and why some patients die as a result highlights the need for robust audit data. Recognition of the importance of audit data is not a new concept. Florence Nightingale described the use of a standard format to report deaths after surgery as early as 1859, and it was her pioneering use of piecharts to illustrate that the majority of deaths in British army hospitals during the Crimean War were due to poor sanitation that helped persuade the British government to improve hygiene in hospitals (Figure 1.1). John Snow (1815–1858), the physician renowned for administering the novel inhalational agent chloroform to Queen Victoria, was the forefather of modern epidemiology and has been credited with promoting quality assessment among his anesthetic colleagues. Leading Boston surgeon Ernest Codman (1869–1940) was one of the earliest to monitor the outcomes of all his surgical patients and, although some

of his plans to evaluate the competency of surgeons proved unpopular among his colleagues, his drive for hospital improvement through monitoring outcomes led him to be one of the founders of the American College of Surgeons (ACS).

In more recent times, the voluntary reporting of surgical deaths for peer review has been a popular method of audit. Examples include the Australian and New Zealand Audit of Surgical Mortality (ANZASM), and the Scottish Audit of Surgical Mortality (SASM), which examine all specialties with the exceptions of cardiac, thoracic, and obstetric surgery. However, while these audits report the absolute numbers of deaths of patients who have undergone an operation during a hospital admission, they are limited by the fact that they do not place these deaths in the context of the volume of surgical procedures performed. Recognizing that improving surgical outcomes requires cooperation between all health care professionals involved in the care of surgical patients, a joint initiative began in the UK in the 1980s, now known as the National Enquiry into Patient Outcome and Death (NCEPOD). Through the voluntary return of questionnaires into perioperative deaths and peer review, reports have been published since 1987 and have led to recommendations to improve practice. Notable examples are the creation of operating lists led by senior anesthetists and surgeons during the day for potentially sicker patients undergoing emergency surgery, and introduction of regular departmental morbidity and mortality meetings. The effect of these changes on outcome, however, is less easy to quantify, since the annual number of deaths identified has changed little between 1989 and 2003.

The initiatives of audits and national registries to peer review surgical deaths have enhanced our understanding of the contributing factors and have resulted

Perioperative Hemodynamic Monitoring and Goal Directed Therapy, ed. Maxime Cannesson and Rupert Pearse.
Published by Cambridge University Press. © Cambridge University Press 2014.

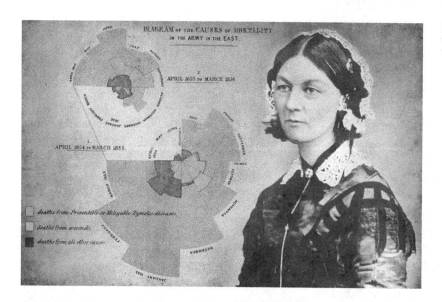

Figure 1.1. Florence Nightingale and the diagram of the cause of mortality in the Army in the East.

in some improvements to clinical practice. However, reporting of absolute numbers of deaths does not yield easily to interpretation. Without a denominator, a mortality rate cannot be calculated. Publications of rates of death and morbidity are much more useful in monitoring standards of surgical and anesthetic care and auditing the effectiveness of planned interventions.

Mortality rates and complication rates

Mortality rates

Our understanding of the epidemiology of surgical outcomes is far from complete. For many surgical specialties, the continuous, prospective collection of accurate data is not yet in place, and mortality rates are estimated from intermittent audits or epidemiological studies. Confusion has arisen from these estimates due to differences in the population studied in terms of geographical boundaries, age exclusions, types of surgery, and the timeframe at which the audit or study was undertaken to obtain the rate of patient deaths.

In the UK, the process of data collection has been pioneered in cardiac surgery, providing robust public audit data on short and medium term mortality not only by hospital, but also by individual surgeons. Risk-adjusted mortality figures are freely available to the public online and these have demonstrated an improvement over time, with a typical hospital mortality rate of 2% or less. Non-cardiac surgery, on the other hand, is less well studied and arguably more important, as the volume of surgery involved is much

greater than cardiac surgery and in many cases mortality rates are higher. Although individual registries for specialties such as vascular, bariatric, bowel cancer, and orthopedic surgery report outcomes for certain key procedures, they represent only an individual part of a care pathway and not of the general system of a hospital with a shared perioperative care pathway of standard facilities for preoperative assessment, anesthesia, operating rooms and postanesthetic recovery.

There have been a number of publications of national mortality rates from retrospective analyses of registries and prospective epidemiological studies showing 30-day to 70-month mortality rates for non-cardiac surgery of between 1% and 3%.[1–3] These, however, describe only a small number of health care systems, or parts of a national health care system. In a recent study, investigators have attempted to study a larger number of health care systems. The European Surgical Outcomes Study was an international prospective study of 46 000 adult patients from 28 European countries undergoing non-cardiac surgery over a 1-week period. It showed a higher overall 60-day mortality of 4%.[4] Although the overall mortality in non-cardiac surgery appears relatively low, mortality may exceed 12% in older patients undergoing emergency surgery (Figure 1.2). A small group of high-risk patients has been shown to be responsible for 84% of deaths and significantly longer hospital stays, despite making up only 12.5% of hospital admissions for surgery.[1] The significance of identifying and caring for this group of patients is highlighted in the next section.

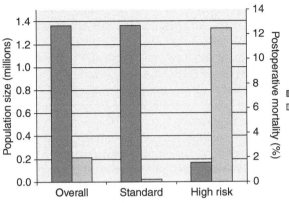

Figure 1.2. Mortality rates for different surgical populations in the UK.

Complication rates

A precise estimate of perioperative complications is difficult to provide, but they may occur following 15% to 27% of all surgical procedures.[5,6] The wide range in complication rates reflects variable reporting and also the large number of possible anesthetic or surgical complications covering many organ systems, including cardiovascular, pulmonary, renal, hematological, and gastrointestinal, as well as infections. Models have been devised to help classify these broad categories of surgical complications. Clavien proposed a model in the 1990s,[7] which has since been updated and validated in a large cohort of patients by an international survey to allow grading of severity of postoperative complications, regardless of the initial surgery.[3] Another model is the Postoperative Morbidity Survey (POMS), which is a validated questionnaire developed to record postoperative complications in non-cardiac surgery.

Collecting information on postoperative complications is important not only for audit purposes, but there has also been an increasing recognition that developing complications increases a patient's risk of death. Patients who develop complications but survive may suffer a substantial reduction in functional independence and long-term survival. Analysis of data from the United States' National Surgical Quality Improvement Program (NSQIP) showed that not only did the occurrence of 30-day postoperative complication reduce patient survival by 69%, but it was more important than preoperative and intraoperative factors in determining survival after major non-cardiac surgery.[3] Another large North American study showed that mortality in an unselected population of surgical patients doubled from 2% to 4% after surgery and by 1 year, 47% of surviving patients had been readmitted to hospital.

Why are mortality and morbidity so high?

Advances in surgical techniques, training, and increased subspecialization have led to significant improvements in care. Concurrently, mortality directly attributable to anesthesia has declined steeply. Despite such improvements in patient treatments during surgery, mortality after surgery has not declined. There is increasing recognition that the care of the patient after an operation is equally important in determining outcomes, and growing concern that it is the quality of this postoperative care that is not of a high enough standard. More surgery is being performed on patients with higher risk as a result of an aging world population with more co-morbid disease, as well as more operations in younger patients who have a higher illness burden. It is estimated that there is a subgroup of high-risk patients that accounts for 80% of all postoperative deaths.[1,8] Epidemiological data suggest that clinicians often fail to identify these high-risk patients preoperatively in order to plan appropriate perioperative care. It is estimated that 170 000 of high-risk patients will undergo non-cardiac surgery in the UK and that 60% of these patients will develop complications after non-cardiac surgery, leading to over 25 000 deaths.[1,8]

There is evidence that critical care-based cardiorespiratory interventions can improve outcomes in high-risk patients. Cardiac surgery in traditionally high-risk patients will routinely admit the majority of its patients to critical care postoperatively. However, critical care provision is low for patients undergoing non-cardiac surgery. Unplanned admissions to critical care are associated with higher mortality rates than planned admissions, yet only 5% of patients undergoing non-cardiac surgery have a planned admission to critical care.[9] A review of Medicare data reveals that the differences in mortality between hospitals are related to the ability of a hospital to effectively rescue patients from complications.[10] This suggests a failure to recognize the sick and high-risk patient and perhaps the lack of availability of critical care resources.

Risk assessment

Identifying the patients who are most likely to suffer postoperative complications or mortality allows informed decisions on whether to operate and to help target postoperative care and critical care provision for these patients. The majority of patients are evaluated prior to surgery solely according to the physician's assessment of clinical history, physiology, and extent of surgery. Several tools have been developed to assist the clinician in predicting the response of a patient to the tissue injury induced inflammatory state of surgery, but many of these are not yet in routine use due to cost, ease of use and a developing evidence base. These tools include risk scores, serum biomarkers, and assessment of functional capacity.

Risk scores

General scores are used to estimate population risk. One of the earliest systems proposed is the American Society of Anesthesiologists (ASA) classification,[11] which stratifies a patient's ability to withstand surgery into one of five classes depending on the presence and severity of co-morbid disease. Although initially developed as a tool for audit and research, the individual ASA classes may be used as predictors of mortality, while the rate of postoperative morbidity varies with class. The ASA system is popular because it is easy to use, but scoring can be subjective and it does not allow consideration of individual specific information or the type of surgery. Hence, the system has poor sensitivity and specificity when used to assess the risk in an individual patient.

The Acute Physiology and Chronic Health Evaluation (APACHE) scores were developed in the 1980s for use in critical care. Of the four versions, the APACHE II score is the most validated for use in preoperative risk prediction. It is based on 12 physiological variables, with additional points for age and chronic health.[12] While the type of surgery is not accounted for, APACHE II can provide an individualized risk of morbidity and mortality. It performs better in predicting outcome than the ASA classification[13] and may be used to predict severity of surgical complications. However, the requirement to measure all variables over the first 24 hours of critical care stay before an operation is a barrier to the regular use of this score.

Goldman and Lee have produced well-validated scoring systems to predict the likelihood of cardiac complications after non-cardiac surgery,[14,15] and Arozullah has provided a model for predicting postoperative respiratory failure.[16] However, these focus on a single organ system and cannot make assessment of the severity of each contributing factor.

The Physiological and Operative Severity Score for the Enumeration of Mortality and Morbidity (POSSUM) score was designed for use in preoperative risk prediction, whilst taking into consideration both individual physiological risk and the type of surgery performed.[6] This scoring system uses 12 physiological and six operative variables to predict mortality and morbidity via two separate equations. POSSUM may overestimate or underestimate risk in specific populations, but it remains the most validated and used scoring system for non-cardiac surgery.

In cardiac surgery, the European System for Cardiac Operative Risk Evaluation (EuroSCORE) is one of the most validated for hospital and long-term mortality.[17] It is calculated using clinical data either in an additive or logistic calculation, the former being easier to derive but less accurate in high-risk patients. It is widely used in research and audit, but caution has been recommended for comparisons and for surgeons with different case mixes.

Biomarkers

There has been a growing interest in biochemical markers with the goal of finding an inexpensive biochemical test that either alone or in combination with existing clinical tools can improve the accuracy of perioperative risk prediction. Several systemic reviews and meta-analyses and observational studies[18–20] suggest that elevated serum concentrations of high-sensitivity C-reactive protein (hs CRP) and N-terminal pro-B-type natriuretic peptide (NT pro-BNP) prior to surgery may be independent predictors of adverse cardiac events in medium or short term following major non-cardiac surgery. Moreover, these preoperative values can be used to prognosticate cardiac complications and mortality after high-risk surgery. Serum concentrations of troponin taken during the postoperative period have also been shown to be a strong independent predictor of short-term mortality in non-cardiac surgery.

Measurement of cardiac troponin levels for the first 3 days after surgery may substantially improve the accuracy of 30-day mortality risk stratification compared with assessment limited to preoperative risk factors.[21] Markers for neurological damage such as S100B, Tau, and the enzyme neurone-specific enolase have been assessed in cardiac and non-cardiac surgery, but results are conflicting.[22]

Functional capacity

Low exercise tolerance is associated with poor outcomes.[23] Preoperative assessment of functional capacity aims to predict an individual's ability to increase oxygen delivery during the perioperative period. Tests such as echocardiography and spirometry are useful but limited as they are performed at rest. The European Society of Cardiology (ESC) and the American College of Cardiology/American Heart Association (ACC/AHA) guidelines recommend using the metabolic equivalent task (MET) as an estimate of functional capacity. One MET is the metabolic requirement of an activity such as walking around indoors or doing light housework and is equivalent to 3.5 ml O_2/kg. The threshold of acceptable functional capacity is given as four METs, which is equivalent to climbing a flight of stairs. It is important to recognize there are inaccuracies in this method of estimation because the definition of MET is derived from the measurement of resting oxygen consumption from a single 70 kg, 40-year-old man. Thus an accurate assessment of functional capacity requires the knowledge of an individual's resting oxygen uptake, as well as reliable reporting of functional activity from the patient.

Cardiopulmonary exercise testing (CPET) is the gold standard method for assessing an individual's functional capacity by measuring oxygen uptake and carbon dioxide elimination while performing incremental, symptom-limited physical exercise up to the patient's maximal level. Incorporating ECG monitoring, it provides an integrated look at both a patient's cardiac and respiratory function during exercise. The main values of interest are the body's peak oxygen consumption (VO_2 peak) and anaerobic threshold (AT). Patients are classified as being at increased risk if VO_2 peak is less than 15 ml O_2/kg and AT is less than 11 ml O_2/kg/min.[23] CPET testing has a good predictive value for postoperative complications in pulmonary resection surgery, and there is increasing evidence of benefit in predicting morbidity and mortality in general surgery. However, CPET requires investment into costly equipment and skilled personnel to perform and interpret the tests, and for some surgical subspecialties there are still doubts over the evidence base, and this has prevented its routine use.

Large international trials are planned to define the optimal approach to evaluate risk assessment prior to surgery. It can be envisaged that all patients may be offered initial screening, based on simple factors such as age, type of surgery, serum biomarkers, and clinical risk scores. Low-risk patients could be offered early surgery following assessment in the community, while complex patients could be offered more sophisticated tests and detailed assessment by a physician. This would improve informed discussions with patients and allow individualized treatment plans with optimal use of postoperative critical care resources.

System-wide strategies to improve surgical outcomes

The design of health care systems significantly impacts on a hospital's ability to detect and manage postoperative adverse events and hence clinical outcomes. Outcome measures are increasingly used to underpin quality improvement frameworks and guide purchasing or commissioning of health care services. In the USA, the Centers for Medicare and Medicaid Services now deny reimbursement to hospitals for specific postoperative adverse events including urinary tract infections, pressure ulcers, and surgical site infections.[5] Such financial penalties may help drive quality improvements in other health care systems.

Various targets along the patient care pathway have been identified for patient safety and quality improvement initiatives. Many of these have been described above, including preoperative risk assessment, and joint clinics involving surgeons, anesthetists, and physicians allowing effective decision making and better communication with community health care teams. Similarly, systems should facilitate effective treatment plans for patients with a delayed recovery after hospital discharge, allowing a prompt return to hospital for review by the surgical team. Important structural factors include availability of critical care beds, staffing levels, and working patterns which influence the specialization of staff involved in the care of the surgical patient. These factors affect the ability of a system to ensure optimal treatment at the time of surgery and to promptly identify and treat those patients who later deteriorate. While there is no direct evidence of the benefits of these systems, they are known to exist more commonly in centers treating large volumes of patients. A clear association exists between hospital volume and clinical outcomes for many complex surgical procedures and high-risk patients.[24] Low-risk patients, however, have been shown to have comparable outcomes in both low-volume and high-volume centers. Hence, it is important to be able to risk-stratify a patient before selecting the most appropriate hospital for an elective operation.

Effective hospital clinical governance is key to delivering high-quality care. This incorporates complete and accurate data collection, internal audit, benchmarking against defined quality standards, and transparent publication of results. The USA has led the way in large-scale quality improvement projects. In the 1990s, data were prospectively collected for major operations in some Veteran Affairs hospitals and used to develop risk-adjusted models for 30-day morbidity and mortality.[25] Hospitals with lower morbidity and mortality were used as a standard against which adjustable factors in individual hospitals with worse outcomes could be identified. Use of data in this way by the National Surgical Quality Improvement Program (NSQIP) resulted in a 45% decrease in morbidity and a 27% reduction in mortality across all the Veteran Affairs hospitals. By 2008, and with funding from the American College of Surgeons (ACS), ACS-NSQIP was expanded to 198 hospitals across the USA. In the UK and in many other countries, clinical benchmarking is only available for selected procedures, and this represents only a small percentage of overall surgical volume. There is therefore an urgent need for investment in effective and widespread audit of surgical care and outcomes.

Conclusions

Rates of mortality and complications postsurgery have been difficult to collect for non-cardiac surgery, with estimates derived from registries and national databases. However, until mortality and morbidity tables for individual hospitals and surgeons are routinely published, hospital managers and clinicians will be limited in their attempts to improve outcomes for their patients. Financial constraints on health services around the world have led to remuneration based on outcome, and this may yet be the driving force for investment into clinical governance and quality improvement programs. At present, we are poor at identifying high-risk patients who are more likely to suffer adverse events. Preoperative scoring has the potential to ensure better informed consent and patient/procedural selection. The possibility of individualized risk prediction based on an individual's physiological response to stress is an exciting area, with the possibility of high predictive value and better use of critical resources to improve patient care

References

1. Pearse RM, Harrison DA, James P, et al. Identification and characterisation of the high-risk surgical population in the United Kingdom. *Crit Care* 2006;**10**(3):R81.

2. Yu PC, Calderaro D, Gualandro DM, et al. Non-cardiac surgery in developing countries: epidemiological aspects and economical opportunities – the case of Brazil. *PLoS ONE* 2010;**5**(5):e10607.

3. Dindo D, Demartines N, Clavien PA. Classification of surgical complications: a new proposal with evaluation in a cohort of 6336 patients and results of a survey. *Ann Surg* 2004;**240**(2):205–13.

4. Pearse R, Moreno RP, Bauer P, et al. Mortality after surgery in Europe – authors' reply. *Lancet* 2013;**381**(9864):370–1.

5. Ghaferi AA, Birkmeyer JD, Dimick JB. Variation in hospital mortality associated with inpatient surgery. *N Engl J Med* 2009;**361**(14):1368–75.

6. Bennett-Guerrero E, Hyam JA, Shaefi S, et al. Comparison of P-POSSUM risk-adjusted mortality rates after surgery between patients in the USA and the UK. *Br J Surg* 2003;**90**(12):1593–8.

7. Clavien PAP, Sanabria JRJ, Strasberg SMS. Proposed classification of complications of surgery with examples of utility in cholecystectomy. *Surgery* 1992;**111**(5):518–26.

8. Jhanji S, Thomas B, Ely A, et al. Mortality and utilisation of critical care resources amongst high-risk surgical patients in a large NHS trust. *Anaesthesia* 2008;**63**(7):695–700.

9. Pearse RM, Moreno RP, Bauer P, et al. Mortality after surgery in Europe: a 7 day cohort study. *Lancet* 2012;**380**(9847):1059–65.

10. Ghaferi AAA, Birkmeyer JDJ, Dimick JBJ. Hospital volume and failure to rescue with high-risk surgery. *Med Care* 2011;**49**(12):1076–81.

11. Saklad M. Grading of patients for surgical procedures. *Anesthesiology* 1941;**2**(3):281.

12. Knaus WA, Draper EA, Wagner DP, Zimmerman JE. APACHE II:

a severity of disease classification system. *Crit Care Med* 1985;**13** (10):818.

13. Goffi L, Saba V, Ghiselli R, et al. Preoperative APACHE II and ASA scores in patients having major general surgical operations: prognostic value and potential clinical applications. *Eur J Surg* 1999;**165** (8):730–5.

14. Goldman L, Caldera DL, Nussbaum SR, et al. Multifactorial index of cardiac risk in noncardiac surgical procedures. *N Engl J Med* 1977;**297**(16):845–50.

15. Lee TH, Marcantonio ER, Mangione CM, et al. Derivation and prospective validation of a simple index for prediction of cardiac risk of major noncardiac surgery. *Circulation* 1999;**100** (10):1043–9.

16. Arozullah AM, Khuri SF, Henderson WG, Daley J. Development and validation of a multifactorial risk index for predicting postoperative pneumonia after major noncardiac surgery. *Ann Intern Med* 2001;**135**(10):847–57.

17. Parsonnet V, Dean D, Bernstein AD. A method of uniform stratification of risk for evaluating the results of surgery in acquired adult heart disease. *Circulation* 1989;**79**(6 Pt 2):I3–12.

18. Karthikeyan G, Moncur RA, Levine O, et al. Is a pre-operative brain natriuretic peptide or N-terminal pro–B-type natriuretic peptide measurement an independent predictor of adverse cardiovascular outcomes within 30 days of noncardiac surgery? A systematic review and meta-analysis of observational studies. *J Am Coll Cardiol* 2009;**54** (17):1599–606.

19. Choi J-H, Cho DK, Song Y-B, et al. Preoperative NT-proBNP and CRP predict perioperative major cardiovascular events in non-cardiac surgery. *Heart* 2009;**96**(1):56–62.

20. Goei D, Hoeks SE, Boersma E, et al. Incremental value of high-sensitivity C-reactive protein and N-terminal pro–B-type natriuretic peptide for the prediction of postoperative cardiac events in noncardiac vascular surgery

patients. *Coron Artery Dis* 2009;**20** (3):219–24.

21. Devereaux PJ, Chan MT, Alonso-Coello P, et al. Association between postoperative troponin levels and 30-day mortality among patients undergoing noncardiac surgery. *JAMA* 2012;**307** (21):2295–304.

22. Cata JP, Abdelmalak B, Farag E. Neurological biomarkers in the perioperative period. *Br J Anaesth* 2011;**107**(6):844–58.

23. Older P, Hall A, Hader R. Cardiopulmonary exercise testing as a screening test for perioperative management of major surgery in the elderly. *Chest* 1999;**116**(2):355–62.

24. Birkmeyer JDJ, Siewers AEA, Finlayson EVAE, et al. Hospital volume and surgical mortality in the United States. *N Engl J Med* 2002;**346**(15):1128–37.

25. Khuri SF, Daley J, Henderson W, et al. The National Veterans Administration Surgical Risk Study: risk adjustment for the comparative assessment of the quality of surgical care. *J Am Coll Surg* 1995;**180**(5):519–31.

Chapter

2

Statistical methods in hemodynamic research

Yannick Le Manach and Gary Colins

Introduction

One of the most common research questions in hemodynamics concerns the comparison of measurement devices, and the determination of specific values in observed parameters. In this chapter, we will provide an overview of the statistical methods used to address them. The cardiac output measurements devices evaluation and the determination of threshold for preload dependency parameters will be used for illustration.

To compare two methods

Hemodynamic research often concerns comparing two methods of measurement. Typically, a new measurement method is being compared with an established method (often referred to as the "gold standard"), to determine whether the two methods can be used interchangeably, or if the new method can replace the established one. Interchangeability refers to the ability of one measurement device to be replaced by another one without affecting clinical interpretation of the observed values. Cardiac output measurement devices are among the most studied and compared devices. They constitute a good support to discuss the methodology, and most of the accumulated knowledge on them can be used to compare other sorts of devices.

Correlations

One of the most commonly used approaches to compare two methods of measurement is to calculate the correlation between the two methods. However, the correlation between two methods of measurement is uninformative and does not actually assess the agreement between the two methods. Correlation measures the strength of linear association between two continuous measurements. A perfect correlation ($r = 1$) occurs when the measurements of the two methods lie on any straight line. However, if we consider the situation whereby the new measurement method outputs a measurement exactly twice that of the standard method, then the correlation is still 1, yet clearly the two methods are not interchangeable. A change of scale in one of the two measurement methods does not affect the correlation, yet it clearly affects the agreement (or lack of). The interpretation of the correlation coefficient between two methods includes some limitations. When a very high correlation (e.g., $r = 0.95$ with $P < 0.001$) is observed, the probability to reject the null hypothesis (e.g., no linear relationship between the two sets of measurements) is very small and we can safely conclude that measurements by both devices are related. However, this high correlation does not mean that the two methods are interchangeable. In fact, as noted earlier, a change in scale of measurement will not affect these correlations, but it certainly affects the agreement and the potential clinical use of the new device. Furthermore, correlation depends on the range of the cardiac outputs in the sample. If the range of observed values is wide, the correlation will be greater than if it is narrow. Since researchers usually try to compare two methods over the whole range of cardiac output values typically encountered, a high correlation is almost guaranteed. Finally, a test of significance may show that the two methods are related, but it would be remarkable if two methods designed to measure cardiac output were not related.[1]

Scatter plots remain useful because they depict the relationship (linear or not) between the devices, as well as the difference in the measure for each level of cardiac output. However, we have to assume that

Perioperative Hemodynamic Monitoring and Goal Directed Therapy, ed. Maxime Cannesson and Rupert Pearse.
Published by Cambridge University Press. © Cambridge University Press 2014.

there is no simple estimator as soon as the statistical relationship is not linear. For this purpose, correlation, and more specifically correlation plots, might be considered in the reporting of studies aiming to compare two cardiac output measurement devices. Nevertheless, non-linear relationships are also identifiable in limit of agreements plots, and the researchers may consider that reporting the two is probably not necessary.

Although widely used in the literature, correlation analyses are not required in most of the cases. Although low correlation reflects low agreements between devices, high correlation doesn't necessarily refer to interchangeability. Correlation plots provide some details about the statistical relationship of interest, but this can be easily read on other analyses. If the inclusion of such analysis in research reports remains disputable, conclusions done only on correlation analyses are not acceptable.

Bland and Altman's graphical representation

In response to the widespread and inappropriate use of the correlation coefficient to assessment method agreement, statisticians Martin Bland and Douglas Altman proposed an alternative approach based on graphical techniques (known as the Bland–Altman plot).[2] This landmark *Lancet* paper by Bland and Altman has to date been cited on more than 22 000 occasions, illustrating its importance in medical research. The primary application of the Bland and Altman agreement plot is in the comparison of two clinical devices that contain error in their measurement. The aim is to determine how much the two measurement methods are likely to differ. If this difference is sufficiently small not to cause problems in clinical interpretation, then it can be considered as a candidate to replace the old method or to be used interchangeably.

The Bland and Altman plot allows us to investigate the existence of any systematic difference between the measurements. It is a plot of the difference against the mean of the two measurements. The mean difference is the estimated bias. If the mean value of the difference differs significantly from 0, this indicates the presence of fixed bias. If the differences lie between the 95% limits of agreement (mean ± 1.96 SD), then they are deemed not important; the two methods may be used interchangeably. Bland and Altman plots have also been used to investigate any possible relationship of the discrepancies between the measurements and the true value (i.e., proportional bias). The existence of

proportional bias indicates that the methods do not agree equally through the range of measurements (i.e., the limits of agreement will depend on the actual measurement). To evaluate this relationship formally, the difference between the methods should be regressed on the average of both methods. When a relationship between the differences and the true value was identified (i.e., a significant slope of the regression line), regression-based 95% limits of agreement should be provided

The presentation of the 95% limits of agreement is for visual judgment of how well two methods of measurement agree. The smaller the range between these two limits the better the agreement. The question of how small is small depends on the clinical context: would a difference between measurement methods as extreme as that described by the 95% limits of agreement meaningfully affect the interpretation of the results?

In the case of cardiac output devices comparison, it has been suggested that the limits of agreement between two methods should approach the precision of the older reference method before accepting the newer technique.[3] Commercial thermodilution devices (i.e., the gold standard for cardiac output measurement) are recognized to have a minimal difference of 12 to 15% (average, 13%) between measurements of cardiac output.[4] Thirteen percent has thus been described as the 95% limits of agreement in studies focusing on cardiac output devices comparison. Nonetheless, a 13% difference should be interpreted differently according to the absolute value of the cardiac output, as this 13% was obtained by averaging three measures, whereas a 22% difference was observed when only one measurement was used per determination. Consequently, 13 is not a magic number and researchers should consider higher variability in their reference measurements, particularly when their protocol does not include an averaging of at least three measurements.

It has also been suggested that the results of such evaluation studies should include the mean cardiac output, the bias, and the 95% limits of agreement.[5] Furthermore, it was suggested to report percentages rather than absolute values. The 95% limits of agreement do not include the variability of the reference method (e.g., 13% for thermodilution). Consequently, the observed disagreement is entirely assigned to the new method. Critchley et al.[5] suggested a corrective method to take into account the variability of the reference methods. Using an error gram, they depicted the relationship between the accuracy of the reference method and the limits of agreement between the new and the reference technique. As an example, they calculated that a limit of agreement of 1.45 L min^{-1} (28.3% of error) represented a clinically relevant disagreement when the reference methods presented variability of 20% and with a mean cardiac output of 5 L min^{-1}. In this setting, they recommended that limits of agreement between the new and the reference technique of up to 30% be accepted.[5]

Although the Critchley et al.[5] demonstration was compelling, the 30% limits of agreement are appropriate only when the variability of the reference method is 20%. This may be the case in most of the studies using averaged thermodilutions as the reference method; however, there is a great risk of rejecting some new methods only because the "reference" method was not as accurate as it should have been (e.g., not averaged thermodilution, alternative method used as reference).

Repeated measurements for each subject are often used in hemodynamic research. When repeated measures data are available, it is desirable to use all the data to compare the two methods. Several alternatives are available for the analysis of repeated measures;[6,7] among them the method described by Bland and Altman appears to be the simplest.[6]

Trend analysis

We described approaches aimed at evaluating the agreement between measures provided by two devices. However, in some clinical settings, these absolute values have limited clinical interest. Instead, the temporal variability of these absolute measures is of interest (referred to as trend analysis). There is no doubt that interchangeable devices would likely present a very high level of agreement in trend analysis. However, some devices presenting a bias in the measurements could be interesting when trends are considered. Repeated measures approaches are not able to evaluate the agreement between trends. The difference between the points of measurement for both methods can be analyzed using a Bland and Altman plot, and absolute or relative variations can be used with this approach. However, absolute variations do not take into account the baseline cardiac output (i.e., mean value before the change) and may not be able to identify clinically relevant disagreements with a wide range of baseline cardiac output. Relative variations do not take basal cardiac output into account; however, the percentage of variation may help the researchers to conclude about the clinical impact.

Critchley et al. have recently introduced a new approach to compare the trends between two cardiac output devices.[8] This new method addresses the magnitude of change between pairs of consecutive readings and the degree of agreement. A circular graph, called a polar plot, is proposed, which requires the changes in measurements given by the two cardiac output measurement devices to be transformed to polar coordinates. The best description of polar plot is given by Critchley:[9]

In the polar plot, the ΔCO data are converted to a radial vector where the degree of agreement between the 2 devices becomes the angle between the radial vector and the horizontal axis (i.e., polar axis). If agreement is perfect, the radial vector will lie along the polar axis and the angle is zero. The mean angle from all the radial vectors is the mean polar angle and is the statistic used to measure agreement. It is continuous rather than binomial variable (i.e., agree or disagree). The distance from the center of the polar plot or radius represents the magnitude of ΔCO in the polar vector and is derived from the average of reference and test ΔCO.

Methodological concerns

Studies evaluating cardiac output measurement devices generally do not specify a clinically meaningful limit of acceptable agreement before the analyses were conducted. Clinical interpretation of the interest of the new device is often done based on the results (i.e., posthoc). This approach is flawed because the width of the 95% limit of agreements confidence interval is mainly determined by the achieved sample size. Although we are dealing with an estimation problem, the estimation of required or desirable sample size is as relevant as it is to inference. Few calculations are needed to demonstrate that the size of confidence interval for the 95% limit of agreement is a function of the standard deviation of the differences between measurements by the two methods and of the sample size.[10] Researchers are thus able to determine the expected width of this confidence of interval. In fact, most of the studies aiming to evaluate cardiac output measurement devices are conducted on small sample sizes (e.g., less than 100 pairs of independent measurements). This impacts considerably on the robustness of the conclusions about the possible interchangeability of the devices. Estimation of the width of confidence interval for the 95% limit of agreement should be calculated a priori and used to determine the number of patients needed to get a robust estimation of the device.

Missing data is ubiquitous in medical research including in studies of cardiac output measurement (e.g., due to technical failures). Unfortunately, the existence of any missing values are rarely reported, including whether there are technical concerns regarding the measurement capability of the device. The ability of the device to produce a measurement is crucial if the device is to be considered interchangeable with the current measurement device. Devices able to produce unbiased measurement in 10% of the cases and no measurement in the 90% other cases should not be described as a perfect device. The statistical methods used to describe the agreement between two devices do not incorporate strategy to take account for this major limitation. Consequently, it is useful to report these unsuccessful measurements in a flowchart describing which method fails to estimate the cardiac output and for which reason.

Checklist for a better reporting of devices' comparisons

Planning the study

- Description of the reference method.
- The 95% limit of agreement should be determined according to the clinical setting of interest. It should also include the variability of the reference methods as suggested by Critchley et al.[5]
- The number of measurements/patients needed should be determined during the study design and not based on the observed data. The 95% limit of agreement defined as clinically relevant should be used to determine the number of measurements/patients to be included in the study.

Reporting the results

- Missing values for one or the other devices should be reported in detail. The percentage and the causes of missing values should be reported and explained for each device.
- The Bland and Altman plot should be presented. The confidence of interval of the 95% limit of agreement should be presented to demonstrate that the sample size was large enough to conclude.

To define thresholds

From a statistical point of view, the dichotomization of continuous variables is a "bad idea."[11] The simplicity achieved with such approaches is gained at a cost; dichotomization of continuous variables may create rather than avoid problems, notably a loss of information, considerable loss of power, and residual confounding. However, from a clinical point of view, continuous variables are often viewed as impractical, because clinicians need to take decisions, and because thresholds are required to define and standardize strategies. Furthermore, the ability to take rapid decisions on observed measurements characterizes clinical practice in the perioperative hemodynamic field. Physicians have a limited access to calculation devices and need to react quickly. Since computer assisted decision making systems are not yet included in all hemodynamic monitors, there is a need for cutoffs for perioperative hemodynamic parameters.

Several methods for selecting optimal cut-points in diagnostic tests have been proposed in the literature depending on the underlying reasons for this choice. However, these methods do not produce the same results for all situations. Clinical researchers need thus to choose the most appropriate method depending on the clinical setting. This choice implies a good knowledge of the advantages and of the weaknesses of the available methods, as well as a clear definition of the expected objectives of these thresholds in clinical practice.

In this chapter, we discuss the different approaches available to define thresholds using preload dependency parameters (i.e., pulse pressure variability) as an example. The aim is not to discuss the predictive value or the interest of preload dependency parameters, but to describe the advantages and the weaknesses of some of the most commonly used methods to define thresholds.

Rules to determine the cutoffs

The receiver operating characteristic (ROC) curve is undoubtedly the most common method to determine a clinical cutoff to make a clinical discrimination between sick or healthy patients or between those requiring a treatment or not. When the situation is only one continuous measurement (predictor), ROC curves provide a graphical representation of the relationship between sensitivity and specificity for each observed value of the continuous variable. The area under the ROC curve (often referred to as the AUC or c-statistic) measures discrimination, that is, the ability of the test to correctly differentiate between those with and without the endpoint. AUC can be also interpreted as a probability that in a randomly drawn pairs of individuals (one with the outcome event, the other one without the event), the individual with the outcome event will have a higher observed value (in the continuous measure) compared with the individual without the outcome.

A frequently neglected parameter of the ROC curves is the number of outcome events included in the discrimination and cutoff evaluation. Determining cutoffs using a small number of patients with outcome event does not provide robust and reliable results. In this situation, the cutoffs obtained may be largely influenced by only a few observations, and replicating the study is highly unlikely to yield similar values for the cutoff. While this is clearly concerning for a clinical use of cutoffs determined in such conditions, there is no clear guidance regarding how many patients with the outcome event are required to determine clinical cutoffs. Cutoffs determined with fewer than ten patients with outcome event are likely to be biased. A sample which includes 30 outcomes may be reasonable; however, this number is influenced by the distribution of the parameter of interest. An appropriate strategy to address this concern is to use bootstrapping.

Another point of major importance in the cutoff determination procedure is the approach to determine the optimal cutoff. Unfortunately, this is often not reported in published studies. Several approaches have been described and two of them are frequently used. The first one (I) is based on the minimum distance between the ROC curve and the top left corner on the ROC plot (coordinates 0,1) and thus intuitively minimizes misclassification. This point that minimizes the distance is the optimal values of the sensitivity and specificity of the measurement. The second approach (J) maximizes the Youden index (sensitivity+(specificity–1)) and thus intuitively maximizes appropriate classification. J point (i.e., the second method) should be preferred, because I does not solely rely on the rate of misclassification, but also on an unperceived quadratic term that is responsible for observed differences between I and J. However, both methods use an equipoise decision, which does not prioritize either sensitivity or specificity; such an approach makes sense in the case of a prevalence of 0.50; in other situations, the prevalence should be taken into account.

In some situations, we do not wish to (or could not) prioritize either sensitivity (identifying diseased patients) or specificity (excluding control patients), and thus, the cutoff point is chosen as the one that minimizes misclassification. However, in many clinical situations, the researcher could prioritize either sensitivity or specificity because the consequence of false-positive or false-negative results are usually not equivalent in terms of a cost–benefit relationship.

No single approach is suitable for all scenarios. An equipoise decision may represent the best approach for most of the studies. Clear reporting including a justification of the chosen approach for cutoff determination is recommended to allow replication and interpretation of the study results.

Gray zone approach[12,13]

Surprisingly, although the cutoff point has a crucial role in the decision process, it is provided in most (if not all) studies without a confidence interval. This may constitute a major methodological (and reporting) flaw, particularly in small sample studies, because this cutoff point is likely to be highly influenced by the values of very few patients, although the confidence intervals of sensitivity and specificity associated with that cutoff are usually reported.

The reason for the absence of a confidence interval is probably related to the fact that more sophisticated statistical methods should be used. All these methods should perform some form of resampling (e.g., bootstrapping) of the study population to provide a reasonable estimate and its associated 95% confidence interval.

Another option for clinical discrimination is to avoid providing a single cutoff that dichotomizes the population, but rather to propose two cutoffs separated by the "gray zone." The first cutoff is chosen to exclude the diagnosis with near-certainty (i.e., prioritize specificity). The second cutoff is chosen to include the diagnosis with near-certainty (i.e., prioritize sensitivity).

When values of the biomarker fall into the gray zone (i.e., between the two cutoffs), uncertainty exists, and the physician should pursue a diagnosis using additional tools. This approach is probably more useful from a clinical point of view and is now more widely used in clinical research. Moreover, the two cutoffs and gray zone comprise three intervals of the biomarker that can be associated with a respective likelihood ratio. In that case, the positive likelihood ratio of the highest value of the biomarker in the gray zone is considered to include the diagnosis and the negative likelihood ratio of the lowest value to exclude the diagnosis. This option results in less loss of information and less distortion than choosing a single cutoff, providing an advantage in interpretation over a binary outcome. This allows the clinician to more thoroughly interpret the results thereby improving clinical decision making.

Checklist for a better reporting of cutoffs' determination

Population's characteristics

- The number of patients with the endpoint included in the cutoff determination should be clearly presented. When this number is below ten, its impact on the final result should be discussed.
- The number of missing values for the parameter of interest should be reported.

Parameter discrimination

- The ROC curves should be provided. The area under the ROC curves should be calculated and presented.

- Ideally, bootstrapped ROC curves should be presented with the average area under the curve for the bootstrapped curves. In the case where a large difference is observed, limitations about the robustness of the analysis should be discussed.

Threshold determination

- The rule of decision used to define the "optimal" cutoff should be presented. Whatever the most appropriate rule is, it seems reasonable also to present the results obtained with an equipoise rule.
- The confidence interval around the "optimal" cutoffs should be presented. The proportion of patients with a parameter value within the confidence interval should be reported.

References

1. Bland JM, Altman DG. Statistical methods for assessing agreement between two methods of clinical measurement. *Int J Nursing Studies* 2010;**47** (8):931–6.

2. Bland JM, Altman DG. Statistical methods for assessing agreement between two methods of clinical measurement. *Lancet* 1986;**1** (8476):307–10.

3. Lamantia KR, O'Connor T, Barash PG. Comparing methods of measurement – an alternative approach. *Anesthesiology* 1990;**72** (5):781–3.

4. Stetz CW, Miller RG, Kelly GE, Raffin TA. Reliability of thermodilution method in the determination of cardiac-output in clinical-practice. *Am Rev Respiratory Dis* 1982;**126** (6):1001–4.

5. Critchley LAH, Critchley J. A meta-analysis of studies using bias and precision statistics to compare cardiac output measurement techniques. *J Clin Monit Comput* 1999;**15**(2):85–91.

6. Bland JM, Altman DG. Agreement between methods of measurement with multiple observations per individual. *J Biopharmaceut Stat* 2007;**17** (4):571–82.

7. Myles PS, Cui J. Using the Bland-Altman method to measure agreement with repeated measures. *Br J Anaes* 2007;**99**(3):309–11.

8. Critchley LA, Lee A, Ho AMH. A critical review of the ability of continuous cardiac output monitors to measure trends in cardiac output. *Anesth Analg* 2010;**111**(5):1180–92.

9. Critchley LA. Validation of the MostCare pulse contour cardiac output monitor: beyond the Bland and Altman Plot. *Anesth Analg* 2011;**113**(6):1292–4.

10. Bland JM, Altman DG. Measuring agreement in method comparison studies. *Stat Meth Med Res* 1999;**8** (2):135–60.

11. Royston P, Altman DG, Sauerbrei W. Dichotomizing continuous predictors in multiple regression: a bad idea. *Stat Med* 2006;**25** (1):127–41.

12. Ray P, Le Manach Y, Riou B, Houle TT. Statistical evaluation of a biomarker. *Anesthesiology* 2010;**112**(4):1023–40.

13. Cannesson M, Le Manach Y, Hofer CK, et al. Assessing the diagnostic accuracy of pulse pressure variations for the prediction of fluid responsiveness: a "gray zone" approach. *Anesthesiology* 2011;**115** (2):231–41.

Chapter 3

New trends in perioperative medicine

Gautam Kumar, David Walker, and Michael Mythen

Introduction

In recent years, greater attention has been placed on improving quality and safety in perioperative health care. Minimally invasive surgery has become more prevalent, and considerable enthusiasm has arisen around robotic-assisted techniques, day-case surgery and regional anesthesia. In the USA, inpatient mortality at 30 days has decreased from 1.68% in 1996 to 1.32% in 2006 with an estimated continued improvement in this trend.[1]

In a 1954 review of surgical procedures, 0.64% of patients died directly as a result of anesthesia. This rate has steadily improved and, in 1989, perioperative death directly attributable to anesthesia was approximately 0.001% for healthy patients, with modern mortality rates now quoted to be as low as 1.4 per 1 000 000 surgical interventions. Significant improvements in survival were witnessed in the 1980s, where rapid improvements in anesthesia safety were made, primarily through the implementation of new clinical practice guidelines, improvements in monitoring technology, and the introduction of new therapies.[2]

Thus improvements in anesthesia safety have evolved with surgical technique and have resulted in more complex surgery being performed on older, less well patients who may have been considered unsuitable for surgery in the past. This large subgroup of high-risk patients account for 12.5% of total patients, but 80% of perioperative deaths. This compares with the total incidence of 0.4 to 0.8% of permanent disability or mortality in all surgical patients in the developed world. The short-term postoperative mortality for this group is estimated at approximately 6% for elective procedures and approaching 30% for those having urgent or emergency surgery.[3] It is estimated that, over the next 10 years, the population in the UK over the age of 65 will increase by a quarter and, by the year 2040, the over 65s will constitute approximately 24% of the world's population, with half requiring a surgical procedure during this period.[4]

Despite an overall improvement, there is considerable geographical variation in postoperative survival. For any given risk level, perioperative mortality rates are higher in the UK than in the USA and the median interval from surgery to death was longer in patients who underwent surgery in the USA compared with the UK. This difference may reflect better elective use of surgical high-dependency areas, as it is recognized that patients admitted directly to ward-based care and who are subsequently admitted to ICU with a complication survive less often, but have reduced length of hospital stay.[5] Perioperative medical practice must therefore develop to meet the needs of a changing patient population, an expanding surgical program, and an identifiable population of patients who require enhanced care pathways.

The rise of the perioperative physician

A study analyzing complications and mortality in an older surgical population conducted in Australia and New Zealand showed that 68% of patients undergoing surgery had pre-existing co-morbidities with 20% suffering perioperative complications and 5% dying within 30 days of surgery.[6] It has therefore been argued that further training leading to skills in risk reduction, patient optimization, and knowledge in perioperative medicine would reduce the disparity in outcomes, and an extended role of the anesthetist as "the perioperative physician" has emerged and is gaining momentum internationally. Utilizing skills developed at the front line of clinical medicine, anesthetists as perioperative

Perioperative Hemodynamic Monitoring and Goal Directed Therapy, ed. Maxime Cannesson and Rupert Pearse.
Published by Cambridge University Press. © Cambridge University Press 2014.

physicians are now delivering clinical leadership to improve outcomes for high-risk surgical patients from admission to discharge. UK-based anesthesia is an example where further definition of the high-risk perioperative episode is taking place, primarily through national audit and quality improvement activity. This is exemplified by projects such as the National Emergency Laparotomy Audit, the Hip Fracture Perioperative Network, and the National Confidential Enquiry into Patient Outcome and Death (NCEPOD).

Such projects seek standardization of perioperative processes, focus on outlying morbidity and mortality, and optimize resource utilization, quality of care, and patient safety. In the USA the perioperative surgical home has been established by the American Society of Anesthesiologists as an innovative, patient-centered, surgical continuity of care model.[7] An anesthetist-led, multidisciplinary system of coordinated and managed perioperative care throughout the entire surgical continuum has been achieved with the aim of utilizing best evidence to inform practice, patient centeredness, and accountable management by a single coordinating service. Eliminating overuse, underuse, and misuse of care, will likely lead to better outcomes at a lower cost – the definition of added value. This new system also seeks to drive performance improvement and outcomes research to promote improved surgical care for all patients.[8]

Central to the debate about a perioperative surgical home are:

- holding the gains made in anesthesia-related patient safety
- impacting surgical morbidity and mortality
- achieving health care outcome metrics
- assimilating comparative effectiveness research into the model
- establishing necessary audit and data collection.

The concept of the anesthesia-led surgical home is in direct comparison to the hospitalist model in the USA, where the co-management of surgical patients is by internal medicine specialists. In an expanded role as perioperative physician, anesthetists play a key role in compliance with broader sets of process measures, thus becoming a more vital and valuable health care provider to the patient, administrators, and financiers. The perioperative surgical home is not intended to replace the surgeon's care responsibility, but rather to leverage the abilities of the entire perioperative team toward patient care.[8]

Improvements in patient assessment

The anesthetist working as a perioperative physician in a surgical Preassessment Clinic (PAC) is now commonplace in the UK, and is considered to have central importance in patient optimization, risk assessment, and supporting informed decision making. Linking to primary care services plays an important function in preparing patients' fitness before surgery by offering advice on smoking cessation, exercise, and weight reduction and by optimizing treatment of chronic conditions such as diabetes and anemia. This closer working relationship may help improve survival, decrease perioperative morbidity, and shorten duration of hospital admission.

The goal of a well-conducted PAC is to minimize risk for all patients, identify patients at high risk of perioperative morbidity and mortality, and establish clear pathways to allow the allocation of individualized resources to patients' needs. It is recognized that patient failure to access PAC results in higher costs, ICU utilization, and mortality.[9,10] Improved triage of patients to nurse and/or physician assessment better allows the targeting of risk assessment and prediction tools to individualize risk. Close liaison with secondary care groups such as diabetes and medical outreach teams can be particularly helpful and may prevent protracted hospital stays, both pre- and postoperatively. Today, it should be standard care that all patients presenting for surgery should undergo adequate preoperative evaluation.

It is useful for perioperative physicians to be able to predict generic morbidity and all-cause mortality so that a patient's care may be modified if they are identified as high risk. The American College of Cardiology/American Heart Association (ACC/AHA) and the European Society of Cardiology/European Society of Anaesthesiology (ESC/ESA) provide consensus guidelines for preoperative cardiac risk assessment and management for non-cardiac surgery.[11] These categorize patients into risk groups using patient characteristics, co-morbidities, functional capacity, and type of surgery as discriminators. Supplementary to this, three of the most commonly used risk stratification tools are the American Society of Anesthesiologists' Physical Status Score (ASA-PSS), Charlson Age-co-morbidity index (CACI), and the Physiological and Operative Severity Score for the enUmeration of Mortality and morbidity (POSSUM). There are also a number of validated assessment tools in use that have been developed purely for the prediction of cardiovascular morbidity and mortality, the most widely used and recommended being the Lee Revised Cardiac Risk Index (RCRI).[12]

Today's perioperative assessment includes measures of dynamic function to identify patients at risk of functional heart failure, inducible myocardial ischemia, or both. An acknowledgment of the limited value of *static* investigations such as echocardiography have less influence, with a recent retrospective analysis of 40 000 patients having resting echocardiography for preoperative assessment showing no evidence of improvement in 1-year survival or hospital stay compared with matched controls. However, graded exercise testing, exercise or dipyridamole myocardial perfusion scan, and stress echocardiography are sensitive to assess dynamic cardiac performance and are associated with improved 1-year survival and shortened postoperative hospital stay. This observation is possibly related to the resultant closer monitoring of patients' hemodynamics in the perioperative period.[13]

Since the clinical utility of cardiopulmonary exercise testing (CPET) was demonstrated in 1999, much attention has focused on it as a measure of perioperative fitness and a predictor of surgical outcome. In the UK, the use of CPET has risen by over 40% in the last 2 years, with an estimated 15 000 tests performed annually for preoperative assessment in England with the majority for patients undergoing vascular surgery. Performed as an incremental workload stress test and providing an objective characterization of an individual's "functional capacity," the role of CPET in the prediction of adverse perioperative outcome remains controversial. However, CPET is now a widely used tool in perioperative risk assessment, but there is little consensus on who should be tested, which variables should be used to identify high-risk patients, and how this should affect patients' subsequent perioperative pathway.[14] These inconsistencies are likely to be related to limitations in the current evidence base and the subsequent piecemeal adoption of technology in the absence of generally accepted practice guidelines. It is acknowledged that such tests have utility to identify low-risk patients, but lack predictive power in determining intermediate to high-risk patients, since the occurrence of a major adverse outcome may depend on concomitant factors. A large randomized controlled study of CPET use in a high-risk, non-cardiac surgery population reported its findings in 2013.[15]

Physiological markers of organ dysfunction may significantly improve surgical risk stratification and there is much on-going research to assess its clinical benefit. Natriuretic peptides (NP) are primarily released by cardiac myocytes in response to ventricular wall stretch or myocardial ischemia, and this may be central to NP becoming one of the strongest and consistent predictors of postoperative cardiac complications. Evidence from patients undergoing vascular surgery has shown that NP level significantly improves the prognostic power of the RCRI risk score.[16] Preoperative NP may soon become useful as a screening tool to stratify risk of postoperative functional heart failure, followed by CPET for objective characterization of functional capacity in problem cases.

Preoperative C-reactive protein (CRP) and troponins (Tn) may also be useful for risk stratification. Peak postoperative Tn in the first 3 days after surgery is significantly associated with 30-day mortality, making it a useful postoperative surveillance test, but it only represents the final common pathway of myocardial injury. CRP only addresses cardiovascular complications attributable to an associated inflammatory pathophysiology, thus making both of these biomarkers inferior to NP. Genotype may also play an important role in the magnitude of the inflammatory response in addition to biomarkers, but preoperative genetic testing is not currently available. Both biomarkers and genetic profiling remain interesting areas of research, which to date have not translated into available bedside tests with true clinical utility.[17]

Patients and the surgical experience

It remains the ideal of surgical care that patients undergoing operative procedures do so cognisant of the associated attendant risks. The history of clinical decision making has to date been one of paternalism, where important decisions have been taken about patients in isolation by health care professionals. Shared decision making (SDM), as outlined in the Salzburg statement of 2010 and representing the view of 18 participating countries, identifies both the ethical and practical benefits of patient involvement in decisions which affect them.[18,19] Thus a concept of "no decision about me without me" has grown to signify that, at any stage of diagnosis, referral, and after treatment, patient empowerment to achieve realistic outcomes should be the desired goal. Further, it is recognized that poor communication between health care providers and patients represents a risk to patient safety. Postoperative patient outcomes can be adversely affected by poor communication between patient and provider and can result in patient dissatisfaction and complaints in the aftermath of an adverse outcome, producing health system costs for complaint resolution.[20]

SDM is an acknowledgment that clinicians and patients bring their own agenda to the consultation process. The patient is able to assess surgical intervention risk in the context of their beliefs, cultural values, and personal experience of their illness. It is not unusual for there to be no decision, but rather an agreement reached based on a process of mutual respect and understanding. The aim is for a partnership whereby clinicians and patients work together and share information to facilitate the clarification of realistic goals and the construction of a mutually satisfactory management plan. Facilitating patient involvement will be a vital area of quality improvement, as there is evidence of an association with improved coping skills and health outcomes, even in those who initially expressed a preference for not partaking in decision making.[21]

Benefits of SDM include a reduction in "decisional regret," less patient anxiety, improved patient satisfaction and increased medical accountability to society.[22] Despite this, there is insufficient evidence to recommend any educational strategies to improve the adoption of SDM by health professionals. Further work is required to engage clinicians and teach the attitudes and skills required to embrace SDM.[21] The recent trend appears to be in the local development of various informative, patient-friendly, peer-reviewed, shared decision making tools for patients undergoing surgery and anesthesia, based on local logistical and management policies. These tools detail the nature and character of anesthetic and surgical procedures, risks, benefits, and alternative treatments and follow-up care. An improved understanding of patient priorities perioperatively is dependent on patient inclusion in the research process and the measurement of patient-reported outcomes.

Opportunity for Quality Improvement

Lacking in demonstrable Quality Improvement (also known as Health care Improvement Science), the process of medical audit has, until recently, been seen as relatively ineffective for improving care for patients. More recently, a new generation of health care worker supported by highly influential professional bodies (for example, The Institute for Healthcare Improvement and the King's Fund) have embraced quality improvement science and, using a structured approach to change, exhibited measurable improvement and reliability of

health care delivery. Anesthesia has led the way in this transformation, and many examples of sustainable high-quality improvement projects are now finding their way into the perioperative medicine area.

The Scottish Audit of Surgical Mortality is one such example and represents a nationwide safety program aimed at improving perioperative outcomes. Highlighting the 2000 perioperative deaths and 10 000 major complications associated with surgery in Scotland each year, the working group called for consensus guidelines to be developed from audit data; these addressed failure to recognize patient deterioration in a timely manner and deficiencies in clear care escalation policies. Similarly, the Scottish Patient Safety Programme (SPSP) has employed a methodology of developing primary and secondary drivers to incorporate quality improvement in order to improve perioperative outcomes.[23] In this example the primary drivers (the key areas that can be worked on to "drive" change) are preventing surgical site infections, creating a team culture, and reducing adverse cardiac events. The primary drivers are then linked to secondary drivers that are specific processes or interventions, which can be addressed and improved by the team. The secondary drivers can be combined as a "bundle" of care to achieve the desired outcomes. This quality improvement process has seen an introduction of a safety culture, surgical checklists, and bundles of care to reduce ventilator-associated pneumonias and catheter-related bloodstream infections. By following these and similar interventions, the SPSP has delivered a 12.4% reduction in hospital standardized mortality with 8497 fewer than expected deaths.[23]

The effective use of quality indicators in health care is long established and, within perioperative care, may hold the potential for a broad range of improvement. Implementing Donabedian principles, analysis of structures, processes, and outcomes with robust data-sets offers a quantitative understanding of variations in perioperative health care. Local data can be used to inform local practice by regular monitoring and feedback with a spotlight on selected performance targets. These data nationally aligned with similar regional data result in adequately powered quality improvement studies, which enable relatively infrequent events to be analyzed and reported on with a degree of certainty. The resulting establishment of commonly agreed national standards may then form national guidance for safer and improved standards of perioperative care.

One current national example in the UK is the National Emergency Laparotomy Audit (NELA),[24] a project with the aim of improving quality of care for patients undergoing an emergency laparotomy through the provision of high-quality comparative data from all providers of this operation. It represents a huge opportunity for perioperative medical specialists to bring about improvements in quality of patient care in virtually every trust in England and Wales. Similarly, the NHS Hip Fracture Perioperative Network which is running a national audit to explore whether an association exists between co-morbidities and anesthetic techniques and the detection of preoperative anemia, intraoperative hypotension, Bone Cement Implantation Syndrome and 30-day mortality in patients undergoing a fractured neck of femur fixation.[25]

Improvement science has a crucial role to play in benefiting individual patients and developing reliable health systems by bridging the worlds of academia and health service delivery. It is based on scientific principles and provides a mechanism to drive continuous improvement in the quality and efficiency of care. As the Perioperative Physician emerges, leads, and ultimately shapes the delivery of future perioperative care, it will be imperative they understand and engage in improvement science activity. Resisting "knee-jerk" service developments, they must align to share data, understand complex problems across geographically diverse areas, and seek to reduce variance in practice and outcomes.

Protocolizing perioperative care

The concept of enhanced recovery (ER) is a proactive patient management pathway, which adopts multimodal "care bundles" in which the patient has an active role and is recognized as an example of high-quality care improvement. The evidence base for ER is clear and continues to strengthen; the evolving philosophy is now extending beyond surgical ER and is being readily adopted for a wide range of hospital services. In the UK, surgical ER has been supported by the National Health Service drive to Quality, Productivity and Prevention in Practice (QIPP), bringing demonstrated quality benefits for patients and reducing the length of hospital stay with no increase in surgical readmission rates.[26]

The perioperative physician is well placed to readily adopt ER culture. By crossing both functional and organizational boundaries, they are able to influence, orchestrate, and monitor quality care improvements for surgical patients. This begins in the aforementioned PAC, which facilitates more appropriate use of investigations, and has closer links to primary care services, allowing optimization of care and effective communication prior to determining a date for surgery.

The operative care bundle is well understood and in gastrointestinal surgery includes core elements such as avoidance of bowel preparation and nasogastric tubes, goal directed fluid therapy, immediate postoperative feeding, and early mobilization facilitated by short acting anesthetic agents and regional analgesia (Figure 3.1). The body of evidence supporting ER is constantly changing and is expected to continue to evolve as evidence-based techniques and therapies emerge. In the UK, ER represents a best-practice model of care for colorectal, urological, gynecological, and orthopedic procedures and has been endorsed by professional organizations including the Royal Colleges of Surgeons and Anesthetists. ER improves the planned care pathway for patients, reducing both the length of hospital stay and postoperative complications.

The ER model defends equity in health care provision by broadly treating all patients in the same way. Recent focus on increased weekend mortality rates and inferred disparities in care compared with weekday activity have been highlighted, and ER may be seen as a way of maintaining optimal care regardless of this parameter.[28]

Due to the benefits of ER, many UK health care trusts now receive payment to incentivize the adoption of best practice. The Commissioning for Quality and Innovation (CQUIN) payment framework enables health care commissioners to reward excellence by linking a proportion of providers' income to the achievement of local quality improvement goals. Since the first year of the CQUIN framework (2009/10), many CQUIN schemes have been developed and more recently published national goals for 2011/12 have detailed enhanced recovery payment schemes. In London, the enhanced recovery CQUIN payment covers eight elective procedures across the four specialties mentioned and covers four components, each reflecting best practice in perioperative care.[29]

1. Recording of comprehensive information about enhanced recovery patients on the national database to allow trusts to better understand ER implementation.
2. To ensure that the majority of patients admitted for colorectal surgery receive goal directed fluid therapy, the trusts qualify for full payment if $\geq$ 80% of patients undergoing

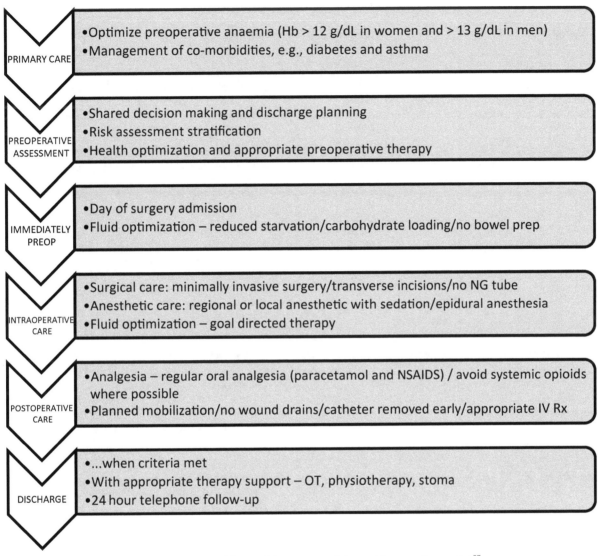

PRIMARY CARE
- Optimize preoperative anaemia (Hb > 12 g/dL in women and > 13 g/dL in men)
- Management of co-morbidities, e.g., diabetes and asthma

PREOPERATIVE ASSESSMENT
- Shared decision making and discharge planning
- Risk assessment stratification
- Health optimization and appropriate preoperative therapy

IMMEDIATELY PREOP
- Day of surgery admission
- Fluid optimization – reduced starvation/carbohydrate loading/no bowel prep

INTRAOPERATIVE CARE
- Surgical care: minimally invasive surgery/transverse incisions/no NG tube
- Anesthetic care: regional or local anesthetic with sedation/epidural anesthesia
- Fluid optimization – goal directed therapy

POSTOPERATIVE CARE
- Analgesia – regular oral analgesia (paracetamol and NSAIDS) / avoid systemic opioids where possible
- Planned mobilization/no wound drains/catheter removed early/appropriate IV Rx

DISCHARGE
- ...when criteria met
- With appropriate therapy support – OT, physiotherapy, stoma
- 24 hour telephone follow-up

Figure 3.1. Enhanced recovery pathway (adapted from NHS Improvement Enhanced Recovery Partnership).[27]

planned colorectal surgery performed receive goal directed fluid therapy.

3. Targeted day of surgery admission. The trusts qualify for full payment only if ≥ 80% of eligible patients were admitted on the day of surgery.

4. Targeted length of stay for patients undergoing the eight specified operations. The target for each procedure was to equal the national median from the previous year.

In the USA, a model of enhanced recovery is also favored with detailed information given to patients before their surgery and anesthesia to diminish anxiety,

enhance postoperative recovery, and hasten hospital discharge. Preoperative psychological intervention including personal counselling, pamphlets, and multi-media information is aimed at decreasing patient anxiety and improving recovery from surgery.

As ER programs evolve, it is expected that future trends (and possible CQUIN payments) will focus on improved preoperative assessment, shared decision making, and the ready adoption of novel techniques shown to provide benefit (for instance, esophageal Doppler to guide perioperative fluid management, as recently approved by the National Institute for Health and Clinical Excellence).

Table 3.1. Examples of large trials in perioperative practice and intensive care affecting outcome.

Clinical trial	Journal and year	Trial size	Key findings
The NICE-SUGAR trial: intensive blood glucose control significantly increases mortality in ICU patients	*NEJM* 2009	6104	1. Tight glycemic control (81–108 mg/dL) in critically ill patients is associated with higher mortality when compared to conventional glycemic control (≤ 180 mg/dL).
A surgical safety checklist to reduce morbidity and mortality in a global population	*NEJM* 2009	7688	1. Introduction of the WHO Surgical Safety Checklist into operating rooms was associated with marked improvements in surgical outcomes. Postoperative complication rates fell by 36% on average, and death rates fell by a similar amount.
The LACTATE trial: early lactate-guided therapy in intensive care patients	*AJRCCM* 2010	348	1. Therapy aimed at reducing lactate levels by 20% every 2 hours during the first 8 hours of ICU admission led to decreased in-hospital mortality and shorter ICU stays. 2. Patients in the early lactate-guided therapy group received more fluids and started on vasopressors earlier than in the control group, but did not have a faster reduction rate of lactate levels.
The PIVOT trial: radical prostatectomy vs. observation	*NEJM* 2012	731	1. Prostatectomy did not significantly reduce all-cause mortality or prostate-cancer mortality when compared to observation. 2. These findings support conservative management for men with localized prostate cancer, especially for those with PSA values less than 10 ng/mL and low-risk disease.
The CREST trial: stenting vs. endarterectomy for carotid stenosis	*NEJM* 2010	2522	1. The rate of stroke, myocardial infarction or death did not differ significantly between patients treated with carotid artery stenting compared to carotid endarterectomy. 2. The periprocedural rate of stroke was higher with stenting while the rate of myocardial infarction was higher with endarterectomy.
The EVAR II trial: endovascular approach when unfit for open aortic aneurysm repair	*NEJM* 2010	404	1. The EVAR II trial compared endovascular abdominal aortic aneurysm repair with no intervention in patients unsuitable for the open procedure. 2. There were significantly fewer aneurysm-related deaths in the endovascular group, compared with no intervention. 3. The rates of complication and re-intervention were similar to the rates observed in EVAR I.
The Scandinavian starch for severe sepsis/septic shock (6S) trial[33–37]	*NEJM* 2012	804	1. Hydroxyethyl starches for fluid resuscitation significantly increased 90-day mortality by 8%. 2. There was an increased likelihood of these patients receiving renal replacement therapy (RRT) although this has no effect on the incidence of end-stage renal failure

Table 3.1. (cont.)

Clinical trial	Journal and year	Trial size	Key findings
The CHEST trial: crystalloid vs. hydroxyethyl starch trial	*NEJM* 2012	7000	1. There was no difference in 90-day mortality between patients in intensive care given HES and those given 0.9% NaCl. 2. There was a significant increase in the need for renal replacement therapy in those who had been given hydroxyethyl starches.

Perioperative medicine defining best practice

Anesthesia and surgery as hospital specialties historically have made little use of the randomized controlled trial (RCT) methodology to inform their clinical practice or to form the basis for quality improvement. Until recently, most studies involving surgical procedures were retrospective case series with RCTs accounting for less than 10% of the total. RCTs declined from 14% of research articles in the *British Journal of Surgery* in the 1980s to 5% in the 1990s. In addition, the treatments in general surgery and anesthesia have been shown to be half as likely to be based on RCT evidence as treatments in internal medicine.[30]

Many of the current clinical trends in perioperative practice have not resulted from high-quality research and, in the absence of rigorously conducted research, important controversies remain. One such controversy is the debate surrounding the perioperative use of beta-blockers in non-cardiac surgery. 2009 joint ESC and AHA guidelines, which were based mainly on evidence including data from the DECREASE trials, advocated their preoperative use in patients with clinical risk factors for perioperative cardiovascular complications.[31] However, these trials have been found to be fraudulent and, in conjunction with data from the POISE trial[32] (a large, double-blinded RCT with over 8000 patients recruited which showed a significant increase in mortality and stroke in patients started on beta-blocker therapy preoperatively), the evidence suggests the use of beta-blockers preoperatively cannot be advocated. Nonetheless, the perioperative community has been slow to adapt with the ESC guidelines still to be withdrawn and a revision of them is not expected before August 2014.

There are suggestions that perioperative medicine is, however, emerging from an evidence base built largely on retrospective case series, consensus opinion, and an over-reliance on surrogate end-markers of questionable clinical significance. The challenge for the perioperative academic community now is to evolve and build its foundations in more solidly rooted science fact. Green shoots are appearing and, in recent years, landmark papers assessing types of surgery and anesthesia, as well as prominent trials assessing interventions in the intensive care setting that have been extrapolated to perioperative care, have become prominent and are beginning to shape modern practice (Table 3.1).

References

1. Semel ME, Lipsitz SR, Funk LM, et al. Rates and patterns of death after surgery in the United States, 1996 and 2006. *Surgery* 2012;**151** (2):171–82.

2. Lagasse RS. Anesthesia safety: model or myth? A review of the published literature and analysis of current original data. *Anesthesiology* 2002;**97(6)**:1609–17.

3. Pearse RM, Holt PJ, Grocott MP. Managing perioperative risk in patients undergoing elective non-cardiac surgery. *Br Med J* 2011;**343**:734–9.

4. Asouhidou I, Asteri T, Sountoulides P, et al. Early postoperative mortality in the elderly: a pilot study. *BMC Research Notes* 2009;**2(1)**:118.

5. Bennett-Guerrero EJ, Hyam S, Shaefi DR, et al. Comparison of P-POSSUM risk-adjusted mortality rates after surgery between patients in the USA and the UK. *Br J Surg* 2003;**90** (12):1593–8.

6. Story DA, Leslie K, Myles PS, et al. Complications and mortality in older surgical patients in Australia and New Zealand (the REASON study): a multicentre, prospective, observational study. *Anaesthesia* 2010;**65(10)**:1022–30.

7. *American Society of Anesthesiologists. The Perioperative or Surgical Home.* Washington, DC: American Society of Anesthesiologists, 2011.

8. Vetter TR, Goeddel LA, Boudreaux AM, et al. The Perioperative Surgical Home: how can it make the case so everyone wins? *BMC Anesthesiol* 2013;**13(1)**:6.

9. Swart M, Carlisle JB. Case-controlled study of critical care or surgical ward care after elective open colorectal surgery. *Br J Surg* 2012;**99(2)**:295–9.

10. National Confidential Enquiry into Patient Outcome and Death, and G.P. Findlay. Knowing the risk: a review of the peri-operative care of surgical patients. *NCEPOD* 2011.

11. Eagle KA, Berger PB, Calkins C, et al. ACC/AHA guideline update for perioperative cardiovascular evaluation for noncardiac surgery – executive summary. A report of the American College of Cardiology/American Heart Association Task Force on Practice Guidelines (Committee to Update the 1996 Guidelines on Perioperative Cardiovascular Evaluation for Noncardiac Surgery). *J Am Coll Cardiol* 2002;**39(3)**:542–53.

12. Moonesinghe SR, Mythen MG, Grocott MPW. High-risk surgery: epidemiology and outcomes. *Anesth Analg* 2011;**112 (4)**:891–901.

13. Pearse RM, Holt PJ, Grocott MPW. Managing perioperative risk in patients undergoing elective non-cardiac surgery. *Br Med J* 2011;**343**:734–9.

14. Older P, Hall A, Hader R. Cardiopulmonary exercise testing as a screening test for perioperative management of major surgery in the elderly. *Chest* 1999;**116**:355–62.

15. Cardiopulmonary exercise testing and preoperative testing. http://clinicaltrials.gov/show/NCT00737828 (Accessed October 9, 2013).

16. Biccard BM, Naidoo P. The role of brain natriuretic peptide in prognostication and reclassification of risk in patients undergoing vascular surgery. *Anaesthesia* 2011;**66(5)**:379–85.

17. Beattie WS, Wijeysundera DN. Perioperative cardiac biomarkers: the utility and timing. *Curr Opin Crit Care* 2013;**19(4)**:334–41.

18. Charles C, Whelan T, Gafni A. What do we mean by partnership in making decisions about treatment? *BMJ* 1999;**319**:780–2.

19. Elywn G. Analysis: Salzburg statement on shared decision making, *BMJ* 2011;**342**: d1745.

20. Duclos CW, Eichler M, Taylor L, et al. Patient perspectives of patient–provider communication after adverse events. *Int J Quality Health Care* 2005;**17(6)**:479–86.

21. Say R, Thomson R. The importance of patient preferences in treatment decisions – challenges for doctors. *BMJ* 2003;**327**:542–5.

22. O'Connor A, Stacey D, Entwistle V, et al. Decision aids for people facing health treatment or screening decisions. *Cochrane Database Syst Rev* 2009;**1**.

23. Haraden C, Leitch J. Scotland's successful national approach to improving patient safety in acute care. *Health Affairs* 2011;**30 (4)**:755–63.

24. Saunders DI, Murray D, Pichel AC, et al. Variations in mortality after emergency laparotomy: the first report of the UK Emergency Laparotomy Network. *Br J Anaesth* 2012;**109(3)**:368–75.

25. Griffiths RJ, Alper A, Beckingsale D, et al. Management of proximal femoral fractures 2011. *Anaesthesia* 2012;**67(1)**:85–98.

26. Ford SR, Pearse RM. Do integrated care pathways have a place in critical care? *Curr Opin Crit Care* 2012;**18(6)**:683–7.

27. NHS Enhanced recovery partnership. Fulfilling the potential. http://www.improvement.nhs.uk/documents/er_better_journey.pdf (Accessed October 5, 2013).

28. Aylin P, Alexandrescu R, Jen MH, et al. Day of week of procedure and 30 day mortality for elective surgery: retrospective analysis of hospital episode statistics. *BMJ* 2013;**346**:f2424.doi:10.1136/bmj. f2424.

29. Mythen MG, Swart M, Acheson N, et al. Perioperative fluid management: consensus statement from the enhanced recovery partnership. *Perioperative Med* 2012;**1(1)**:2.

30. McCulloch P, Taylor I, Sasako M, et al. Randomised trials in surgery: problems and possible solutions. *BMJ* 2002;**324(7351)**: 1448.

31. Fleisher LA, Poldermans D. Perioperative β blockade: where do we go from here? *Lancet* 2008;**371(9627)**: 1813–14.

32. Devereaux PJ, Yang H, Yusuf S, et al. Effects of extended-release metoprolol succinate in patients undergoing non-cardiac surgery (POISE trial): a randomised controlled trial. *Lancet* 2008;**371 (9627)**:1839–47.

33. Perner A, Haase N, Guttormsen AB, et al. Hydroxyethyl starch 130/0.42 versus Ringer's acetate in severe sepsis. *N Engl J Med* 2012;**367(2)**:124–34.

34. Myburgh JA, Finfer S, Bellomo R, et al. Hydroxyethyl starch or saline for fluid resuscitation in

intensive care. *N Engl J Med* 2012;**367**(20):1901–11.

35. Gattas DJ, Arina D, Myburgh J, et al. Fluid resuscitation with 6% hydroxyethyl starch (130/0.4) in acutely ill patients: an updated systematic review and meta-analysis. *Anesth Analg* 2012;**114** (1):159–69.

36. Haase N, Perner A, Hennings LI, et al. Hydroxyethyl starch 130/0.38–0.45 versus crystalloid or albumin in patients with sepsis: systematic review with meta-analysis and trial sequential analysis. *BMJ* 2013;**346**:f839. doi:10.1136/bmj.f839.

37. Patel A, Waheed U, Brett SJ. Randomised trials of 6% tetrastarch (hydroxyethyl starch 130/0.4 or 0.42) for severe sepsis reporting mortality: systematic review and meta-analysis. *Intens Care Medi*, 2013;**39**(5)811–12.

38. Van Der Linden P, James M, Mythen M, Weiskopf RB. Safety of modern starches used during surgery. *Anesth Analg*, 2013;**116** (1):35–48.

39. Martin C, Jacob M, Vicaut E, et al. Effect of waxy maize-derived hydroxyethyl starch 130/0.4 on renal function in surgical patients. *Anesthesiology* 2013;**118** (2):387–94.

The surgical home: a paradigm shift toward perioperative practice

Shermeen B. Vakharia, Zeev N. Kain, and Leslie M. Garson

Introduction

Currently, care of the surgical patient in the United States (USA) is highly variable during all phases of the perioperative period. Preoperative care varies from assessing the patient on the day of surgery to often inappropriate and excessive laboratory work and consults. Intraoperative anesthesia and fluid management strategies vary among providers, often depending on personal training, experience, and comfort level. Likewise, in few health care institutions is postoperative care standardized. Often, a significant portion of the practitioner's time is occupied in completing documentation to meet regulatory requirements rather than in providing direct patient care. Multiple providers make unilateral health care decisions without unified oversight of care.[1] Lack of coordination and standardization of care pathways in the perioperative period lead to fragmentation of care along many dimensions. In its narrowest dimension, fragmentation of perioperative processes during a single surgical episode can lead to errors, complications, suboptimal patient satisfaction, possibly increased mortality, and ultimately, increase in the cost of care. In a broader perspective, fragmentation from misaligned consumer–provider–payer incentives and lack of information infrastructure perpetuates the problem and drives up the total cost of health care. The economic burden of fragmented perioperative care on the health care system is substantial, considering surgical care accounts for 65% of all hospital expenses, and that in 2011 alone, 850.6 billon US health care dollars were spent on hospital care.[2]

Deficiency in perioperative care is a part of the larger health care crisis in the USA. Consider that the USA spends nearly 18% of its gross domestic product (more than any other developed country) on health care costs, and yet ranks poorly in terms of quality of health care, lifespan and mortality rates compared with peer countries.[3] One of the several approaches to address this problem has been to change the reimbursement structure from volume-based (fee for service) to a value-based approach. Value in health care is generally defined as health outcomes achieved per dollar spent.[4] Moving toward better value for health care dollars spent, payment initiatives like value-based purchasing, pay-for-performance, and other more collaborative risk sharing models such as accountable care organizations and bundled payments for hospital and physicians have evolved.

In response to the changing health care environment, the American Society of Anesthesiologists (ASA) proposed a concept of the "Perioperative Surgical Home" for redesigning the delivery of perioperative care.[5] The following section attempts to illustrate the clinical, financial, and public health impact of existing surgical practices in support for much needed changes in perioperative care.

Clinical and financial impact of gaps in perioperative care

An estimated 30 million major inpatient surgeries and 50 million ambulatory outpatient surgeries are performed annually in the USA.[6-9] Preoperative and postoperative care for a large number of these patients is provided by non-anesthesia practitioners with no formal training in perioperative medicine. Often non-evidence-based arbitrary tests and care plans are executed, creating significant waste in the health care system.[10] In fact, it has been shown that the incidence of unindicated preoperative screening tests is still more than 50%, and no previously unidentified benefit was found to support this persistence of unwarranted testing.[11] This is particularly prevalent

Perioperative Hemodynamic Monitoring and Goal Directed Therapy, ed. Maxime Cannesson and Rupert Pearse. Published by Cambridge University Press. © Cambridge University Press 2014.

during the preoperative phase when preoperative consultations and tests are often done in low-risk patients undergoing low-risk procedures,[12–15] thereby presenting an enormous opportunity for cost savings.

The Institute of Medicine has recognized the specialty of anesthesiology for its achievements in patient safety.[16] Anesthesia-related severe morbidity and mortality are rare. In fact, most perioperative complications are not related to the anesthetic management or the surgical technique, but rather to medical complications that occur during the postoperative period.[17] These complications are frequently a result of lack of preoperative optimization or lapses in postoperative management. Kassin et al. also showed an increased risk of 30 day readmission in patients who had postoperative complications.[17] The financial ramifications of hospital readmissions go beyond that of providing medical care, as a decreased number of hospital free beds interferes with the opportunity to treat other patients. Similarly, treatment of postoperative complications is costly, for example, a retrospective study of 13 292 patients with hospital-acquired pneumonia following abdominal surgery showed an increase in hospital charges by $31 000, an increase in hospital length of stay by 11 days, and a fourfold increase in rate of discharge to skilled nursing facility.[18] Likewise, data from another health care system showed that the cost of treating a postoperative urinary tract infection is $32 866.[19] Besides hospital costs, there is evidence to indicate that postoperative complications may also decrease long-term survival, independent of the patient's pre-existing co-morbid condition. Based on the American College of Surgeons National Surgical Quality Improvement (ACS-NSQIP) data on veteran population, the occurrence of postoperative complications and not preoperative patient risk factors reduced median 30-day survival by 69%.[20] Moreover, the opportunity costs of postoperative complications for the patient, the family, and the society (loss of productivity and quality of life as a result of illness and treatment) are unaccounted for by clinical studies.

Significant variation in postoperative mortality rates among US hospitals has also been attributed to delayed recognition and ineffective management of postoperative complications.[21,22] ACS-NSQIP data on 105 951 patients undergoing different non-cardiac surgeries showed mortality rates ranging from 3.5% low mortality hospitals to 6.9% high mortality hospitals, although both hospital groups had a similar rate of postoperative complications.[23] Another study

in Medicare beneficiaries undergoing six major surgeries found similar results. The authors attributed higher mortality rates to failure to rescue among the worst performing hospitals, thereby suggesting a lack of organized strategies for managing postoperative complications.[24]

Prevention of postoperative complications has received a lot of attention from payers and regulatory agencies. As part of the new value-based purchasing strategy of the Affordable Care Act, a portion of the hospital reimbursement is tied to achieving a certain performance level on process-of-care-measures, aimed at decreasing postoperative complications. These measures include timely administration of preoperative antibiotics, correct antibiotic choice, maintenance of perioperative normothermia, venous thromboembolism prophylaxis, timely discontinuation of foley catheter, and postoperative glycemic control in cardiac surgery patients.[25] However, as the system shifts to outcome-based bundled payment, these efforts alone will be insufficient to address the gaps in surgical care. Major improvements will only be affected by restructuring the delivery of perioperative health care.

Surgical home: a model of coordinated patient-centered perioperative care

The American Society of Anesthesiologists (ASA) has proposed a new construct of integrated perioperative care, the "Perioperative Surgical Home (PSH)."[5] The concept was based on the American Academy of Pediatrics' Patient Centered Medical Home, which has been endorsed by CMS as "A primary care model that aims to improve patient outcomes by adopting a patient-centered rather than disease-centered approach, with the aim of improving quality of care, lowering costs, and improving the patient experience."[26] The ASA Committee on Future Models of Anesthesia Practice has defined PSH as "a patient-centered and physician-led multidisciplinary and team-based system of coordinated care that guides the patient throughout the entire surgical experience, from decision for the need for surgery to discharge from a medical facility and beyond.[27] The goal is to create a better patient experience and make surgical care safer, efficient, and aligned in order to promote a better medical outcome at a lower cost."[24]

A PSH model of coordinated care is depicted in Figure 4.1. Some essential features of the PSH are described below.

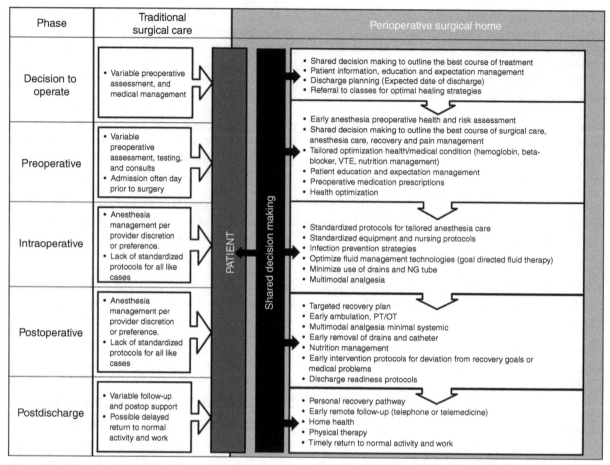

Phase	Traditional surgical care	Perioperative surgical home
Decision to operate	• Variable preoperative assessment, and medical management	• Shared decision making to outline the best course of treatment • Patient information, education and expectation management • Discharge planning (Expected date of discharge) • Referral to classes for optimal healing strategies
Preoperative	• Variable preoperative assessment, testing, and consults • Admission often day prior to surgery	• Early anesthesia preoperative health and risk assessment • Shared decision making to outline the best course of surgical care, anesthesia care, recovery and pain management • Tailored optimization health/medical condition (hemoglobin, beta-blocker, VTE, nutrition management) • Patient education and expectation management • Preoperative medication prescriptions • Health optimization
Intraoperative	• Anesthesia management per provider discretion or preference. • Lack of standardized protocols for all like cases	• Standardized protocols for tailored anesthesia care • Standardized equipment and nursing protocols • Infection prevention strategies • Optimize fluid management technologies (goal directed fluid therapy) • Minimize use of drains and NG tube • Multimodal analgesia
Postoperative	• Anesthesia management per provider discretion or preference. • Lack of standardized protocols for all like cases	• Targeted recovery plan • Early ambulation, PT/OT • Multimodal analgesia minimal systemic • Early removal of drains and catheter • Nutrition management • Early intervention protocols for deviation from recovery goals or medical problems • Discharge readiness protocols
Postdischarge	• Variable follow-up and postop support • Possible delayed return to normal activity and work	• Personal recovery pathway • Early remote follow-up (telephone or telemedicine) • Home health • Physical therapy • Timely return to normal activity and work

(Center column vertical labels: PATIENT / Shared decision making)

Figure 4.1. Comparison of traditional perioperative patient care to perioperative surgical home. Integration of care in perioperative surgical home throughout all perioperative phases, with incorporation of shared decision making at each phase.

Shared decision making

Shared decision making (SDM) is a collaborative process between clinicians and patients to arrive at the best treatment options after considering all available evidence. It takes into account patient's values, preferences, and autonomy, especially when diverging treatment plans may have important and lasting implications. It is a crucial element of patient-centered care.[28] In fact, it has been shown that patient perception of patient-centeredness is associated with positive health outcomes and lower levels of postencounter discomfort.[29] This model actively engages patients and their families in every aspect of their care.

Anesthesia-led integrated team

Anesthesiologists by the virtue of their profession have more expertise in perioperative medicine than any other medical specialty. Critical care and pain medicine are a natural extension of anesthesia training. Also, anesthesiologists are knowledgeable in operating room management and working in care teams. Therefore, anesthesiologists are the most suitable physicians to lead the PSH team. The PSH leverages the unique training, skills, and perspectives of the anesthesiologists allowing them to coordinate and manage the perioperative care of patients by integrating surgeons and other health care providers, family members, as well as hospital administrators and ancillary personnel, in achieving the shared vision of value-based care.

Integrated care pathway

The pathway should allow for evidence-based, protocol-driven seamless integration of all phases of perioperative care, starting with the preoperative phase all the way to smooth transition to postdischarge phase (Figure 4.1). Streamlining preoperative preparation of the patient, allowing optimization of the patient's health and medical condition, early discharge planning, protocol driven strategies for fluid therapy (including goal directed fluid management) and prevention of complications, early detection of and rescue from complications, and smooth transition of care to discharge setting are integral to PSH.

Quality management

The program and care pathways should be audited regularly, and any cause for variation should be addressed immediately. Data collection should include data on operational efficiency, processes of care, outcomes, and cost. The data should be mined for comparative research.

Since the inception of the PSH concept, several prototypes have been implemented at a number of hospitals across the USA. Not surprisingly, several of these PSH bear similarities to the Enhanced Recovery After Surgery (ERAS) program; both PSH and ERAS having the same basic fundamental framework of evidence-based, standardized, patient-centered coordinated perioperative care. (The reader is referred to chapter 3, *New Trends in Perioperative Medicine*.) Judging from the success of the ERAS in the United Kingdom, the US model of the PSH appears promising. Although yet to be proven in large-scale demonstrations, the preliminary reports are encouraging. The University of Alabama at Birmingham has established a PSH model based on performance-based, integrated team model of anesthesiologists and mid-level providers for achieving desired outcomes.[30] An anesthesiologist-intensivist serves as the "Perioperativist." At the University of California in Irvine,

the authors have implemented a PSH for joint surgery. A multidisciplinary team consisting of anesthesiologists, surgeons, nurses, pharmacists, physical therapists, case-managers, social workers, and information technology experts met weekly during the implementation phase. LeanSigma techniques and evidence-based protocols were used to streamline and standardize care pathways and reduce variability. Patient education, shared decision making, goal oriented personal recovery pathway/diary, and performance benchmarks were incorporated at every phase. The anesthesia regional/acute pain team followed the patients daily and a "surgical home call system" was established by the Department of Anesthesiology and Perioperative Care to ensure continuity of care. A nurse navigator working with the PSH team ensured smooth transitions of care between home, hospital and post-discharge facility. A 24-hour call center was established for patients, families and home health agencies. Preliminary results for 170 cases show a very high patient–physician satisfaction; an average hospital length of stay of 2.6 days, a low case cancellation rate of 0.4%, and a low all-cause readmission rate of 1.7%.

The development and implementation of surgical homes will depend on the individual institution's needs and resources, and will probably evolve with changes in local, political, and economic climate. Owing to its fundamental framework of evidence-based, standardized, coordinated, patient-centered care, it will likely improve patient outcomes and decrease cost of care. Future observational and comparative studies on appropriately selected and relevant metrics will likely determine the real impact and success of the perioperative surgical home at the local and national level.

References

1. Elhauge E. Why should we care about health care fragmentation and how to fix it: causes and solutions. In Elhauge E, ed. *The Fragmentation of U.S. Health Care*. Oxford University Press, 2010.

2. National Health Expenditures 2011 Highlights. http://www.cms.gov. (Accessed September 8, 2013).

3. Institute of Medicine. *US Health in International Perspective;*

Shorter Lives, Poorer Health. National Academy Press, 2013.

4. Porter ME. What is value in health care? *N Engl J Med* 2010;**363** (**26**):2477–81.

5. Warner M. Surgical Home Draft Proposal. Report [310–3.2] to the American Society of Anesthesiologists House of Delegates 2011.

6. Centers for Disease Control and Prevention: National Hospital Discharge Survey 2010 http://www.cdc.gov/nchs/fastats/

insurg. (Accessed September 8, 2010).

7. Kehlet H, Wilmore DW. Evidence-based surgical care and the evolution of fast-track surgery. *Ann Surg* 2008;**248**:189–98.

8. Cullen KA, Hall MJ, Golosinskiy A. Ambulatory surgery in the United States, 2006. *Natl Health Stat Report* 2009:1–25.

9. Hall MJ, DeFrances CJ, Williams SN, Golosinskiy A, Schwartzman A. National Hospital Discharge

Survey: 2007 summary. *Natl Health Stat Report* 2010:1–20, 24.

10. Berwick DM, Hackbarth AD. Eliminating waste in US healthcare. *JAMA* 2012;**307** (**14**):1513–16.

11. Mantha S, Roizen MF, Madduri J, et al. Usefulness of routine preoperative testing: a prospective single-observer study. *J Clin Anesth* 2005;**17**(**1**), 51–7.

12. Newman MF, Matthew JP, Aronson S. The evolution of anesthesiology and perioperative medicine. *Anesthesiology* 2013;**118**:1005–7.

13. Thilen SR, Bryson CL, Reid RJ. Patterns of preoperative consultation and surgical specialty in an integrated healthcare system. *Anesthesiology* 2013;**118**(**5**):1028–37.

14. Kuma A, Srivastava U. Role of routine laboratory investigation in preoperative evaluation. *Anaesthesiol Clin Pharmacol* 2011;**27**(**2**):174–9.

15. Practice advisory for pre-anaesthesia evaluation: a report by American Society of Anesthesiologists Task Force on Preanaesthesia evaluation. *Anesthesiology.* 2002;**96**:485–96.

16. Donaldson MS, Kohn LT, Corrigan J. *To Err is Human: Building a Safer Health System.* Washington: National Academy Press, 2000.

17. Kassin TM, Owen RM, Parez SD, et al. Risk factors for 30-day hospital readmission among general surgery patients. *J Am Coll Surg* 2012;**215**;322–30.

18. Thompson DA, Makary MA, Dorman T, et al. Clinical and economic outcomes of hospital acquired pneumonia in intra-abdominal surgery patients. *Ann Surg* 2006;**243**:547–52.

19. Kain ZN, Vakharia SB, Garson L. The perioperative surgical home as a future perioperative model. *Anesth Analg* 2013; (in press).

20. Khuri SF, Henderson WG, DePalma RG, et al. Determinants of long-term survival after major surgery and the adverse effects of postoperative complications. *Ann Surg* 2005;**242**(**3**): 326–43.

21. Silber JH, Williams SV, Krakauer H, Schwartz JS. Hospital and patient characteristics associated with death after surgery: a study of adverse occurrence and failure to rescue. *Med Care* 1992;**30**:615–29.

22. Taenzer AH, Pyke JB, McGrath SP. A review of current and emerging approaches to address failure to rescue. *Med Care* 1993;**30**(**7**):615–29.

23. Ghaferi AA, Birkmeye JD, Dimik JB. Variation in Hospital mortality associated with inpatient surgey. *N Engl J Med* 2009;**361**(**14**):13688–75.

24. Ghaferi AA, Birkmeye JD, Dimik JB. Complications, failure to rescue and mortality with major inpatient surgery in Medicare patients. *Ann Surg* 2009;**250** (**6**):1029–34.

25. Hospital value-based purchasing program. *Department of Health and Human Services, Centers for Medicare and Medicaid.* Medicare Learning Network, 2013.

26. Rittenhouse DR, Shortell SM. The patient centered medical home: will it stand the test of health reform? *JAMA* 2009;**301** (**19**):2038–40.

27. American Society of Anesthesiologists Perioperative Surgical Home Brief. ASA Committee on Future Models of Anesthesia Practice; 2013.

28. Barry MJ, Edgman-Levitan S. Shared decision making – pinnacle of patient-centered care. *N Engl J Med* 2012;**366**; 780–1.

29. Oates J, Weston W, Jordan J. The impact of patient-centered care on outcomes. *Fam Pract* 2000;**49**;796–804.

30. Vetter RT, Goeddel LA, Boudreaux AM, et al. The perioperative surgical home: how can it make the case so that everyone wins. *BMC Anesthesiology* 2013. http://www.biomedcentral.com/1471-2253/13/6.(Accessed September 9, 2013).

Overview of the circulation

5

Michael R. Pinsky

Introduction

Maintaining cardiovascular stability and reserve are fundamental in minimizing complications, morbidity, and mortality in the critically ill. Titration of therapies aimed at supporting the cardiovascular system, respiratory gas exchange, and internal homeostasis form the basis for acute care management. Diagnostic approaches, such as therapeutic trials and functional hemodynamic monitoring, or therapies, such as preoptimization and other goal directed therapies, are based on data derived from hemodynamic monitoring. These analyses and treatments are tightly linked to physiological monitoring. Although specific combinations of hemodynamic variables often reflect certain disease states and their intrinsic physiologic adaptive responses, there may be considerable overlap among markedly different pathological states, which often require different therapies. This diagnostic confusion can be minimized by examining the specific hemodynamic responses to a specific therapy, often referred to as a therapeutic trial. For example, both unresuscitated severe sepsis and acute heart failure present with hypotension, a low cardiac output, mixed venous O_2 saturation (SvO_2), and pulmonary artery occlusion pressure (Ppao). However, septic shock patients are usually fluid responsive, whereas acute heart failure patients usually are not. Why these differences occur is a function of baseline cardiac function and reserve, vascular tone and reactivity, blood flow distribution, and the effective circulating blood volume. The information needed to identify which of these processes is driving a given pathological state requires hemodynamic monitoring targeted on the most likely pathological processes involved. Although the cardiovascular system is a tightly integrated system, one can artificially separate out the determinants of cardiovascular homeostasis into those that primarily are determined by: (1) ventricular pump function, (2) arterial vasomotor tone and blood flow distribution, and (3) effective circulating blood volume and venous return.

Ventricular pump function

Ventricular systolic and diastolic function can be linked or separated, but carry a common determinant in adequate energy stores and delivery, calcium trafficking, and structural changes in response to ischemia and either pressure or volume overload. Although most studies of ventricular function revolve around left ventricular (LV) function, right ventricular (RV) function is now getting more attention as a primary determinant of cardiovascular state. Still, understanding LV physiology is essential to diagnosing and managing critically ill patients.

Frank, a German physiologist, noted that, unlike skeletal muscle strips, when cardiac muscle strips were stretched, they increased their force of contraction. Starling reasoned that, since the LV cavity approximated a sphere, increases in LV end-diastolic volume (EDV) should proportionally increase LV myocardial fiber stretch. Thus, he modified Frank's observations to say that force of LV contraction was related to LV EDV. According to this rule, increasing LV EDV will increase LV stroke volume, and for a constant heart rate, increase cardiac output. If LV pump function is impaired, then for the same increase in LV EDV, stroke volume will increase much less (Figure 5.1a). This concept is central to most diagnostic and therapeutic protocols used to assess cardiac function.[1] The immediate treatment of acute cardiovascular insufficiency and arterial hypotension is usually to increase intravascular volume with the goal of increasing LV stroke volume via the Frank–Starling mechanism. If arterial pressure increases, then the subject is said to be

Perioperative Hemodynamic Monitoring and Goal Directed Therapy, ed. Maxime Cannesson and Rupert Pearse.
Published by Cambridge University Press. © Cambridge University Press 2014.

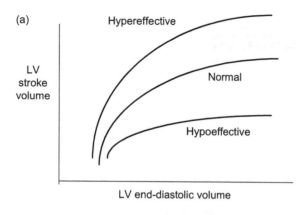

(a)

Hypereffective

Normal

Hypoeffective

LV stroke volume

LV end-diastolic volume

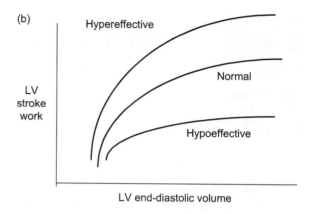

(b)

Hypereffective

Normal

Hypoeffective

LV stroke work

LV end-diastolic volume

Figure 5.1a. Graphic representation of the Frank–Starling relationship defining left ventricular (LV) function, showing the relation between LV end-diastolic volume and stroke volume for normal hyper-, and hypo-functioning ventricles.

Figure 5.1b. Same relation as shown in Figure 5.1a, except left ventricular (LV) stroke work is substituted for stroke volume.

"preload-responsive" and the presumptive diagnosis of hypovolemia is made. The relation between LV EDV and either stroke volume is referred to as the Frank–Starling relationship. However, focusing on stroke volume as the measure of LV responsiveness when treating patients with presumed hypovolemia and preserved ventricular pump function is potentially misleading and dangerous. First, the Frank–Starling mechanism primarily operates on a beat-to-beat basis to match LV and RV outputs over relatively short time intervals (e.g., 5–10 seconds) as venous return varies with ventilation. However, with sustained increase in venous return, the left ventricle adapts with increased contractility, such that LV stroke volume remains elevated but LV EDV returns to baseline values. This phenomenon, referred to as the Anrep effect, can be demonstrated in isolated perfused hearts, demonstrating that it is intrinsic to the myocardium.[2] Presumably, increased myocardial wall stress increases local calcium flux causing increased contractility. In fact, we can define patients as having systolic heart failure if they can only increase their LV stroke volume through the Starling mechanism.

However, with either the Frank–Starling or Anrep mechanisms in play, we still model the left ventricle as a pump. The mechanical correlate of volumes moved under pressure is work, or stroke work. LV stroke volume will vary inversely with outflow pressure (arterial pressure) for a constant LV EDV and LV contractility. To account for this important influence, LV stroke work, rather than stroke volume is often

used to assess LV function. If stroke work is less for the same LV EDV, then LV contractility is also said to be less under this condition as well (Figure 5.1b). The measure of LV function used to assess cardiovascular status is highly dependent on the question being asked. If the physician is wishing to assess the adequacy of LV output to meet the metabolic demands of the body, the cardiac output is most important, because it reflects blood flow. On the other hand, if the physician wishes to understand the level of myocardial contractile reserve, independent of the level of blood flow, then the change in LV stroke work relative to the change in LV EDV is a better index.

The Frank–Starling relationship only describes superficially the mechanical quality of LV ejection, which is better characterized by the rate of increase in myocardial wall stiffness or elastance over systole, described by time-varying elastance.[3] Graphically, this distinction is better illustrated by displaying LV performance as plotting the relation between LV pressure and volume loop during the cardiac cycle.

The left ventricular pressure–volume loop

When displayed as the changes in LV pressure and volume during a cardiac cycle, time is not seen (Figure 5.2). Traditionally, LV volume is on the *x*-axis and LV pressure on the *y*-axis. Filling occurs during diastole when LV chamber pressure decreases to less than left atrial pressure. The slope of the passive LV distention is diastolic compliance. Right before the end of diastolic filling, the atria contract, rapidly

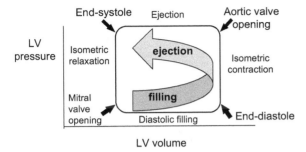

Figure 5.2. Stylized representation of the left ventricular (LV) pressure–volume relation over a complete cardiac cycle, referred to as the LV pressure–volume loop. Note that filling, contraction, emptying, and relaxation proceed in a counterclockwise fashion.

increasing LV pressure at end-diastole. This results in a higher EDV, but a lower overall filling pressure, because LV end-diastolic pressure only increases rapidly at the end of diastole. At end-diastole, defined by the electro-mechanical coupling of contraction, there exists the minimal pressure–volume ratio. This point is often used to assess diastolic compliance, but is influenced by the pericardium, lungs, and right ventricle. Thus, measures of LV end-diastolic pressure to LV EDV often vary widely without any actual changes in LV diastolic compliance. LV EDV is often used synonymously with LV preload as applied to the Frank–Starling relationship. However, LV preload by the Frank–Starling relationship is LV myocardial wall stress. If LV diastolic compliance changes from one beat to the next, as can easily occur with acute RV overload or hyperinflation, then for the same LV myocardial fiber stress, LV EDV will be less. Thus, the bedside clinician is often left with the confusing situation of seeing increasing LV end-diastolic pressures without an increase in LV stroke volume and inferring that LV contractility is depressed. Although contractility may well be depressed, it is more likely that the decreased LV stroke volume reflects RV overload or hyperinflation in a non-cardiac patient. This process by which increased RV EDV or RV end-diastolic pressures limit LV filling is referred to as ventricular interdependence and occurs commonly in both health and disease, making estimates of LV function by plotting the Frank–Starling curse using Ppao and LV stroke volume or stroke work inaccurate at best and often misleading.

With systolic contraction, LV intra-cavitary pressure rises causing a passive closing of the mitral valve, changing the shape of the LV from an ellipsoid into a sphere. Once intracavitary pressure exceeds aortic pressure, the aortic valve passively opens and ejection begins with continued LV contraction but now decreasing LV volume. In normal subjects, the point where ejection occurs represents the maximal LV wall stress. Wall stress is the product of radius of curvature and developed pressure. Thus, diastolic arterial pressure is a major determinant of LV wall stress. LV wall stress is LV afterload and is often (but inaccurately) referred to as LV ejection pressure. This concept is important because any therapy that selectively decreases diastolic arterial pressure will reduce LV afterload more than therapies that selectively decrease systolic arterial pressure. Similarly, if a vasodilator therapy, for example, induced both vasodilation and increased LV stroke volume, then diastolic arterial pressure will decrease, but systolic arterial pressure may either remain constant or increase. If the clinicians were specifically targeting systolic arterial pressure as LV afterload, then they would incorrectly presume that the vasodilator therapy paradoxically increased afterload. This presumption potentially could lead to an incorrect decision to either increase vasodilator therapy, further promoting coronary ischemia or stop vasodilator therapy altogether, despite the fact that such patients who increase their arterial pulse pressure in response to vasodilator therapy are actually showing a positive response to this treatment.

Importantly for the LV pressure–volume loop, we see that LV ejection occurs as LV volume decreases and both LV pressure and aortic pressure rise. As ejection increases the transfer of blood into the thoracic aorta, it distends becoming stiffer. Thus, arterial pressure rises more toward the end of ejection, even though the actual amount of volume being ejected at the end is much less than in the beginning. Accordingly, most of the increase in arterial pressure occurs when the LV volume is already small. That the left ventricle unloads itself during ejection has important clinical implications. First, systolic hypertension is reasonably well tolerated on a short-term basis without much increase in myocardial O_2 demand (MVO_2), whereas diastolic hypertension immediately increases MVO_2 and stimulates the development of LV hypertrophy. However, if the left ventricle is dilated and at end-ejection still has a large volume, then systolic pressure will be a major contributor to both LV wall stress and MVO_2. This systolic reduction of LV afterload only works if the LV cavity gets much smaller during ejection. So, in dilated heart failure states, ejection only minimally decreases LV volumes. Accordingly, such patients are very sensitive to changes in systolic arterial pressure.

Interestingly, LV end-ejection occurs at a pressure–volume ratio that appears to be only minimally altered by ejection history, but highly influenced by end-ejection pressure and intrinsic contractility. If arterial resistance is high, then LV end-systolic pressure and end-systolic volume (ESV) increase, whereas if arterial resistance is low, both decrease. However, they do so along an end-systolic elastance line, called the end-systolic pressure–volume relationship (ESPVR) that is independent of the actual pressure or volume. Importantly, the ESPVR slope varied in proportion to changes in contractility: increasing with increased contractility and decreasing with decreased contractility.[3] Thus, one can say that LV ESV then is a function of both after-load and contractility. As such increases in afterload will increase ESV, whereas decrease in afterload will decrease ESV, but the slope of the ESPVR remains unchanged.

Once end-ejection has occurred, the left ventricle actively relaxes. Diastolic relaxation or lusitropy is the energy-dependent part of the cardiac cycle, causes LV intra-cavitary pressure to decrease faster than would be predicted by passive relaxation alone (i.e., sucking action occurs) and is impaired by myocardial ischemia. Thus, impaired active diastolic relaxation is the earliest manifestation of myocardial ischemia. Once LV intracavitary pressure decreases below aortic pressure, the aortic valve passively closes, allowing LV pressure to continue to decrease as aortic pressure remains elevated, creating a coronary artery pressure gradient needed to support LV coronary flow during diastole. Since coronary artery blood flow occurs primarily in diastole, when LV wall stress is low whereas perfusion pressure is high, any process which impairs diastolic relaxation will decrease coronary blood flow.

Expanding the ESPVR to encompass all of systole: time-varying elastance

The entire LV contractile process can be understood better from the perspective not of a single pressure–volume loop, but from the pressure–volume domain of contraction across many potential LV pressure–volume loops that might potentially be created for the same level of contractility. By varying preload and afterload, one may describe increasing LV stiffness as an increasing slope of a theoretical LV pressure–volume domain identical to the LV ESPVR but at earlier points during systole. Thus, as time progresses from the start of contraction to end-ejection, the left ventricle becomes

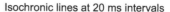
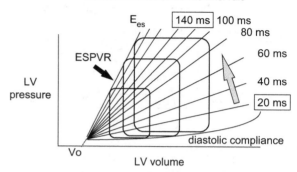

Figure 5.3. Stylized representation of three left ventricular (LV) pressure–volume loops at differing volumes showing how diastolic compliance, end-systolic elastance, and the isochronic (same point in time following the start of systole) time-varying elastance are calculated. The estimated zero LV pressure residual volume of the heart is called V_0.

progressively more stiff, such that the slope of the unique LV elastance curves for each time past the start of contraction will become progressively greater until they merge with the ESPVR curve. Since stiffness is also referred to an elastance, this time-dependent increase in stiffness is referred to as time-varying elastance (Et). In essence, time-varying elastance describes the progressive stiffening of the left ventricle through systole and then its relaxation in diastole within the pressure–volume domain.[3] Time-varying elastance can be calculated as a plot of the slopes of the isochronic (similar point in time) pressure–volume relations during ejection as the end-diastolic volume is rapidly varied (Figure 5.3). The slopes of these sequential pressure–volume lines reflect the obligatory LV pressure–volume domain that must be followed during systole. Importantly, Et defines the LV systolic function with the slope of the ESPVR defining end-systolic elastance (E_{es}). E_{es} is usually calculated from the regression line of the ESPVR data pairs of repetitive LV pressure–volume loops. Importantly, the Et behavior of the heart has direct clinical applications and explains many of the previously unexplained physiological determinants of LV systolic function. Recall that the Frank–Starling relationship maintains that, as LV EDV increases, LV stroke work also increases. Indeed, any ejection phase index, like stroke volume, velocity of circumferential fiber shortening, ejection fraction, and LV dP/dt will all show an increase with increasing LV EDV. But why? Time-varying elastance explains all these phenotypic outputs as epi-phenomena of time-varying elastance. Note that, as systole progresses, Et also increases.

Since E_{es} is greater than end-diastolic elastance, any increase in LV EDV will create a lesser increase in ESV and EDV, if LV ejection pressure does not also increase significantly. Since the Et is always increasing up to E_{es}, the resultant stroke volume, stroke work, LV dP/dt, and velocity of circumferential fiber shortening must also increase for a given diastolic compliance and Ees. When does this not happen? When does increasing LV EDV not increase stroke volume or other ejection phase indices? This occurs when LV contractile function is depressed or LV diastolic compliance reduced so much that the slopes of the two lines become equal.

Applying cardiac physiology at the bedside

The preload-dependent nature of LV performance is a primary characteristic of normal ventricular function. Demonstrating that LV EDV is above some minimal value, despite cardiac output and stroke work both being depressed, and with increases in LV EDV further, neither cardiac output or LV stroke work increase are fundamental attributes of the phenotype of systolic heart failure. Regrettably, the opposite is not true. Documenting that LV EDV is reduced in the setting of hemodynamic instability does not identify hypovolemia because reduced LV EDV is also seen commonly in conditions associated with diastolic dysfunction, such as tamponade, cor pulmonale, hyperinflation, and pulmonary hypertension. These conditions are common in the critically ill, making finding a reduced LV EDV not synonymous with volume responsiveness. These points are addressed further in the chapter on Functional hemodynamic monitoring.

Right ventricular function: the forgotten ventricle

Traditionally, cardiovascular chapters would now switch to discussing peripheral circulation, which is appropriate if the major aspects of ventricular pump function have already been covered. Regrettably, they have not been. The right ventricle behaves in a very different manner when presented with increased volume (preload) or ejection pressure (afterload).

Under normal conditions, it is extremely difficult to document that RV filling pressure changes during RV filling. When RV filling pressure, defined as right atrial pressure minus pericardial pressure, was directly measured in patients undergoing open chest operations as RV volume was varied by acute volume loading, RV filling

pressure is insignificantly altered.[4] Although right atrial pressure increases with volume loading, pericardial pressure also increases, such that RV filling pressure, defined as right atrial pressure minus pericardial pressure, remains unchanged. Similar data are seen when RV volumes are reduced by the application of PEEP in postoperative cardiac patients.[5] Thus under normal conditions, RV diastolic compliance is very high and most of the increase in right atrial pressure seen during volume loading reflects pericardial compliance and cardiac fossa stiffness. If RV wall stress is not increased during filling, then RV sarcomere length remains constant. Conformational changes in the RV more than wall stretch are responsible for RV enlargement.[6] Accordingly, changes in right atrial pressure do not follow changes in RV end-diastolic volume, as has recently been validated to define why measures of right atrial pressure, or central venous pressure, cannot predict either intravascular volume status or RV preload.[7] When cardiac contractility is reduced and intravascular volume is expanded, RV filling pressure does increase as a result of either decreased RV diastolic compliance, increased pericardial compliance, increased end-diastolic volume, or a combination of all three. RV over-distention has important clinical consequences. As RV EDV increases, the absolute volume remaining in the cardiac fossa decreases, making LV diastolic compliance less, by a process referred to as ventricular interdependence.[2] Lung expansion if causing hyperinflation, compresses the heart within the cardiac fossa in a fashion analogous to pericardial tamponade, but in this setting, it is the expanding lungs that increase intrathoracic pressure, and not pericardial restraint, limiting ventricular filling.[5]

As will be described further below, venous return, the primary determinant of cardiac output,[8] is maintained near maximal levels at rest[9] because RV filling occurs with minimal changes in filling pressure. This is because right atrial pressure is the back pressure to venous return. Accordingly, the closer right atrial pressure remains to zero relative to atmospheric pressure, the maximal is the pressure gradient for systemic venous blood flow.[10] For this mechanism to operate efficiently, RV output must equal venous return, otherwise sustained increases in venous blood flow would overdistend the RV, increasing right atrial pressure. Fortunately, under normal conditions of spontaneous ventilation this is not a problem because most of the increase in venous return is in phase with inspiration, decreasing again during expiration as ITP increases. Likewise, the pulmonary arterial inflow circuit is highly compliant and can accept large increases in RV stroke volume without changing pressure. Thus, any increase in venous return is proportionally delivered to the pulmonary circuit without forcing the RV to increase its force of contraction or myocardial oxygen demand.

This normal adaptive system will rapidly become dysfunctional if RV diastolic compliance decreases or if right atrial pressure increases independently of changes in RV EDV. Clinical examples of states where this usually occurs include acute RV dilation or cor pulmonale (pulmonary embolism, hyperinflation, and RV infarction), which induce profound decreases in cardiac output not responsive to fluid resuscitation. Dissociation between right atrial pressure and RV EDV also occurs during either cardiac tamponade or positive-pressure ventilation. Thus, positive pressure ventilation impairs circulatory adaptive processes normally occurring during spontaneous ventilation. Since the primary effect of ventilation on cardiovascular function in normal subjects is to alter RV preload via altering venous blood flow, the detrimental effect of positive pressure ventilation on cardiac output can be minimized either by fluid resuscitation to increase venous return or by keeping PEEP and tidal volumes as small as possible. Finally, over-resuscitation causes transient acute right heart failure and though often underappreciated, it probably occurs more often than not with aggressive resuscitation scenarios not targeted as limited resuscitation to only preload responsive subjects.

Arterial pressure and blood flow distribution

Arterial pressure is a primary determinant of organ perfusion. The other factor determining organ blood flow is intraorgan vascular resistance. Importantly, organ perfusion is independent of cardiac output. Cardiac output is only important within this context so as to maintain an adequate organ perfusion pressure, which allows autoregulation of organ blood flow. Thus, hypotension directly reduces organ blood flow and is synonymous with cardiovascular instability. Since a fundamental goal of hemodynamic monitoring is to identify cardiovascular instability,[11] documenting systemic hypotension is essential in defined profound circulatory shock. Operationally, mean arterial pressure (MAP) is presumed to be the input pressure to the organs. However, LV perfusion occurs primarily during diastole, and brain and intra-abdominal organs also see intracranial and intra-abdominal pressures as

their back-pressures to flow, respectively. Thus, actual organ perfusion pressure may be quite different among vital organs for the same MAP.

So if MAP is the primary pressure defining organ perfusion, can a patient be in circulatory shock and not be hypotensive? The answer is yes. In normal homeostatic mechanisms, functioning carotid body baroreceptors vary arterial peripheral vascular tone through sympathetic nerves to maintain MAP relatively constant despite varying cardiac output. This is done to maintain cerebral and coronary blood flow at the expense of the remainder of the body. In an otherwise healthy subject, this reflex response can totally mask hypotension. For example, in the postoperative period, if occult hemorrhage causes progressive hypovolemia, the initial findings are usually hypertension and tachycardia, not hypotension, as the increased sympathetic drive causes marked peripheral vasoconstriction. Thus, MAP is a remarkably stable measure and relatively insensitive as a marker of cardiovascular instability. Indirect measures of sympathetic tone, such as heart rate, respiratory rate, and peripheral capillary filling and peripheral cyanosis reflect better estimates of cardiovascular status than does MAP. Still, hypotension is a medical emergency because its presence defines that tissue hypoperfusion must exist.

Nevertheless, MAP monitoring is essential in the assessment and management of hemodynamically unstable subjects for several reasons. Measures that specifically increase MAP will also increase organ perfusion pressure. Vasoconstrictor therapies may increase vasomotor tone in non-vital peripheral organs, but will maintain flow to the cerebral and coronary beds because their arteries have little or no alpha adrenergic receptors, whereas the gut, kidneys, muscles, and skin demonstrate a marked reduction in blood flow in response to marked sympathetic stimulation. Accordingly, short-term survival of the host is closely linked to MAP through the maintenance of cerebral and coronary blood flows. If profound hypotension persists for even a brief period of time, irreversible cerebral and cardiac damage can occur. Thus, the initial priority in resuscitation of a hypotensive patient is to restore MAP above a level that will ensure coronary and cerebral perfusion, usually >60 mmHg, and then to restore cardiac output once MAP is stabilized to restore vital organ blood flow.

The primary method of increasing vascular tone is to infuse vasopressor agents, like norepinephrine. Regrettably, vasopressor support in the absence of fluid resuscitation will improve transiently both global blood flow and MAP, despite worsening local non-vital blood flow and hastening tissue ischemia. Thus, initial resuscitative efforts should always include a volume expansion component and fluid challenge so as to identify preload-responsive shock states, prior to relying on vasopressors alone to support the unstable patient.

Arterial pressure is created by the ejection of LV stroke volume into the aorta causing it to distend. Since LV ejection is rapid, absolute arterial blood volume increases with each systole and then decreases slowly during diastole as the arterial blood runoff into the organs continues. Since neither arterial pressure nor blood flow are constant during life, it is fundamentally difficult to assess arterial vasomotor tone. Simplistically, one can estimate MAP and plot the relation between changes in MAP and changes in cardiac output over time. The inverse slope of this relationship, with flow on the y-axis, defines arterial tone (Figure 5.4). With increased arterial vascular tone, a great increase in arterial pressure is needed to cause the same increase in blood flow as would be the case if tone was less. Importantly, the zero flow pressure intercept intersects the y-axis at a pressure significantly higher than right atrial pressure. In otherwise healthy individuals, this zero flow intercept pressure is approximately 40–50 mmHg. This is because that zero flow pressure is the actual back pressure to arterial blood flow and reflects the mean weighted critical closing pressure of the arterial circuit below which arterial vasomotor tone causes the arterioles to collapse. The other implication of this reality is that the artificial calculation of systemic vascular resistance as the ratio of the difference between MAP and right atrial pressure to cardiac output, grossly overestimates vasomotor tone and places an inappropriately important value on the role right atrial pressure plays in defining arterial tone.[12] Another way to analyze arterial tone is to assess the dynamic changes in arterial pressure and flow during ejection, as quantified by measures of aortic input impedance. Although this approach may seem daunting, if dynamic changes in arterial pulse pressure and stroke volume can be simultaneously recorded, as is often the case with the use of minimally invasive hemodynamic monitoring techniques, then the ratio of the pulse pressure variation to stroke volume variation will reflect central arterial elastance or stiffness. The greater the arterial elastance, the greater the variance of pulse pressure relative to stroke volume. Since these changes are relative, elastance measured using this approach is unitless. Normal subjects have a dynamic arterial elastance

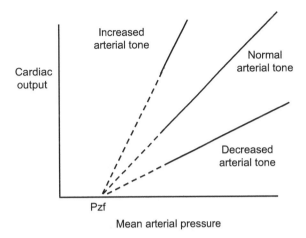

Figure 5.4. Relation between mean cardiac output and mean arterial pressure, as cardiac output is varied over a normal physiological range for a normal, increased, and decreased arterial vasomotor tone state. The zero cardiac output–mean arterial pressure intercept reflects arterial pressure at zero flow (Pzf) and is the effective back pressure to arterial blood flow.

of between 2 and 1.2, whereas a dynamic arterial elastance <0.8 reflects profound loss of arterial vasomotor tone.[13]

Blood volume and mean systemic pressure

Although ventricular pump function and arterial tone are extremely important in defining blood flow distribution once the blood is delivered to the heart, it is axiomatic that the heart can only pump the blood that it receives. In fact, up to the end of severe heart failure, the heart pumps 100% of the blood it receives back into the circulation. Clearly, as ventricular pump function decreases, increased filling pressures for the left ventricle can cause pulmonary edema and increased filling pressure for the right ventricle can cause peripheral edema. Furthermore, when vascular pressures are measured along the route of blood flow from the heart, through the aorta into the arteries, arterioles, capillaries, venules, and veins, one sees that most of the intravascular pressure generated by the ejecting heart is held constant down to the level of the small arteries, then drops quickly over the next 0.5 cm of vessel length as the circuit passes through the arterioles and precapillary sphincters into the capillaries. This vascular waterfall occurs at a pressure measured as the zero flow pressure (Figure 5.4) described above. That pressure drops beyond these vascular loci means that systemic capillaries are spared from seeing high hydrostatic pressures that would otherwise

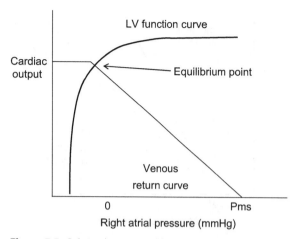

Figure 5.5. Relation between cardiac output and right atrial pressure when right atrial pressure (Pra) is independently varied defines two separate curves. The LV function curve is also displayed in Figure 5.1, but with cardiac output and not stroke volume as the flow unit; and the venous return curve. The intersection of the two curves defines steady-state cardiac output and is referred to as the equilibrium point. The zero cardiac output Pra intercept of the venous return curve is the mean systemic pressure (Pms); the slope of the cardiac output to Pra line is inversely proportional to the resistance to venous return.

promote edema formation. However, the low capillary pressure demands that the resistance to venous return from the capillaries to the right side of the heart must remain very low or the pressure gradient for venous return will be inadequate to sustain flow.

The blood flow back to the heart from the circulation is venous return and is the primary determinant of cardiac output.[10] Since the pressure in the periphery draining the organs is much lower than arterial pressure, the resistance to venous return is much lower than arterial resistance and flow much more dependent on small changes in downstream pressure. Guyton described this interaction over 50 years ago as the venous return curve (Figure 5.5) wherein cardiac output or venous return is plotted on the *y*-axis against right atrial pressure (Pra) on the *x*-axis. The summed weighted average systemic pressure in all the vascular reservoirs is referred to as mean systemic pressure (Pms) and is the subject of its own chapter later in this volume. Under steady-state conditions Pms is a function of blood flow distribution among all the vascular reservoirs, their stressed and unstressed volumes, and their vasomotor tone of the blood in their circuits within their stressed volume. Since vasomotor tone and unstressed volume can be rapidly changed by increasing intra-abdominal pressure, muscle contraction or changes in sympathetic tone, Pms is a highly

dynamic variable under normal conditions. However, during rest, general anesthesia, and critical illness where little changes in metabolic demand or blood flow distribution usually occur, Pms remains relatively constant over minutes, whereas Pra changes dynamically over the ventilatory cycle as changes in intrathoracic pressure artificially alter Pra relative to atmosphere. Spontaneous inspiration causes Pra to decrease, while positive pressure inspiration increases Pra. Thus, the blood flow back to the right ventricle can vary considerably throughout the ventilatory cycle. As mentioned above, one of the primary reasons for the Frank–Starling mechanism is to balance LV output to this changing RV output over a few heart beats. Still sustained and rapid increases in Pra will markedly decrease venous return inducing hypovolemic shock. This is the mechanism for cardiovascular collapse from an acute massive pulmonary embolism. The immediate pulmonary vascular obstruction blocks RV ejection, rapidly increasing Pra and stopping blood flow. By examining the venous return curve shown in Figure 5.5, this effect can be clearly understood. The normal Pra of healthy individuals is zero to 2 mmHg. This very low Pra ensures a maximal venous return with minimal peripheral edema. If an acute obstruction of >50% of the pulmonary vasculature were to occur as is often the case with massive pulmonary embolism, then RV ejection will be markedly impeded resulting is rapid RV dilation, intraventricular septal shift into the left ventricle decreasing LV diastolic compliance, and a sudden and sustained increase in Pra decreasing the pressure gradient for venous return. Thus, the underfilled left ventricle cannot adjust and, unless the pulmonary vascular obstruction is eliminated, profound circulatory shock and death ensue. Importantly, increasing venous return by fluid resuscitation alone will only cause further RV dilation compromising LV function further. The treatment of this condition is to give systemic vasopressors to maintain coronary perfusion and Pms while instituting thrombolytic therapy to lyse the intravascular clot.

The determinants of venous return are Pms, Pra, and the resistance to venous return. Although we discussed Pra and Pms and will discuss Pms in greater detail in a later chapter, the resistance to venous return is often dismissed. This is a mistake. Since the pressure gradient for venous return is low and all of cardiac output must be defined by venous return, the small changes in the resistance to venous return will have profound effects on venous return for the same Pra and Pms. Importantly, venous resistance is not due to changes in downstream venomotor tone as seen in the arterial circuit, but due to changes in the total cross-sectional area of vascular outflow resistance. Since the splanchnic circulation drains through a second organ, the liver, before returning to the heart, splanchnic blood flow carries with it twice the venous resistance of systemic vascular beds. Similarly, increasing sympathetic tone decreases unstressed volume, increasing Pms for the same blood volume, but also decreases the number of parallel venous conduits draining that organ, thus causing Pms to increase, but also increasing the resistance to venous return. The results of vasopressor therapy on cardiac output are thus hard to predict beforehand unless one knows baseline contractile reserve, circulating blood volume and vasomotor tone. However, if vasopressor therapy while increasing MAP also increases cardiac output, then LV contractile reserve and circulating blood volume are adequate, whereas if the same increase in MAP causes cardiac output (CO) to decrease, then LV contractile reserve is limited. Accordingly, knowing the response to vasopressor therapy on cardiac output also allows the bedside clinician to know the patient's underlying cardiovascular reserve.

Cardiac output, oxygen delivery, and oxygen consumption

A central goal of normal homeostasis is to continually maintain delivery of oxygenated blood and nutrients to the metabolically active tissues in amounts adequate to sustain normal function overall and tissue viability in the short run without wasting energy or overstressing the cardiovascular circuit. The O_2 carrying capacity of the blood is the product of the hemoglobin times the O_2 saturation times the cardiac output. If one assumes an adequate O_2 carrying capacity, then O_2 delivery to the tissues is dependent on cardiac output and blood flow distribution. Clearly, cardiac output and O_2 delivery may vary independently if arterial O_2 tension, hemoglobin levels, or hemoglobin affinity for O_2 vary rapidly, as may occur during hemorrhage or rapid resuscitation with or without red blood cell infusions. Given this limitation, however, it is useful to consider the two together because cardiac output is relatively easy to measure and, in stress states, cardiac output and O_2 delivery share common determinants. Recall, however, that normal homeostasis allows for local metabolic demand to determine local blood flow and thus local O_2 delivery. Thus, loss of the ability to auto-regulate blood flow distribution relative to regional metabolic demands will also result in regional tissue hypoperfusion and tissue ischemia even if cardiac output and O_2 delivery are in a range that would otherwise ensure adequate tissue O_2 delivery. This is the scenario present in systemic hypotension, wherein local vasodilation in response to increased metabolic demand does not equate with increased flow. The clinical example of this is severe sepsis, wherein cardiac output is either in a normal or elevated range, and mixed venous O_2 saturation (SvO_2) is increased, but clear evidence of tissue ischemia co-exists (e.g., lactic acidosis and organ dysfunction).

Since metabolic demand is ever changing even in the critically ill patient on mechanical ventilation and sedation, cardiac output usually co-varies with O_2 uptake.[14] O_2 supply and O_2 demand must co-vary as a normal and expected aspect of homeostasis. In cardiovascular insufficiency states, such as cardiogenic shock or hypovolemic shock, cardiac output is often limited and cannot increase in response to increasing metabolic demand. Under these conditions, O_2 consumption tends to remain constant despite minimal increases in cardiac output by increasing O_2 extraction. Different organs have different abilities to extract O_2 to low levels and still maintain function. Muscular activity effectively extracts O_2 from the blood because of the setup of the microcirculatory flow patterns and the large concentration of mitochondria in these tissues. Thus, sustained muscular activity is often associated with a marked decrease in SvO_2 despite a normal circulatory system. Trained athletes can push their SvO_2 to very low levels during exercise. Muscular activities, such as moving in bed, physical therapy, or being turned, "fighting the ventilator," and breathing spontaneously can double resting O_2 consumption.[15–16] In the patient with an intact and functioning cardiopulmonary apparatus, this will translate into an increase in both cardiac output and O_2 consumption.

There is no level of cardiac output which is "normal," but there are thresholds of O_2 delivery below which normal metabolism can no longer occur.[17] Taking global measures first, if SvO_2 is less than 50%, then some vascular beds somewhere are at the brink of dysoxia because tissue O_2 extraction becomes inefficient at maintaining O_2 flux when end-capillary blood has little O_2 to unload.[9] Regrettably, the converse is not always true. A higher level of SvO_2 does not ensure adequate end-capillary O_2 levels because SvO_2 reflects the mix of all venous blood. Thus, some areas with low extraction may mix with areas of lesser extraction to create a "normal" SvO_2 of $>70\%$ despite the co-existence of tissue ischemia. Thus, measures of SvO_2 are useful only in defining the risk for ischemia and, by extension, circulatory insufficiency and not in excluding the presence of tissue ischemia.[18]

Conflicts of interest

Consultant: Edwards LifeSciences, Inc; LiDCO Ltd. Research support: NIH, DoD, Edwards Lifesciences, Inc.

References

1. Ross J, Jr., Peterson KL. On the assessment of cardiac inotropic state. *Circulation* 1973;**47**:435–8.

2. Rosenblueth A, Alanis J, Lopez E, Rubio R. The adaptation of ventricular muscle to different circulatory conditions. *Arch Int Physiol Biochim* 1959;**67**(3):358–73.

3. Suga H, Sugawa K. Instantaneous pressure–volume relationships and their ratio in the excised supported canine left ventricle. *Circ Res* 1983;**53**:306–18.

4. Tyberg JV, Taichman GC, Smith ER, et al. The relationship between pericardial pressure and right atrial pressure: an intraoperative study. *Circulation* 1986;**73**(3):428–32.

5. Pinsky MR, Vincent JL, DeSmet JM. Effect of positive end-expiratory pressure on right ventricular function in man. *Am Rev Respir Dis* 1992;**146**:681–7.

6. Kingma I, Smiseth OA, Frais MA, Smith ER, Tyberg JV. Left ventricular external constraint: relationship between pericardial, pleural and esophageal pressures during positive end-expiratory pressure and volume loading in dogs. *Ann Biomed Eng* 1987;**15**(3–4):331–46.

7. Marik PE, Cavallazzi R. Does the central venous pressure predict fluid responsiveness? An updated meta-analysis and a plea for some common sense. *Crit Care Med* 2013;**41**:1774–81.

8. Goldberg HS, Rabson J. Control of cardiac output by systemic vessels: circulatory adjustments of acute and chronic respiratory failure and the effects of therapeutic interventions. *Am J Cardiol* 1981;**47**:696–704.

9. Scharf SM, Brown R, Saunders N, Green LH. Effects of normal and loaded spontaneous inspiration on cardiovascular function. *J Appl Physiol* 1979;**47**(3):582–590.

10. Guyton AC, Lindsey AW, Abernathy B, Richardson T. Venous return at various right atrial pressures and the normal venous return curve. *Am J Physiol* 1957;**189**(3):609–15.

11. Wiedemann HP, Matthay MA, Matthay RA. Cardiovascular–pulmonary monitoring in the intensive care unit (Part 1). *Chest* 1984;**85**:537–49.

12. Geerts BF, Maas JJ, Aarts LP, Pinsky MR, Jansen JR. Partitioning the resistances along the vascular tree: effects of dobutamine and hypovolemia in piglets with an intact circulation. *J Clin Monit Comput* 2010;**24**(5):377–84.

13. Monge García MI, Gil Cano A, Gracia Romero M. Dynamic arterial elastance to predict arterial pressure response to volume loading in preload-dependent patients. *Crit Care* 2011;**15**(1):R15.

14. Mohsenifar Z, Goldbach P, Tashkin DP, Campisi DJ. Relationship between O_2 delivery and O_2 consumption in the adult respiratory distress syndrome. *Chest* 1983;**84**:267–71.

15. Annat G, Viale JP, Percival C, Froment M, Motin J. Oxygen delivery and uptake in the adult respiratory distress syndrome. Lack of relationship when measured independently in patients with normal blood lactate concentrations. *Am Rev Respir Dis* 1986;**133**(6):999–1001.

16. Weissman C, Kemper M, Elwyn DH, et al. The energy expenditure of the mechanically ventilated critically ill patient. An analysis. *Chest* 1986; **89**(2):254–9.

17. Pinsky MR. The meaning of cardiac output [editorial]. *Intens Care Med* 1990;**16**:415–17.

18. Miller MJ, Cook W, Mithoefer J. Limitations of the use of mixed venous pO_2 as an indicator of tissue hypoxia. *Clin Res* 1979;**27**:401A.

Chapter

6

Cardiac function and myocardial perfusion

Jason H. Chua, Rudolph Nguyen, and Aman Mahajan

Introduction

The heart functions to serve the metabolic needs of the entire body; while receiving blood from the low pressure venous system, it imparts mechanical work to eject the blood into the arterial system at high pressure. This pressure, in conjunction with the peripheral vascular system, drives perfusion to deliver oxygen to, and remove metabolic waste from, peripheral tissues. Each beat of the heart is the culmination of a sophisticated interaction of electrical excitation and mechanical contraction. Coronary perfusion itself is intricately related to the very beats that drive corporeal perfusion. These intricacies therefore require a focused, goal directed approach to the management of patients with cardiovascular disease in the acute care setting.

ACC/AHA Guidelines on perioperative cardiovascular care

The American College of Cardiology Foundation and American Heart Association have frequently collaborated to address pertinent issues regarding the acute care of patients with cardiovascular disease since 1980. The latest guidelines addressing perioperative care focus primarily on risk stratification and optimization prior to elective, non-cardiac surgery.[1] Patients with active cardiac conditions, poor functional capacity, or multiple clinical risk factors for perioperative cardiac morbidity necessitate further risk stratification. Clinical risk factors include a history of ischemic heart disease, heart failure, diabetes requiring insulin use, renal insufficiency, and a history of cerebrovascular disease. The type of procedure is also considered, as more intensive preoperative evaluations are recommended for intermediate and high-risk surgeries. Additional studies to assess cardiac

function and stratify risk for perioperative myocardial infarction include echocardiography, electrocardiogram (ECG), and stress testing.

It is recommended that beta-blockade continue in the perioperative period for all patients already taking such medications. Additionally, heart rate control is encouraged in patients with multiple clinical risk factors proceeding to surgery. Intraoperative management is deferred to the anesthesia team providing care; however, a comprehensive plan including the potential use of invasive monitors, ventilation strategies, and analgesic regimens is recommended. Postoperatively, the judicious use of surveillance methods for myocardial ischemia is encouraged.

Review of cardiac physiology

Naturally, all living cells require metabolic substrates in order to perform their designated function. There must also be a mechanism by which metabolic waste is removed. In the human body, the heart assumes the role of providing the driving pressure for the circulatory system to meet these metabolic needs. By combining an intricate electrical system with a complex array of muscular mechanics, the heart generates pulsatile flow and provides the driving pressure for perfusion of every cell of the body.

Each heartbeat is the result of an electrical impulse translated into a mechanical process. Electrical changes in the sinoatrial (SA) node are conducted to the ventricles and result in organized, electromechanically efficient contraction. Pacemaker cells in the SA node are able to generate spontaneous action potentials to set the heart rate when in sinus rhythm. Other pacemaker cells exist in the atrioventricular (AV) node and ventricular conduction system, but as the intrinsic rate

Perioperative Hemodynamic Monitoring and Goal Directed Therapy, ed. Maxime Cannesson and Rupert Pearse.
Published by Cambridge University Press. © Cambridge University Press 2014.

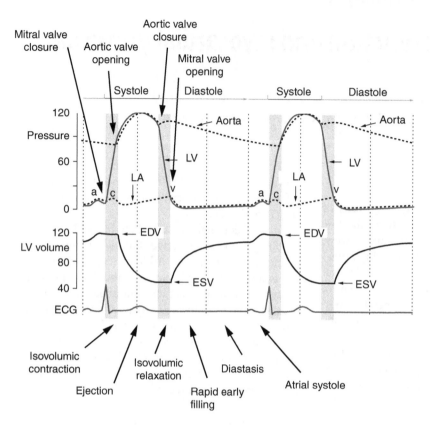

Figure 6.1. Pressure and volume in the atria and ventricles throughout the cardiac cycle. LA = left atrium; LV = left ventricle; EDV = end-diastolic volume; ESV = end-systolic volume; ECG = electrocardiogram.

of these cells is significantly slower than that of the SA node, they are therefore overdrive-suppressed. In contrast to the non-pacemaker cells of the heart, pacemaker cells have no true resting potential – they generate regular action potentials by way of slow, inward calcium currents through L-type calcium channels.

The cardiac cycle is divided into systole and diastole. Systole encompasses ventricular contraction and ejection, while diastole includes ventricular relaxation and filling. The cardiac cycle begins at end-systole when the semilunar valves close. Relaxation of the ventricles and a closed AV valve define the first phase of diastole, isovolumic relaxation. "Relaxation" is a classic misnomer, in that it is caused by the inactivation of contractile proteins by re-entry of calcium into the sarcoplasmic reticulum, which is an active and energy-requiring process. Indeed, one of the earliest signs of myocardial ischemia is new or worsening diastolic dysfunction, as during this phase, the left ventricular myocardium is appreciated to actively untwist in an energy-dependent manner, generating negative pressure to pull blood forward from the atrium. When ventricular pressure falls below atrial pressure, the atrioventricular valve opens, allowing forward flow from the atrium into the

ventricle. The time between opening of the AV valve and pressure equalization is termed the rapid filling phase of diastole, and it comprises 80% of ventricular filling under normal, resting conditions. A brief period of diastasis occurs, when active myocardial "relaxation" has ended, and further filling is dependent on the passive compliance of the ventricle. The final phase of diastole occurs when a depolarization impulse is transmitted from the sinus node across the atrium, resulting in organized atrial systole.

Ventricular contraction is initiated when an SA nodal impulse is conducted by the AV node to the ventricles via the His–Purkinje system. When atrial contraction has ended and ventricular pressure exceeds atrial pressure by way of organized contraction, the atrioventricular valve closes abruptly and systole begins with isovolumic contraction of the ventricle against a closed outflow valve. When intraventricular pressure exceeds the pressure in the outflow vessel (aorta or pulmonary artery), the semilunar valve opens and blood is ejected, thus completing the cardiac cycle with the ejection phase (Figure 6.1).

Both normal physiologic as well as pathologic states can alter the balance of the normal cardiac cycle. In the setting of tachycardia, the rapid filling phase of diastole is cut short and the ventricle is more reliant on atrial contraction to fill. Pathologic states that decrease ventricular compliance, such as ventricular hypertrophy and diastolic dysfunction, also shift the balance of ventricular filling more toward a dependence on organized atrial contraction. In such instances, over 40% of ventricular filling (and ultimately cardiac output) may be dependent upon atrial contraction. Sinus rhythm is particularly important to maintain in these patients, and a non-sinus rhythm may precipitate hemodynamic collapse.

Left and right ventricular mechanics are quite different and rely upon one another. Both ventricles are composed of complex matrices of myocardial fibers in multiple orientations that combine to generate mechanically efficient contraction. While both ventricles generate pulsatile flow, the right ventricle has been described as peristaltic in its contractions and the left ventricle exhibits a unique torsional motion in its normal, contractile state. This torsional motion is attributed to the helical arrangement of myocardial fibers as they progress from the base of the heart to the apex. Due to the right ventricle's unique mechanism of contraction, as well as its lower generated pressures, its perfusion occurs throughout the cardiac cycle; in contrast, the left ventricle is almost entirely perfused during diastole.[2] In the setting of right ventricular dysfunction or failure, its normal mechanics are obliterated and its perfusion can be compromised during systole such that it is only perfused during diastole, significantly compromising its perfusing time during the cardiac cycle. The left ventricle also suffers in the setting of right heart failure by way of ventricular interdependence. Left ventricular filling is impaired due to decreased right ventricular cardiac output in a process referred to as series interaction. Also, left ventricular contraction mechanics are disrupted by the distorted shape of the right ventricle in two ways. First, muscle fiber orientation is altered such that left ventricular contraction is less efficient.[3] Second, the right ventricle's increased volume decreases left ventricular size in a fixed pericardial space in a process referred to as direct, or pericardial, interaction.

Coronary circulation

The left and right coronary arteries arise from the aortic root above the left and right cusps of the aortic valve. The left coronary artery bifurcates near its origin to form the left anterior descending and circumflex arteries. The right coronary artery travels down the right atrioventricular groove and forms the posterior descending artery in most patients. Venous drainage occurs predominantly by way of the coronary sinus, which drains into the right atrium. Venous communications (Thebesian veins) also exist between the vessels of the myocardium and the cardiac chambers, draining deoxygenated blood directly into the left atrium and ventricle and contributing to physiologic right-to-left shunt.

The driving pressure for myocardial perfusion is the pressure in the aortic root, which is generated by the heart itself. Coronary perfusion is unique due to the contractile nature of the heart; with each beat of the heart, the pressure generated by myocardial contraction is imparted upon the coronary vasculature, thus determining the resisting pressure to forward flow in the coronary arteries. Given the inherent differences in contractile mechanics, perfusion to the left and right ventricles are not the same. As the contractile force of the left ventricle determines both the driving and resisting forces to coronary perfusion during systole, no pressure gradient exists, and therefore no coronary perfusion occurs during that phase of the cardiac cycle. Indeed, it has been appreciated that coronary blood flow in the large, left ventricular arteries is actually reversed during early systole. Maximal forward flow in the coronary arteries occurs during early diastole, when extravascular compression is minimal. As intramural pressure in the left ventricle is greatest in the endocardium and least in the epicardium, myocardial blood flow is greater in the epicardium, while the endocardium is at greater risk for ischemia. As mentioned previously, the right ventricle generates much lower pressures, and does not create reversal of flow in the right coronary arteries during systole. Systolic flow comprises a much greater portion of total coronary flow in the right ventricle due to less extravascular compression and a greater perfusion gradient.

The physiologic state of the heart has a great impact on myocardial perfusion. A higher inotropic state results in greater extravascular compression and greater resistance to coronary flow during systole. With regards to the cardiac cycle, increases in heart rate are primarily accommodated by shortening diastole and effectively decreasing the time of maximal coronary forward flow.

Autoregulation of coronary blood flow is mediated by the metabolic demands of the heart. While α- and β-adrenergic receptors do exist on coronary vessels, autoregulation is primarily mediated by non-adrenergic means. Muscarinic acetylcholine receptors on endothelial cells cause vasodilation via release of nitric oxide. However, local metabolic factors are the primary determinants of autoregulation of coronary flow; changes in myocardial oxygen demand effect the required changes in coronary blood flow. Vasodilating substances, including nitric oxide and adenosine, are released in response to supply–demand mismatch to increase coronary blood flow via coronary arterial dilation.

Oxygen supply to the myocardium is primarily determined by flow, as oxygen is maximally extracted in a single passage through the coronary capillaries. Frequency and strength of myocyte contraction determine myocardial oxygen consumption (MVO_2). A normal resting MVO_2 is 8 mL O_2/100 mL of myocardial tissue per minute; during heavy exercise this can increase to 70 mL O_2/100mL per minute or higher. Increasing heart rate increases MVO_2 in a near-linear fashion as the heart must generate an increasing number of contractions. An increased inotropic state will also increase MVO_2, as an increased magnitude and rate of development of tension in the myocyte generates greater energy expenditure. Thus, myocardial wall tension and oxygen consumption are closely related. As wall tension also determines extravascular compression of coronary arteries, it is a keystone factor in the determination of oxygen supply and demand. The Laplace relationship as applied to the heart states that myocardial wall tension is proportional to the product of pressure and volume. As afterload increases, cardiac myocytes must develop more tension to generate forward flow, and oxygen consumption increases. A higher preload increases ventricular volume throughout the cardiac cycle, which also increases wall tension and myocardial oxygen consumption.

Coronary atherosclerotic disease disrupts the normal balance of oxygen supply and demand, leaving the heart susceptible to ischemia and infarction. The classic clinical finding of a deficit in myocardial oxygenation is *angina pectoris*. As coronary artery disease progresses, more myocardium is subject to relative hypoxemia, resulting in less mechanically efficient contraction. Surrounding myocytes must compensate by increasing their contractile force which results in further increases in MVO_2. Plaque disruption or an embolic event can result in severe or complete disruption of coronary perfusion and subsequent myocardial infarction.

Assessment and monitoring

Defining hemodynamic goals is vital to the care of patients in the perioperative and critical care settings. A comprehensive assessment of a patient's hemodynamic status includes an evaluation of preload, afterload, intrinsic cardiac function, and structural disease. Traditionally, central venous pressure and pulmonary capillary wedge pressure have been used to evaluate the preload state of the right and left heart, respectively. However, the clinical reliability of these pressures is often poor. Further, these parameters have also proven to be unreliable in the setting of concurrent pathology, including pulmonary vascular disease and valvular dysfunction. Recently, evaluations of intra-arterial catheter waveforms have yielded parameters such as stroke volume variation (SVV), pulse pressure variation (PPV), and systolic pressure variation (SPV) as representatives of volume responsiveness.[4] In mechanically ventilated patients, these analyses have proven to be reliable predictors of "volume responsiveness" (increased stroke volume after volume challenge). The increasing pleural pressure of positive pressure ventilation creates cyclic changes in left ventricular stroke volume, and subsequently in arterial pulse pressure. A high pulse pressure variation indicates that a patient's volume status lies on a steeper portion of the preload–stroke volume relationship (Frank–Starling curve); in such patients, a fluid challenge is likely to shift their preload status rightward and improve hemodynamics (Figure 6.2).

By determining the preload dependence of stroke volume, the clinician may optimize cardiac function by providing volume when clinically appropriate. There are many benefits to using this mechanism to determine a patient's preload state. These methods allow for evaluation independent of variation of any given patient's Frank–Starling curve, with respect to the norm. They also provide dynamic feedback during and after specific interventions such as a fluid challenge, thus allowing for continuous assessment and optimization of further management. Indeed, patients with SVV >10% or PPV >12% have been found to respond to a volume challenge with a rise in stroke volume >10%.[5]

However, one must also be aware of the limitations of these indices when used to guide fluid therapy. Only mechanical ventilation provides the stable, consistent variations in intrathoracic pressure necessary to make arterial waveform analysis meaningful. Also, these indices are validated in studies where

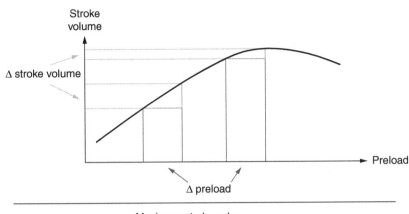

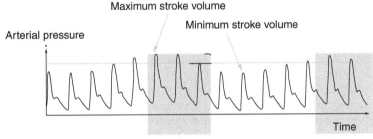

Figure 6.2. The same increase in preload will result in different increases in stroke volume, based on where a patient resides on the Frank–Starling curve (top). Stroke volume variation (SVV) may be demonstrated on arterial line tracing (bottom). SVV is calculated by the equation: SVV = SVmax − (SVmin/SVmean).

patients are mechanically ventilated with >8 mL/kg tidal volumes, the threshold at which some believe the intrathoracic pressures are great enough to have a consistent, meaningful effect on stroke volume variation. Additionally, patients must have a regular heart rate and adequate stroke volume for these analyses to be effective. These indices, therefore, are meaningless in the setting of advanced heart failure with pulsus alternans, atrial fibrillation or right ventricular dysfunction, all physiologic states where stroke volume will vary from beat to beat.

In the absence of LVOT obstruction or aortic stenosis, systemic vascular resistance (SVR) comprises the majority of the heart's afterload. SVR can vary dramatically in the perioperative and intensive care settings. Most anesthetic agents inherently decrease SVR to varying degrees, while the fluctuating balance between depth of anesthesia and surgical stimulation over the course of an operation can result in large swings in SVR. Additionally, patients exhibiting a systemic inflammatory response or those in frank sepsis will typically present in a low SVR state. In such instances, invasive monitoring is necessary in order to quantify SVR, which is calculated by the equation:

$$\text{SVR (dyn} \cdot \text{s} \cdot \text{cm}^{-5}) = 80 \times (\text{mean arterial pressure} - \text{central venous pressure}) \div \text{cardiac output}$$

Clearly, intrinsic cardiac function has a dramatic effect on systemic circulation and, as such, systolic and diastolic function must be carefully considered in the evaluation of the acute care patient. Systolic function may be imaged via echocardiography or measured in real time as cardiac output via dye dilution, thermodilution, or the Fick principle. Dilution techniques require an indicator – dye or blood temperature – measured at two separate points in the circulation and a subsequent calculation of the flow rate responsible for the difference in concentration. The Fick principle relies upon calculating the difference in inflow and outflow of a substance, usually oxygen, and knowledge of the consumption of the substance. Knowing inflow and outflow rates as well as the rate of consumption allows one to solve for overall flow rate, or cardiac output:

$$\text{CO} = \text{VO}_2 \div (\text{Ca} - \text{Cv})$$

Echocardiography is widely used to evaluate systolic and diastolic function. Multiple ejection phase indices have been described that can be used to estimate systolic function by measuring the difference between end-systolic and end-diastolic parameters and dividing by the end-diastolic value. Of these parameters, ejection fraction (EF) is the most common. EF uses ventricular volumes as the measure of function, estimating the percentage of blood at end-diastole that is ejected during systole. The left ventricular end-diastolic and end-systolic volumes may be measured using various echocardiographic techniques; EF may be calculated as follows:

$$EF = (EDV - ESV) \div EDV$$

EF is a composite parameter that reflects the contractile state of the heart as well as the preload and afterload at a given time. Upon closer evaluation of this equation, one will note that in a volume-depleted state both EDV and ESV are diminished. This results in a minimally changed numerator and a smaller denominator, thus increasing overall EF even though this state does not in fact lead to improvement in intrinsic systolic function. This is a classic example of the justification for load-independent parameters, which may be better, true assessments of systolic function, as the preload and afterload states of the heart are very dynamic, particularly in the acute care setting. In patients with mitral regurgitation, for example, the maximum rate of rise of pressure in the left ventricle can be estimated by utilizing continuous-wave Doppler. A greater contractile force will develop a greater rate of rise of pressure in the ventricle. Newer technology has allowed for sophisticated evaluations of ventricular function by way of strain analysis by utilizing Doppler tissue imaging or speckle tracking.[6] Strain is a dimensionless index that measures a change in length produced by the application of stress. Quantification of strain, strain rate (the rate of development of strain), and rotational motion of the heart as load-independent assessments of ventricular function is rapidly evolving in its utility in clinical practice.[7]

While systolic function has classically received far more clinical attention, the impact of diastolic dysfunction should not be overlooked as it is an independent risk factor for adverse clinical outcomes. As mentioned previously, diastole is an energy-dependent process and diastolic dysfunction an early sign of myocardial impairment. Transthoracic and transesophageal echocardiography remain exceedingly popular modalities for evaluation of diastolic function. Echocardiographic diastology consists of varying indices used to quantify the physiologic disturbances of impaired relaxation and compliance of the ventricle. Doppler tissue imaging of the mitral annulus and transmitral inflow are used to grade the presence and severity of diastolic dysfunction. As diastolic dysfunction progresses, ventricular filling

becomes more reliant upon atrial contraction, and the peak mitral inflow velocity during atrial contraction becomes greater than the peak velocity during early diastolic filling. Eventually, left atrial pressures rise to restore the relative atrioventricular pressure balance, and peak velocity during early diastolic filling again predominates in a process referred to as pseudonormalization.

The myocardial performance index (MPI), or Tei index, was developed in 1995 as a singular index to evaluate both systolic and diastolic function. The MPI may be calculated as the sum of time in the cardiac cycle spent in isovolumic contraction and relaxation divided by the ejection time. All markers may be derived from echocardiography. Initially validated for the left ventricle, studies have also demonstrated utility in the evaluation of right ventricular function as well. The MPI increases as myocardial function worsens, as the heart must spend more time in isovolumic contraction in order to generate enough pressure to eject. Also, the heart must spend more time in isovolumic relaxation in the setting of diastolic dysfunction. This index is relatively independent of heart rate as well as preload and afterload and has been shown to correlate well with clinical outcomes.[8]

Goal directed therapy for patients with cardiovascular disease

When managing patients with cardiovascular disease, hemodynamic goals must be defined in order to direct appropriate intervention. Traditional therapy in the acute care setting has relied on an integration of multiple invasive physiologic parameters to help guide fluid therapy as well as dosing of vasopressor and inotrope infusions. Goal directed therapy serves to better organize and optimize the integration of this data. The ultimate objective is the accurate diagnosis of the etiology of a hemodynamic disturbance, ultimately leading to appropriate therapy to ensure adequate and efficient tissue perfusion.

Arterial waveform analysis has drawn a great deal of interest in the development of goal directed therapy algorithms. Given that arterial catheters are frequently placed in patients at risk for hemodynamic instability, harvesting more information from an in-situ catheter presents little risk and great benefit. Goal directed therapy simply designed to continuously monitor and maintain pulse pressure variation <10% with fluid boluses has been shown to reduce duration of hospital stay, intensive care stay, duration of mechanical ventilation, and rate of postoperative complications.[9]

Oxygen delivery index (DO_2I), expressed in mL/min/m^2, is also a subject of repeated study as a target for goal directed therapy. DO_2I is the calculated amount of oxygen delivered per minute, indexed to the patient's height. A goal $DO_2I > 600$ mL/min/m^2 has been established in prior studies as a reliable target to improve clinical outcomes. DO_2I may be used to guide pressor therapy when clinical signs indicate that euvolemia has been established. Pearse et al. studied goal directed therapy to target euvolemia via central venous pressure versus maximizing stroke volume in patients following major general surgery. They found that the DO_2I goal of >600 mL/min/m^2 could be reached in a significantly higher proportion of patients in whom stroke volume was maximized and dopexamine was infused via a goal directed protocol targeting DO_2I.[10] Additionally, they found a decreased number of total postoperative complications and a shorter hospital stay in the goal directed therapy group.

Goal directed therapy may also have a long-term impact when implemented in the acute setting. Rhodes et al. performed a 15-year follow-up on previously randomized patients to goal directed versus conventional therapy, finding that median survival was significantly longer in the goal directed therapy group.[11] Additionally, among surviving patients, the three independent factors predicting survival were age, avoidance of major adverse cardiac events, and having been randomized to the goal directed treatment arm. The authors attribute the improved survival mostly to the reduced number of perioperative complications, as established in other studies.

The search for newer, more accurate, and less invasive goal directed parameters continues. Drawn from the same vein as analyses of the arterial waveform, recent advances in plethysmogram waveform analysis have yielded the variation in pulse oxymeter plethysmographic waveform amplitude (delta-POP) or pleth variability index (PVI). Both indices examine the difference between the maximal and minimal amplitudes of the plethysmogram's waveform. Similar to pulse pressure variation (PPV), these parameters rely on beat-to-beat changes in stroke volume that occur during mechanical ventilation. Delta-POP has been shown to correlate well with PPV. A PPV $>13\%$ correlates very well with a delta-POP $>15\%$,[12] implying that delta-POP may reliably be used as a surrogate for volume-responsiveness in patients without an arterial catheter. A prospective, randomized investigation of the use of PVI to guide intraoperative fluid therapy demonstrated less intraoperative fluid administered and lower postoperative lactate levels in the OR and on postoperative day two.[13] Further investigation continues on these and other novel monitoring modalities.

Conclusions

Complex interactions between preload, intrinsic cardiac function, and afterload mediate cardiac function and systemic perfusion. The clinician must use appropriate monitoring modalities integrated with clinical presentation to form an effective treatment plan. Goal directed therapy is critical in the management of patients with cardiovascular disease, as every organ is dependent on cardiac output to maintain viability. Recent studies investigating goal directed therapies suggest that focusing treatment on specific physiologic parameters may allow better optimization of the heart's ability to meet corporeal metabolic demand.

References

1. Fleisher LA, Beckman JA, Brown KA, et al. ACC/AHA 2007 Guidelines on perioperative cardiovascular evaluation and care for noncardiac surgery. *Circulation* 2007;**116**:e418–e500.

2. Chua JH, Nguyen R. Anesthetic management of the patient with low ejection fraction. *Am J Therap* 2013; doi:10.1097/MJT.0b013e31826fc458.

3. Chua JH, Zhou W, Ho JK, et al. Acute right ventricular pressure overload compromises left ventricular function by altering septal strain and rotation. *J Appl Physiol* 2013;**115** (2):186–93.

4. McGee WT, Raghunathan K. Physiologic goal-directed therapy in the perioperative period: the volume prescription for high-risk patients. *J Cardiothor Vasc Anesth* 2013;**S1053–0770(13)**:00256–5.

5. Hamilton MA, Cecconi M, Rhodes A. A systematic review and meta-analysis on the use of preemptive hemodynamic intervention to improve postoperative outcomes in moderate and high-risk surgical patients. *Anesth Analg* 2011;**112**:1392–402.

6. Artis NJ, Oxborough DL, Williams G, et al. Two-dimensional strain imaging: a new echocardiographic advance with

research and clinical applications. *Int J Cardiol* 2008;**123**–3:240–8.

7.   Abraham TP, Dimaano VL, Liang H-Y. Role of tissue Doppler and strain echocardiography in current clinical practice. *Circulation* 2007;**116**:2597–609.

8.   Haddad F, Denault AY, Couture P, et al. Right ventricular myocardial performance index predicts perioperative mortality or circulatory failure in high-risk valvular surgery. *J Am Soc Echocardiogr* 2007;**20**–9:1065–72.

9.   Lopes MR, Oliveira MA, Pereira VOS, et al. Goal-directed fluid management based on pulse pressure variation monitoring during high-risk surgery: a pilot randomized controlled trial. *Crit Care* 2007;**11**: R100.

10. Pearse R, Dawson D, Fawcett J, et al. Early goal-directed therapy after major surgery reduces complications and duration of hospital stay: a randomised, controlled trial. *Crit Care* 2005;**9**; R687–93.

11. Rhodes A, Cecconi M, Hamilton M, et al. Goal-directed therapy in high-risk surgical patients: a 15-year follow-up study. *Intens Care Med* 2010;**36**;1327–32.

12. Cannesson M, Besnard C, Durand PG, et al. Relation between respiratory variations in pulse oximetry plethysmographic waveform amplitude and arterial pulse pressure in ventilated patients. *Crit Care* 2005;**9**;R562–8.

13. Forget P, Lois F, Kock MD. Goal-directed fluid management based on the pulse oximeter – derived Pleth Variability Index reduces lactate Levels and improves fluid management. *Anesth Analg* 2010;**111**:910–14.

Chapter

7

Blood pressure regulation

Sheldon Magder

Introduction

Regulation of arterial blood pressure is one of the most basic homeostatic processes in mammals, and the range of regulated pressures also is very similar among species. Even with a fivefold increase in cardiac output during aerobic exercise, arterial pressure in normal young males does not increase more than 50%. Regulation of blood pressure occurs over the short term, meaning seconds to minutes and over longer time periods, meaning days to months. This chapter deals primarily with acute adjustments. The analysis is based on a global view of the mechanical processes involved in regulating arterial pressure, and emphasizes changes in cardiac output and systemic vascular resistance.

What is arterial pressure?

The potential of blood vessels to be stretched by a force is determined by the elastance of the vessel, which is calculated from the change in pressure for a change in volume. The inverse of elastance is compliance. Measured arterial pressure is primarily the pressure (force per cross-sectional area) created by blood volume on the inside of elastic walls of the arteries relative to the pressure outside their walls. This pressure difference across the wall is called transmural pressure. The resulting tension in the wall can be determined from the pressures on the inside and outside of the wall and the inner and outer radii of the vessel. The analysis is often simplified by using the LaPlace relationship, which is based on the product of the transmural pressure and inner radius. However, this simplification is only valid in very thin-walled structures. Calculation of wall stress by the LaPlace relationship gives a positive value of stress, whereas the use of inner

and outer radii and inner and outer absolute pressures that are not relative to atmospheric pressure gives a negative value.[1,2] The elastic force of the wall is detected by catheters with side holes and by blood pressure cuffs. Flow through a tube is determined by the difference between the inflow and outflow pressure. This drop of pressure along the length of a tube occurs because of friction from the interaction of the fluid and the inner surface of the tube as well as friction between layers that form in an ideal flowing liquid. This energy loss is called resistance and, based on the Poiseuille relationship, is calculated from the length of the tube, the fourth power of the radius, and the viscosity of the fluid as long as the flow is not turbulent.

It might seem at first that flow must always occur from an area of high pressure to an area of low pressure, but this is not true (Figure 7.1). It is the total energy loss of the system that matters and, besides the elastic pressure, there are two other forms of energy that need to be considered.[3] These are kinetic and gravitational energy. Kinetic energy is related to the product of the mass of the fluid and the square of the velocity of the fluid, which is distance per time. Velocity is related to flow, which is liter per time, by multiplying velocity by the cross-sectional area of the tube. The importance of kinetic energy becomes evident if there are variations in the cross-sectional area of a vessel. At a constant flow, the same number of particles that enter the tube must leave the tube. If a middle section of a tube has a narrowed cross-sectional area, the velocity of the particle must increase through this narrowed section so that the same number of particles to pass through (i.e., same "flow"), and thus the kinetic energy of the particles must increase. To maintain the conservation of energy, this means that elastic energy must be converted into

Perioperative Hemodynamic Monitoring and Goal Directed Therapy, ed. Maxime Cannesson and Rupert Pearse.
Published by Cambridge University Press. © Cambridge University Press 2014.

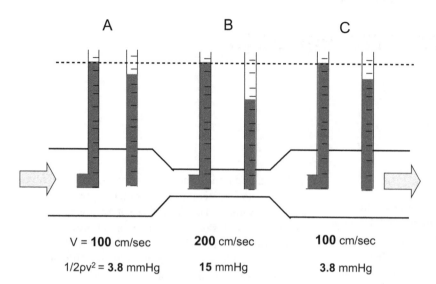

A   B   C

V = **100** cm/sec **200** cm/sec **100** cm/sec

$1/2\rho v^2$ = **3.8** mmHg **15** mmHg **3.8** mmHg

Figure 7.1. Effect of velocity on measured pressure with side-hole versus end-hole. In A the pressure measured with a side-hole is slightly lower than the pressure measured with an end-hole facing the flowing fluid. In the middle section, B, the tube is narrowed by half so that the velocity must double to allow the same flow of particles. The kinetic energy thus rises and the elastic energy decreases. In C the diameter is the same as baseline so the kinetic energy decreases and elastic energy increases again. An assumption is that there is a negligible resistive loss over this short distance.

kinetic energy. Thus elastic energy falls and kinetic energy rises. When the tube again widens, the velocity slows so that the kinetic energy is converted back into elastic energy, which means that the lateral pressure is higher downstream of the narrowed section. This has implications for the measurement of pressure. When pressure is measured with a cannula that faces the flow, the fluid that hits the cannula stops and its kinetic energy is converted into elastic energy, which means that the value measured with this device is greater than that obtained with a side-hole catheter. Kinetic energy contributes about 4 mmHg to normal arterial systolic pressure and 0.35 mmHg to the mean, but the contribution increases with increases in cardiac output and velocity, as occurs during exercise and also in sepsis. The velocity of blood flow in the vena cavae is the same as that in the aorta, so that the kinetic energy on the venous side is the same as in arteries. Since venous elastic pressure is so much lower than in arteries, the kinetic energy is a larger fraction of the total pressure. This is also true in the pulmonary circuit.

In a supine subject the third component of the energy, the gravitational component, has only a minor effect on arterial pressure measurements, but the gravitational component becomes very important in the upright posture. In a 170 cm person, the gravitational component of the pressure in the foot is almost equal to the elastic energy due to vascular volume. The gravitational component must also be considered when using fluid filled catheters to measure pressure. This is because the fluid in the device creates a gravitation force (i.e., weight) that needs to be accounted

for by making sure that pressures are always measured relative to the same fixed level. This is especially important when calculating perfusion pressure in the brain or abdomen. To measure these perfusion pressures properly, the transducers for each measurement must be at the same level and not, as is sometimes suggested, with different levels for the cerebral and abdominal compartments.

Why is arterial pressure regulated at such a high value in mammals?

The right heart is able to pump the same amount of blood as the left heart through the pulmonary circulation with a mean driving pressure of only about 15 mmHg and a systolic pressure of less than 18 mmHg. So why is arterial pressure maintained in such a high range compared with the pulmonary circuit? One possibility might be to allow us to stand up. The hydrostatic gradient from the heart to the head in the upright posture of a 170 cm person is about 40 mmHg, so that the arterial pressures must be high enough to ensure steady cerebral perfusion. However, the arterial pressure of rats and mice is similar to that of humans and they obviously have no significant gravitational challenge! The answer thus is more likely related to physiological advantages. By starting with a relatively high aortic pressure, regional blood flows, such as blood flow to skeletal muscle during exercise, can be increased by lowering local resistances according to local metabolic needs without much change in aortic pressure. Thus other regions of the body do not have to adjust their local resistances to maintain the same perfusion pressure. The alternative strategies would require that all other regions vasoconstrict to redirect flow to the working muscle, or that flow increases to all parts of the body at the same time, which would create an overwhelming demand on the heart. The value of having a constant pressure source works much like the provision of water to homes. A community's water sources are maintained at a constant pressure, often by being in a water tower. Opening taps in individual residences effectively decreases the local resistance in the places where flowing water is wanted. A second reason is that, by keeping arterial pressure relatively constant, the load on the heart remains constant. The importance of this is that pressure work requires much more energy for the heart than volume work and thus by having a relatively constant pressure the energy demands of the heart do not change very much.

What determines blood pressure?

A fundamental principle in cardiovascular physiology is that blood pressure does not determine total systemic blood flow, i.e., cardiac output, but rather that cardiac output and systemic vascular resistance determine arterial blood pressure.[4] Based on the Poiseuille relationship, arterial pressure is approximately the product of cardiac output and systemic vascular resistance. I say approximately because it should be arterial pressure minus a downstream pressure rather than simply arterial pressure, but because the downstream value is relatively constant and low, this simplification is still useful. From the clinical point of view, this simple relationship means that a decrease in arterial pressure must be because there was either a decrease in cardiac output or a decrease in systemic vasculature. Furthermore, since systemic vascular resistance is calculated, the real question for the management of hypotension becomes: did the blood pressure fall with a fall in cardiac output, in which case it is an "output" problem, or did it fall with a normal or elevated cardiac output, in which case it is a "resistance" problem. This allows the clinician to direct diagnostic reasoning to the appropriate physiological mechanism. The same rationale can be applied to the physiological processes that regulate arterial blood pressure and I will use this logic throughout this chapter. The implication is that deviations of arterial pressure from normal must be due to changes in cardiac output or to changes in systemic vascular

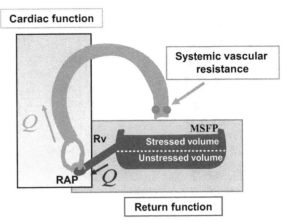

Figure 7.2. Schema for processes that can regulate blood pressure. Return function gives the determinants of venous return and are represented by a tank with an opening on the side. Stressed volume is the volume above the opening and unstressed below the opening. Stressed volume determines the elastic recoil pressure, the mean systemic filling pressure (MSFP). The tank drains through venous resistance (Rv). Cardiac function is based on the Frank–Starling relationship (Q = cardiac output). Systemic vascular resistance is regulated by arteriolar tone.

resistance (Figure 7.2). Furthermore, regulatory mechanisms that restore arterial pressure to normal also must act through changes in cardiac output or through changes in systemic vascular resistance.

Regulation of vascular resistance

There are many factors that regulate the vascular resistance component, each of which could be a separate chapter so my comments will be limited to some broad descriptions of their roles. The factors regulating vascular resistance are easier to understand and usually more evident than the factors regulating cardiac output.

Baroreceptor regulation of arterial pressure is one of the best-studied regulatory mechanisms. These receptors are located in the carotid sinus as well as in the aortic arch but the carotid sinus receptors dominate the control. Because the carotid sinus is located outside the chest, these receptors are not directly affected by changes in pleural pressure. Their proximity to the brain also ensures that the pressure for perfusion of the cerebral vasculature is well regulated, and their location above the heart makes these receptors sensitive to the demands of being in an upright posture. A rise in blood pressure increases distention of the wall of carotid arterial baroreceptors. This increases the afferent activity of the carotid sinus nerve, which runs along with the

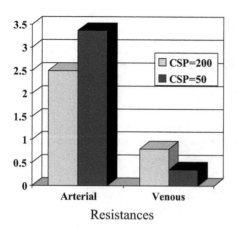

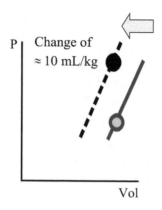

Figure 7.3. Integrated response to carotid sinus pressure (CSP). Pressure in the carotid sinus was decreased from 200 to 50 mmHg. The upper left shows the volume–pressure change in the splanchnic (Spl) region. There was a left shift of the volume–pressure relationship that recruited 10 mL of unstressed into stressed volume. The lower left bar graph indicates the change in splanchnic arterial and venous resistances with CSP hypotension. Arterial resistance increased, whereas venous resistance decreased. The right side shows the integrated response and how each factor alters venous return (VR). V0 = unstressed volume. Rv = venous resistance. Based on reference 23 (Deschamps and Magder).

glossopharyngeal (IX cranial) nerve. Centrally, this activates a vasodepressor zone, which increases vagal activity and inhibits a vasostimulatory zone, which thereby decreases sympathetic activity. The result is decreased heart rate, decreased contractility, and decreased vasoconstriction, so that there are changes in both cardiac output and systemic vascular resistance components of blood pressure.

There are central mechanisms that can result in cardiac activation and systemic vasoconstriction. During exercise, the central commands[5] that activate muscle contraction spill over into thalamic regions and increase sympathetic activity and thus produce vasoconstriction and cardiac stimulation. Neural output from the cerebral cortex such as occurs in anxious states can do the same.

There are important peripheral factors that regulate vascular resistances. Factors related to metabolic activity such as partial pressure of oxygen, oxygen saturation, potassium, osmolality, pH, and adenosine can induce vasodilatation to increase flow to match metabolic needs.[6] This process is especially active in skeletal and cardiac muscles. Vascular smooth muscle in arterioles can contract when arterial pressure is increased, or dilate when arterial pressure is decreased, and thereby maintain constant flow despite differences in arterial pressure. This is called the myogenic mechanism,[7,8] and it is especially important in coronary, cerebral, renal, and gastrointestinal vasculatures where the objective is to maintain constant flow. Increased blood flow increases shear stress on the endothelial lining of blood vessels and this induces the release of nitric oxide, which can dilate downstream resistance;[9,10] the process is called flow-mediated dilatation and acts as a feed-forward mechanism, which would cause progressive vasodilatation if not counteracted by the myogenic

and metabolic regulatory mechanisms. Disease states can also affect vascular resistance. These include loss of vascular tone in sepsis or ischemia reperfusion and obstructive problems due to atherosclerotic disease.

Regulation of baseline cardiac output

Cardiac output is normally tightly related to metabolic needs.[11] For example, during aerobic exercise, cardiac output increases linearly with increasing oxygen consumption. This relationship is so tight that, if the subject's hemoglobin concentration is normal, cardiac output can be predicted within about a 5% accuracy by just knowing the oxygen consumption. Cardiac output itself is regulated by two functions: a return function, which is given by Guyton's venous return analysis and cardiac function, which is given by the Frank–Starling relationship.[4] The actual cardiac output is determined by the intersection of these two functions (Figure 7.3).

Approximately 70% of blood volume resides in small veins and venules of the systemic circulation, so that the analysis of the return function can be simplified with a reasonable approximation by just considering the drainage characteristics of the systemic veins. These create what I have called a large bathtub-like effect[12] in which the arterial inflow to this region alters the outflow not by producing an inflow pressure, but rather by increasing the volume in the region, which increases the elastic recoil in the walls of the vessels in this region. The return function then is determined by four factors: stressed volume, venous compliance, venous resistance, and the outflow pressure of the venous drainage, which is right atrial pressure (RAP).[13] Stressed volume is the volume that stretches the elastic walls of vessels, and under basal conditions in an average-sized male stressed volume is about 1.3 to 1.4 L or approximately 30% of total blood volume. Venous compliance indicates the stretchiness of the venous reservoir and determines the slope of the relationship of stressed volume to venous pressure. This slope is essentially linear in the physiological range, and does not change acutely. Another useful term is capacitance. This refers to the total volume, which includes stressed and unstressed volume at a given pressure. Importantly, stressed volume can be increased by constriction of the walls of small veins and venules so that their unstressed volume becomes stressed volume. Venous resistance is normally only about 5% of arterial resistance but can be increased or decreased by neural input, drugs, and disease states. The high cardiac output of sepsis likely involves dilation of venous resistance vessels.

Cardiac function defines the cardiac output at different preloads considering constant heart rate, contractility, and afterload. An increase in heart rate, contractility, or decrease in afterload shift the cardiac function curve upwards, which indicates an increase in cardiac function. The preload for the heart as a whole is RAP, which should be noted is also the outflow of the return function. An increase in cardiac function allows the heart to put out the same amount at a lower RAP, which means the heart is more "permissive" in that it allows greater venous drainage.

Regulations by the system in response to changes in blood pressure

As already stated, deviations of arterial pressure from normal values must occur through either changes in cardiac output or changes in systemic vascular resistance. Changes in cardiac output must occur through changes in cardiac function or changes in the return function. It follows that regulation of deviations of arterial pressure from the normal value must involve changes in these same parameters, whether through normal physiological mechanisms or through exogenous interventions by the treating health care team.

Responses to increased arterial pressure

Increases in cardiac output or sympathetic activity are an important part of daily activities and these would increase arterial pressure unless there is reflex vasodilatation to keep arterial pressure constant. The baroreceptors play a major role in this regulation under normal physiological conditions. This is supported by the pattern of response of the carotid sinus nerve. Activity of the carotid sinus nerve occurs when distended by increases in arterial pressure and decreases when arterial pressure falls and there is less distension of the carotid sinus. A good example of the physiological need for the systemic vascular resistance to adapt to an increase in cardiac output is aerobic exercise. If there were no adjustments in systemic vascular resistance, there would be a marked rise in arterial pressure with the rise in cardiac output. The marked rise in arterial pressure would increase the afterload on the left ventricle and reduce the expected increase in cardiac output. The consequent increase in left ventricular preload would shift volume from the systemic circulation to the pulmonary circulation and reduce elastic recoil pressure for venous return from peripheral veins.[14] As already noted, during exercise, cardiac output can increase fivefold with only a 50% increase in arterial pressure and only a small increase in mean arterial pressure, which means that there is a large decrease in arterial resistance. An obvious mechanism for the fall in systemic arterial resistance is the metabolically induced vasodilatation in the working muscle, which allows the increase in muscle blood flow and ensures good matching between local blood flow and tissue needs. If there is more blood flow into the muscle, there must be more coming out, but the increase in venous return is likely not sufficient to prevent a fall in arterial pressure, and arterial pressure needs to be sustained by an increase in sympathetic tone.[15] This occurs through a number of pathways, which include afferent signals from the working muscle[16] and what is called central command,[5] which is sympathetic activation that occurs when the cerebral cortex sends motor signals to muscle tissue. If there is any decrease in arterial pressure, the baroreceptors will also contribute and provide fine tuning to the process. The set-point of the pressure range of the carotid sinus is increased during exercise, which allows systolic pressure to rise above the normal value. The increase in sympathetic activity by these mechanisms during exercise raises arterial resistance in non-working areas of the body. This helps redirect more blood to the working muscle. These responses, too, would be modified by baroreceptor feedback.

Pathological increases in arterial pressure are primarily due to an inappropriate increase in arterial resistance and failure of the appropriate vasodilatory response. A good example is essential hypertension. Since the problem is a failure of proper regulation of arterial resistance, and considering again that blood pressure is equal to the product of cardiac output and systemic vascular resistance, the only process that could counter the inappropriate rise in vascular resistance is a decrease in cardiac output. However, cardiac output is too strongly regulated by metabolic activity to allow this to happen. Thus the system has no intrinsic mechanism to correct the problem and the only solution is the use of exogenous substances, that is, pharmacotherapy to decrease vascular resistance. These include centrally acting alpha-2 agonists, inhibition of constriction with calcium channel blockers, angiotensin converting enzyme inhibitors or angiotensin receptor antagonists, or by active dilators such as nitric oxide-releasing substances or drugs inhibiting entry of calcium into cells such as hydralazine. Arthur Guyton proposed that, in the early stages of essential hypertension, arterial pressure could be increased by expansion of vascular volume by retention of sodium with a consequent secondary increase in cardiac output. This would still require failure of normal baroreceptor activity and likely occurs to some extent during excessive salt loading, but can be resolved over a number of days by renal excretion of the excess sodium.

Responses to decreased arterial pressure

Reflex responses to decreases in arterial pressure need to occur rapidly, especially in the upright posture to protect cerebral circulation and normal brain function. The baroreceptors are thus critical for proper postural adaptations. Blood pressure is also decreased with increases in pleural pressure as can be demonstrated with a Valsalva maneuver and the accompanying baroreceptor-mediated increase in vascular resistance. In both these physiological causes of hypotension, the problem is the decrease in cardiac output.

Cardiac output can fall because of decrease in cardiac function or a decrease in return function. In these two examples the problem is the decrease in return function. In the postural stress, there is peripheral pooling of volume because of gravitational stress, and in the Valsalva maneuver the increase in pleural pressure decreases the gradient for venous return. The initial response is most likely familiar to most readers. The fall in blood pressure with the fall in cardiac output decreases distention of the carotid arterial baroreceptors. This decreases activity of the carotid sinus nerve and consequently decreases vagal tone and increases

sympathetic activity. There is thus an increase in systemic arterial resistance, which helps restore blood pressure. Cardiac function, too, improves because of increased heart rate and contractility. However, an increase in cardiac function does not mean that there is restoration of cardiac output, which is the primary problem. Under normal conditions, RAP in the upright posture is at, or below, atmospheric pressure, and lowering RAP further by improving cardiac function will not increase cardiac output. This is because of what is known as the vascular waterfall effect in veins. When the pressure inside collapsible veins is less than their outside pressure, flow limitation occurs in the great veins in that lowering downstream pressure does not increase flow. When there is a vascular waterfall, cardiac output only can be increased by increasing drainage from the venous reservoir except for some other small changes. For example, increased cardiac activity can pump some volume from the thoracic compartment to the systemic circulation, but the magnitude of this is small. The primary physiological processes for increasing venous return is by the recruitment of unstressed into stressed volume by contraction of the venous capacitance vessels.[17] However, this mechanism can only work if there are reserves in unstressed volume. Decreased venous resistance could also contribute as discussed below and could help even if reserves in capacitance are low. There could also be some recruitment of volume from the interstitial space by alterations in pre- and postcapillary resistances and consequent changes in capillary filtration,[18] but this process will act over minutes to hours, whereas changes in capacitance and venous resistance are in seconds.

Two-compartment model of the systemic circulation

At this point it is necessary to add another level of complexity to the systemic circulation. The sympathetic response to hypotension as sensed by the baroreceptors does not increase arterial resistance equally in all arterial beds.[19] Resistance in non-splanchnic circulation, which is primarily muscle, increases more than the resistance in the splanchnic circulation. This increases the fraction of cardiac output going to the splanchnic circulation. From an evolutionary point of view, this makes sense for it means that more of the available blood flow can go to the more vulnerable abdominal organs. However, a shift in the fraction of flow to the splanchnic vasculature by itself will actually decrease cardiac output. As first described by August Krogh in 1912,[20] and later by Permutt and co-workers,[21,22] when there are two parallel venous beds that have different compliances, the fractional distribution of inflow between these two regions affects the rate of return of blood to the right heart. In this model the splanchnic circulation is considered to have a large compliance, whereas non-splanchnic vasculature has a low compliance. Because of its large compliance, drainage from the splanchnic bed has a long time constant, in the range of 20 to 24 seconds, whereas that of the low compliant non-splanchnic bed has a time constant of drainage of 4 to 6 seconds. The consequence of this is that the splanchnic accumulates more of the available volume when it receives a greater fraction of the total flow, and the effective mean circulatory filling pressure (elastic recoil pressure) is reduced. This leads to a decrease in the return function.

To understand how all this could work during baroreceptor activation for hypotension, we conducted an animal experiment in which we created a right heart bypass and kept cardiac output constant with a pump.[23] We then isolated the splanchnic and limb circulations so that we could measure the regional compliance, venous resistance, unstressed volume, and flow draining each region. We isolated the carotid sinuses so that we could produce step changes in carotid sinus pressure and observe the responses in the isolated venous beds. This is called an open loop analysis of a reflex pathway because the reflex adjustments cannot feed back to baroreceptors. Lowering isolated carotid sinus pressure, the equivalent hypotension for the baroreceptors, produced a marked rise in systemic vascular resistance, but as expected increased the fraction of cardiac output going to the splanchnic bed compared with the non-splanchnic bed (Figure 7.3). However, it also resulted in recruitment of unstressed volume into stressed volume in the splanchnic bed with no significant recruitment in non-splanchnic regions. Most surprisingly, although the arterial resistance to the splanchnic bed increased, venous resistance draining this region decreased. This decreased the time constant of drainage from the splanchnic region, which increased the venous return from this region. Together, all these adaptations in an intact animal would have resulted in an increase in cardiac output of ~10%. The decrease in splanchnic venous resistance could be related to a sphincter-like mechanism in the hepatic vein, which dilates in response to beta-adrenergic agonists. On the other hand, venous resistance vessels are constricted by alpha-adrenergic agonists.

Responses to pathological causes of hypotension

Pathological causes of hypotension can be due to loss of vascular tone and decreased systemic vascular resistance, decreased cardiac output due to decreased stressed volume and decreased return function, or decreased cardiac function, or both. Loss of vascular tone is the major factor for the septic shock, for the cardiac output is usually increased. As is the case with essential hypertension, since the problem is one of a loss of vascular tone, the only defense for the body is to increase cardiac output, which is already elevated and further increases are often limited because of sepsis-induced myocardial depression and an exogenous intervention is needed. The initial step is usually an infusion of volume to increase stressed volume, and to use the Starling mechanism to increase cardiac output, but this can only work when the heart still is functioning on the ascending part of the cardiac function curve. When right heart filling is limited, pharmacotherapy is needed to correct the loss of vascular tone or to improve the cardiac response.

If hypotension is due to primary cardiac function, increasing vascular resistance will restore the pressure, but do nothing for tissue perfusion. There is thus no value for the use of pure alpha agonist such as phenylephrine, for it can only increase the load on the left heart and increase the resistance to venous return and thus tend to decrease cardiac output further.[24] Changes in preload are unlikely to be helpful because the problem is depressed cardiac function. The problem can only be resolved by improving cardiac function by an increase in contractility, decrease in afterload, or perhaps an increase in heart rate. In contrast to phenylephrine, norepinephrine can increase cardiac function and does not increase venous resistance and might even decrease it.[25] It is also crucial to determine if there is a cardiac component that can be corrected, such as an obstructed coronary artery or a malfunctioning valve.

Critical closing pressure

It is often not appreciated that there is a critical closing pressure or Starling-resistor mechanism that is active in the arterial vasculature.[26] For the whole body this has been estimated to be around 30 mmHg,[27] but the value can be much higher in skeletal muscle, which contains a major proportion of the vasculature. The significance of this is that RAP is not the downstream pressure for the assessment of resistance in the vasculature. It also adds another control mechanism, which can significantly magnify perfusion changes when arterial resistance is low, as during exercise or in sepsis. Critical closing pressures are regulated by baroreceptor activity and sympathetic tone,[28] local metabolic factors,[26] and myogenic tone.[29] Their tone is likely lost in distributive shock with sepsis.

Starling included a critical closing pressure in his heart–lung preparation because it helped provide a constant afterload for the left ventricle, which he could then adjust and it could serve a similar role in the systemic vasculature.[30]

Distribution of resistances

So far in the discussion, systemic vascular resistance has largely been considered as one variable. However, the important factor is the distribution of resistances, for this is what determines regional flows and is why maintaining a relatively high central pressure is so useful. It needs to be appreciated that it is also not the actual value of the individual resistances, but their relative values compared with other regions as I already discussed under the fractional flow between splanchnic and non-splanchnic vascular beds. The significance of this is that, if there is someone who has an arterial pressure of 90 mmHg, but has the same proportional distribution of regional vascular resistances as someone with a systolic pressure of 120 mmHg, their regional blood flows and cardiac output could be the same, which is why people function normally with different blood pressures. However, there are some limits. One is gravitational. If systolic pressure were only 50 mmHg, the average-sized male would not be able to be sit up. Also physical limits based on the structure of vascular beds limit how low the vascular resistance can be.[31] For example, the kidney starts with a very low resistance and would not be able to decrease it adequately to allow for enough flow at pressures as low as 50 mmHg.

The implication of regional differences in vascular resistance and the variable response to sympathetic activation that I discussed under the two-compartment model is that the response to exogenous vasopressors is not completely predictable. If the vasoconstrictor does not increase cardiac output and increases all regional resistances equally, there will be no increase in blood flow to any region. Thus, an assumption when using a vasopressor is that resistance vessels in vital organs such as the brain, heart, and kidney will not constrict as much as non-essential organs, so that they can get a greater proportion of the limited cardiac output. At high doses of vasopressors, it is very likely that this is not true. The key is not to forget that pressure is not the same as flow.

Limits of the system

It should become apparent from this analysis of the regulation of arterial pressure that the physiological and therapeutic options are quite limited. If there are limited reserves in unstressed volume, sympathetic activation cannot compensate by increasing stressed volume. If the right heart is functioning on the flat part of the cardiac function curve, increasing blood volume cannot correct hypotension. If there is flow limitation to venous return because of low venous pressures, increasing cardiac function cannot increase cardiac output in response to hypotension. If there is already near maximal vasoconstriction, further sympathetic activation cannot increase vascular resistance.

Conclusions

A general approach to understanding the regulation of arterial pressure should begin by considering whether the problem and solutions involve changes in systemic vascular resistance, or changes in cardiac output, and if the problem is changes in cardiac output, is it due to changes in cardiac function or due to changes in the return function. Based on this rationale, some assessment of the status of cardiac output is key. When the primary problem is a change in cardiac output due to a change in the return function, volume status is usually the major variable to be considered. If cardiac function is the problem, choices are more limited. Drugs will be necessary to improve the function, and the cause of decreased cardiac function needs to be addressed. Finally, one must always keep in mind that blood pressure does not indicate flow.

References

1. Shrier I. Critical closing pressures, vascular waterfalls, and the control of blood flow to the hindlimb 1993. PhD thesis McGill University.

2. Azuma T, Oka S. Mechanical equilibrium of blood vessel walls. *Am J Physiol* 1971;**221**:1210–318.

3. Burton AC. *Total Fluid Energy, Gravitational Potential Energy, Effects of Posture. Physiology and Biophysics of the Circulation: An Introductory Text.* Chicago: Year Book Medical Publishers Incorporated, 1965, pp. 95–111.

4. Magder S. An approach to hemodynamic monitoring: Guyton at the bedside. *Crit Care* 2012;**16**:236–43.

5. Mitchell JH, Shephard JT. Control of the circulation during exercise. In Paul McNeil Hill, ed. *Exercise – The Physiological Challenge.* USA: Conference Pub., 1993, pp. 55–85.

6. Berne RM. Metabolic regulation of blood flow. *Circ Res* 1964;**5: Suppl** 8.

7. Johansson B, Mellander S. Static and dynamic components in the vascular myogenic response to passive changes in length as revealed by electrical and mechanical recordings from the rat portal vein. *Circ Res* 1975;**36** (1):76–83.

8. Bayliss WM. On the local reactions of the arterial wall to changes of internal pressure. *J Physiol* 1902;**28**(3):220–31.

9. Dimmeler S, Assmus B, Hermann C, Haendeler J, Zeiher AM. Fluid shear stress stimulates phosphorylation of Akt in human endothelial cells: involvement in suppression of apoptosis. *Circ Res* 1998;**83**:334–41.

10. Fulton D, Gratton J-P, McCabe TJ, et al. Regulation of endothelium-derived nitric oxide production by the protein kinase Akt. *Nat* 1999;**399**:597–600.

11. Guyton AC, Carrier O, Jr., Walker JR. Evidence for tissue oxygen demands as the major factor causing autoregulation. *Circ Res* 1964;**15:Suppl** 9.

12. Magder S, De Varennes B. Clinical death and the measurement of stressed vascular volume. *Crit Care Med* 1998;**26**:1061–4.

13. Magder S, Scharf SM. Venous return. In Scharf SM, Pinsky MR, Magder SA, eds. *Respiratory–Circulatory Interactions in Health and Disease.* 2nd edn. New York: Marcel Dekker, Inc., 2001, pp. 93–112.

14. Magder S, Veerassamy S, Bates JH. A further analysis of why pulmonary venous pressure rises after the onset of LV dysfunction. *J Appl Physiol* 2009;**106**(1):81–90.

15. Rowell LB. *Human Cardiovascular Control.* New York: Oxford University Press, 1993.

16. McCloskey DI, Mitchell JH. Reflex cardiovascular and respiratory responses originating in exercising muscle. *J Physiol (Lond)* 1972;**224**(1):173–86.

17. Rothe CF. Reflex control of veins and vascular capacitance. *Physiol Rev* 1983;**63**(4):1281–95.

18. Mellander S, Johansson B. *Control of Resistance, Exchange, and Capacitance Functions in the Peripheral Circulation.* Pharmacological Reviews. Williams & Wilkins Co., 1968, pp. 117–96.

19. Hainsworth R, Karim F. Responses of abdominal vascular capacitance in the anaesthetized dog to changes in the carotid sinus pressure. *J Physiol London* 1976;**262**:659–77.

20. Krogh A. The regulation of the supply of blood to the right heart. *Skand Arch Physiol* 1912;**27**:227–48.

21. Caldini P, Permutt S, Waddell JA, Riley RL. Effect of epinephrine on pressure, flow, and volume relationships in the systemic circulation of dogs. *Circ Res* 1974;**34**:606–23.

22. Permutt S, Caldini P. Regulation of cardiac output by the circuit: venous return. In Boan J, Noordergraaf A, Raines J, eds. *Cardiovascular System Dynamics.* 1st edn. Cambridge, Mass. and London, England: MIT Press, 1978, pp. 465–79.

23. Deschamps A, Magder S. Baroreflex control of regional capacitance and blood flow distribution with or without alpha adrenergic blockade. *J Appl Physiol* 1992;**263**:H1755–63.

24. Magder S. Phenylephrine and tangible bias. *Anesth Analg* 2011;**113**(2):211–13.

25. Datta P, Magder S. Hemodynamic response to norepinephrine with and without inhibition of nitric oxide synthase in porcine endotoxemia. *Am J Resp Crit Care Med* 1999;**160**(6):1987–93.

26. Magder S. Starling resistor versus compliance. Which explains the zero-flow pressure of a dynamic arterial pressure–flow relation? *Circ Res* 1990;**67**:209–20.

27. Sylvester JL, Traystman RJ, Permutt S. Effects of hypoxia on the closing pressure of the canine systemic arterial circulation. *Circ Res* 1981;**49**:980–7.

28. Shrier I, Hussain SNA, Magder SA. Carotid sinus stimulation influences both arterial resistance and critical closing pressure of the isolated hindlimb vascular bed. *Am J Physiol* 1993;**33**: H1560–6.

29. Shrier I, Magder S. Response of arterial resistance and critical closing pressure to change in perfusion pressure in canine hindlimb. *Am J Physiol* 1993;**265**: H1939–45.

30. Chapman CB. Starling's work. *Ann Int Med* 1962;**57**(**Suppl 2**): 19–43.

31. Magder SA. Pressure–flow relations of diaphragm and vital organs with nitroprusside-induced vasodilation. *J Appl Physiol* 1986;**61**:409–16.

Microcirculation and mitochondrial dysfunction

Daniel De Backer and Diego Orbegozo Cortes

Introduction

Organ dysfunction often occurs in the perioperative setting and in sepsis. Alterations in systemic hemodynamics may play a role, but even when these are within therapeutic goals, organ dysfunction may still occur. Microcirculatory alterations, a key determinant of tissue perfusion and of mitochondrial dysfunction, may play a role in the development of organ dysfunction. In this chapter, we discuss the evidence for alterations in microcirculatory and mitochondrial functions, and their relevance, in circulatory failure and in the perioperative setting.

Microcirculatory alterations in sepsis: where is the evidence?

Multiple experimental studies have found that sepsis induces marked alterations in the microcirculation. Compared with normal conditions where there is a dense network of well-perfused capillaries, sepsis is associated with a decrease in capillary density. More importantly, intermittently perfused or not perfused capillaries are located in close proximity to well-perfused capillaries, which results in shunt.[1–4] Importantly, this is a dynamic process, as the stop flow capillaries may be perfused a few minutes later and vice versa. In addition, there is an increase in heterogeneity in microvascular perfusion between areas separated by a few microns. These alterations have been reported after administration of endotoxin or live bacteria and during bacterial peritonitis,[2,3,5] and have been observed in small[6,7] as well as in large animals.[3,4] In addition, all studied organs are affected, including the skin,[8] muscle,[6,7] eye,[9] tongue,[3] gut,[3,4] liver,[1] heart,[10] and the brain.[5] Hence, these changes seem to be ubiquitous and to have common pathophysiologic mechanisms.

Technical limitations have long impaired the demonstration of microcirculatory alterations in patients. The development of new imaging techniques has enabled direct visualization of the human microcirculation with small handheld microscopes.[11,12] In patients with severe sepsis and septic shock, we observed a decrease in vascular density, together with an increased number of capillaries with stopped or intermittent flow.[13] Typical examples of normal and septic microcirculations are shown in Figures 8.1 and 8.2. These alterations are very similar to those occurring in experimental models of sepsis. Since this initial study, more than 30 studies have shown similar results.

What are the consequences of these alterations?

Tissue oxygenation is impaired as the diffusion distance for oxygen increases as a result of the decreased capillary density.[10] In addition, the heterogeneity in microvascular blood flow with perfused capillaries in close vicinity to non-perfused capillaries, leads to alterations in oxygen extraction capabilities[4,14–17] and heterogeneity in tissue oxygenation.[18] Hence zones of tissue hypoxia may develop, even when total blood flow to the organ is preserved.[19]

Importantly, heterogeneity in perfusion leads to more severe alterations in tissue oxygenation than a homogenous decrease in perfusion.[14,17] During episodes of hypoperfusion, the heterogeneity of microvascular perfusion further increases in sepsis instead of being minimized as in normal conditions.[16]

These alterations play an important role in the development of organ dysfunction and are not just an indication of the severity of sepsis. Microvascular alterations can lead to cellular injury,[20] and reversal of these alterations is associated with improvement in lactate[21]

Perioperative Hemodynamic Monitoring and Goal Directed Therapy, ed. Maxime Cannesson and Rupert Pearse.
Published by Cambridge University Press. © Cambridge University Press 2014.

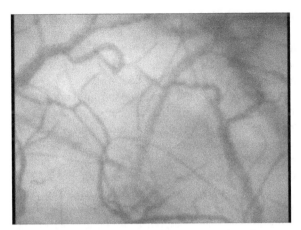

Figure 8.1. Sublingual microcirculation in normal conditions. Photograph of the sublingual microcirculation in a normal individual with septic shock using a sidestream dark field (SDF) imaging device.

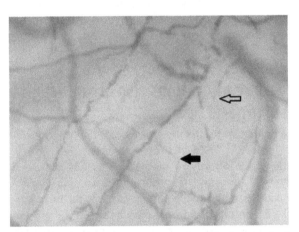

Figure 8.2. Sublingual microcirculation in sepsis. Photograph of the sublingual microcirculation in a patient with septic shock using a sidestream dark field (SDF) imaging device. The solid arrow shows a well-perfused capillary; the empty arrow identifies a stopped flow capillary.

and NADH[22] levels, suggesting that microvascular alterations directly impair tissue oxygenation. In addition, several trials have demonstrated an association between the severity of microvascular dysfunction and the development of organ dysfunction[23–25] and mortality.[13,19,24,26–30]

In 252 patients with septic shock, microvascular perfusion was an independent factor associated with survival[31]. Dividing the population into quartiles of proportions of perfused capillaries, mortality rates markedly increased with alterations in the microcirculation.[31] The proportion of perfused capillaries was the strongest predictor of outcome, but vascular density of perfused capillaries, and heterogeneity index were also associated with outcome.[13,19,31] Of note, the velocity in perfused capillaries was not associated with outcome,[19] illustrating that the diffusive component of oxygen transport seems to be more important at the microcirculatory level than its convective component.

The evolution over time of these alterations also differed in patients with good or poor outcomes.[27,30] Microvascular perfusion rapidly improved in survivors, but remained disturbed in non-survivors, whether these patients died from acute circulatory failure or from organ failure after resolution of shock.[27,30]

Mitochondrial dysfunction: where is the evidence?

Mitochondrial dysfunction is characterized by alteration in mitochondrial electron transport chain by cytochromes I to IV. Several experimental models have reported decreased complex I, II, and/or complex IV activity.[32,33] In a long-term model of sepsis in rodents, mitochondrial dysfunction, mostly characterized by decreased complex I activity, was associated with organ dysfunction and mortality.[32] In late phases of sepsis, administration of exogenous cytochrome C corrected mitochondrial alterations and reversed myocardial depression.[34]

Three publications investigated skeletal muscle mitochondria in septic patients.[35–37] Complex I and IV as well as citrate synthase activity were reduced in septic patients if the enzymatic activity was expressed per tissue weight, and again, no change was observed when normalized to citrate synthase activity.[35,36] Additionally, the muscle ATP content was decreased in septic patients. Brealey et al.[37] observed differences between surviving and non-surviving septic patients and controls: complex I activity decreased compared with controls and ATP content decreased compared with survivors of sepsis and controls. However, complex IV activity increased in non-survivors compared with controls. Overall, skeletal muscle mitochondria and tissue ATP content seem mainly to be reduced in patients who will later die from sepsis.

On the other hand, other studies have demonstrated normal or even increased mitochondrial function. In hearts demonstrating impairment in systolic and diastolic function at the early phase of sepsis, mitochondrial histology and function were normal.[38] In peripheral white blood cells obtained from patients with sepsis, mitochondrial respiratory function was increased, not decreased.[39] Oxidative phosphorylation and electron transfer were increased in patients with sepsis, suggesting integrity of cytochrome pathways.

In a recent systematic review, which included 76 trials, Jeger et al.[40] pointed out the different factors contributing to these different results. In addition to species and organ specificities, the methods used to investigate cellular respiration, in particular the way results were expressed, should be examined carefully. Results can be expressed per tissue weight, mitochondrial protein, or per citrate synthase activity. As citrate synthase activity is down-regulated by ATP content, results of mitochondrial function expressed per citrate synthase activity should be looked at with caution. In addition, it appears to change throughout the course of sepsis. Mitochondrial function seems to be increased in early sepsis, but impaired in later stages;[37,41] mitochondrial dysfunction is more severe in non-resuscitated than in resuscitated models,[42] and more severe in non-survivors than in survivors.[37]

Microcirculatory and mitochondrial dysfunction: a different relevance at different periods?

As alterations in systemic hemodynamics, microvascular perfusion, and mitochondrial function may all occur, it is quite difficult to determine which contributes most to the development of organ dysfunction.

Several factors suggest that the microcirculatory alterations are important at the early stages and act as a primary event leading to cellular dysfunction. First, microcirculatory alterations are co-localized with low PO_2, production of hypoxia-inducible factor[10] or redox potential[22] in experimental conditions. Second, oxygen saturation at the capillary end of well-perfused capillaries is low, suggesting that the tissues are using the delivered oxygen.[15] Third, there is an inverse relationship between microvascular perfusion and tissue to arterial PCO_2 gradient, in the sublingual area[43] and in the ileal mucosal area.[44] This gradient would be normal if flow was matching metabolism, as CO_2 production would be low because the primary alteration is the decrease in metabolism. Fourth, perfusion abnormalities precede alterations in organ function.[45] Fifth, improvement in the sublingual microcirculation in response to initial resuscitation procedures was associated with an improvement of organ function 24 h later.[25] Finally, the decrease in lactate levels is proportional to the improvement of the microcirculation during dobutamine administration.[21] Hence, it seems that, at early stages, flow alterations seem to precede and maybe contribute to cellular alterations.

One may thus raise the following unifying theory: at initial stages, systemic hemodynamic alterations predominate. Once these are within targets (i.e., arterial pressure, cardiac index, and SvO_2), the contribution of microcirculatory alterations becomes predominant. After some time, cellular alterations dominate. This suggests that there is a time window opportunity for therapeutic interventions aiming at improving tissue perfusion. This view is supported by some experimental and clinical data. In animals with sepsis, delayed fluid resuscitation, compared to timely resuscitation was associated with increased levels of inflammatory mediators and impairment of cytochrome function.[42] In patients with septic shock, Finfer et al.[46] reported that patients undergoing early goal directed therapy had lower activation of inflammatory and apoptotic pathways.

Do these alterations also occur in high risk surgery?

Microcirculatory alterations also occur in the perioperative period.[47–49] In patients submitted to high-risk surgery, the severity of the alterations was associated with development of perioperative complications.[49] In patients submitted to cardiac surgery, the microvascular alterations culminated during the surgical procedure and the severity of these alterations correlated with peak levels of lactate and SOFA score in the perioperative period.[47] The impact of anesthesia should not be neglected, but this effect is not sustained and rapidly disappears in the postoperative period.[47]

Mitochondrial dysfunction occurs in organs submitted to clamping, as a consequence of the ischemic process. Hearts submitted to cardioplegic arrest under cardiopulmonary bypass demonstrate a diffuse loss of mitochondrial cytochrome C, and in particular complex I, and a decrease in mitochondrial oxygen consumption.[50,51] Do we also observe similar alterations in remote organs? This issue has not yet been evaluated in humans.

Conclusions

Multiple experimental and clinical trials have shown that microcirculatory alterations occur in sepsis and that they may play a role in the development of organ dysfunction. Similar alterations occur in the perioperative period. In addition, mitochondrial dysfunction also occurs, especially in late stages of sepsis, and is associated with organ dysfunction. The relative contribution of both factors is difficult to determine at this stage.

It seems that temporal factors may play a role and that microcirculatory alterations prevail at early stages, once global hemodynamic variables are within target values, and that mitochondrial dysfunction dominates at later stages.

References

1. Croner RS, Hoerer E, Kulu Y, et al. Hepatic platelet and leukocyte adherence during endotoxemia. *Crit Care* 2006;**10**: R15.

2. Secor D, Li F, Ellis CG, et al. Impaired microvascular perfusion in sepsis requires activated coagulation and P-selectin-mediated platelet adhesion in capillaries. *Intens Care Med* 2010;**36**:1928–34.

3. Verdant CL, De Backer D, Bruhn A, et al. Evaluation of sublingual and gut mucosal microcirculation in sepsis: a quantitative analysis. *Crit Care Med* 2009;**37**:2875–81.

4. Farquhar I, Martin CM, Lam C, et al. Decreased capillary density in vivo in bowel mucosa of rats with normotensive sepsis. *J Surg Res* 1996;**61**:190–6.

5. Taccone FS, Su F, Pierrakos C, et al. Cerebral microcirculation is impaired during sepsis: an experimental study. *Crit Care* 2010;**14**:R140.

6. Hollenberg SM, Broussard M, Osman J, et al. Increased microvascular reactivity and improved mortality in septic mice lacking inducible nitric oxide synthase. *Circ Res* 2000;**86**:774–8.

7. McKinnon RL, Lidington D, Tyml K. Ascorbate inhibits reduced arteriolar conducted vasoconstriction in septic mouse cremaster muscle. *Microcirculation* 2007;**14**:697–707.

8. Ruiz C, Hernandez G, Godoy C, et al. Sublingual microcirculatory changes during high-volume hemofiltration in hyperdynamic septic shock patients. *Crit Care* 2010;**14**:R170.

9. Pranskunas A, Pilvinis V, Dambrauskas Z, et al. Early course of microcirculatory perfusion in eye and digestive tract during hypodynamic sepsis. *Crit Care* 2012;**16**:R83.

10. Bateman RM, Tokunaga C, Kareco T, et al. Myocardial hypoxia-inducible HIF-1α, VEGF and GLUT1 gene expression is associated with microvascular and ICAM-1 heterogeneity during endotoxemia. *Am J Physiol Heart Circ Physiol* 2007;**293**: H448–56.

11. Groner W, Winkelman JW, Harris AG, et al. Orthogonal polarization spectral imaging: a new method for study of the microcirculation. *Nat Med* 1999;**5**:1209–12.

12. Goedhart P, Khalilzada M, Bezemer R, et al. Sidestreal Dark Field (SDF) imaging: a novel stroboscopic LED ring-based imaging modality for clinical assessment of the microcirculation. *Optics Express* 2007;**15**:15101–14.

13. De Backer D, Creteur J, Preiser JC, et al. Microvascular blood flow is altered in patients with sepsis. *Am J Respir Crit Care Med* 2002;**166**:98–104.

14. Goldman D, Bateman RM, Ellis CG. Effect of decreased O_2 supply on skeletal muscle oxygenation and O_2 consumption during sepsis: role of heterogeneous capillary spacing and blood flow. *Am J Physiol Heart Circ Physiol* 2006;**290**: H2277–85.

15. Ellis CG, Bateman RM, Sharpe MD, et al. Effect of a maldistribution of microvascular blood flow on capillary O_2 extraction in sepsis. *Am J Physiol* 2002;**282**:H156–64.

16. Humer MF, Phang PT, Friesen BP, et al. Heterogeneity of gut capillary transit times and impaired gut oxygen extraction in endotoxemic pigs. *J Appl Physiol* 1996;**81**:895–904.

17. Walley KR. Heterogeneity of oxygen delivery impairs oxygen extraction by peripheral tissues: theory. *J Appl Physiol* 1996;**81**:885–94.

18. Legrand M, Bezemer R, Kandil A, et al. The role of renal hypoperfusion in development of renal microcirculatory dysfunction in endotoxemic rats. *Intens Care Med* 2011;**37**:1534–42.

19. Edul VS, Enrico C, Laviolle B, et al. Quantitative assessment of the microcirculation in healthy volunteers and in patients with septic shock. *Crit Care Med* 2012;**40**:1443–8.

20. Eipel C, Bordel R, Nickels RM, et al. Impact of leukocytes and platelets in mediating hepatocyte apoptosis in a rat model of systemic endotoxemia. *Am J Physiol Gastrointest Liver Physiol* 2004;**286**:G769–76.

21. De Backer D, Creteur J, Dubois MJ, et al. The effects of dobutamine on microcirculatory alterations in patients with septic shock are independent of its systemic effects. *Crit Care Med* 2006;**34**:403–8.

22. Kao R, Xenocostas A, Rui T, et al. Erythropoietin improves skeletal muscle microcirculation and tissue bioenergetics in a mouse sepsis model. *Crit Care* 2007;**11**: R58.

23. Doerschug KC, Delsing AS, Schmidt GA, et al. Impairments in microvascular reactivity are related to organ failure in human sepsis. *Am J Physiol Heart Circ Physiol* 2007;**293**:H1065–71.

24. Shapiro NI, Arnold R, Sherwin R, et al. The association of near-infrared spectroscopy-derived tissue oxygenation measurements with sepsis syndromes, organ dysfunction and mortality in emergency department patients with sepsis. *Crit Care* 2011;**15**: R223.

25. Trzeciak S, McCoy JV, Phillip DR, et al. Early increases in microcirculatory perfusion during protocol-directed resuscitation are associated with reduced multi-organ failure at 24 h in patients with sepsis. *Intens Care Med* 2008;**34**:2210–17.

26. De Backer D, Creteur J, Dubois MJ, et al. Microvascular alterations in patients with acute severe heart failure and cardiogenic shock. *Am Heart J* 2004;**147**:91–9.

27. Sakr Y, Dubois MJ, De Backer D, et al. Persistant microvasculatory alterations are associated with organ failure and death in patients with septic shock. *Crit Care Med* 2004;**32**:1825–31.

28. den Uil CA, Lagrand WK, van der Ent M, et al. Impaired microcirculation predicts poor outcome of patients with acute myocardial infarction complicated by cardiogenic shock. *Eur Heart J* 2010;**31**:3032–9.

29. Creteur J, Carollo T, Soldati G, et al. The prognostic value of muscle StO(2) in septic patients. *Intens Care Med* 2007;**33**:1549–56.

30. Top AP, Ince C, de Meij N, et al. Persistent low microcirculatory vessel density in nonsurvivors of sepsis in pediatric intensive care. *Crit Care Med* 2011;**39**:8–13.

31. De Backer D, Donadello K, Sakr Y, et al. Microcirculatory alterations in patients with severe sepsis: impact of time of assessment and relationship with outcome. *Crit Care Med* 2013;**41**:791–9.

32. Brealey D, Karyampudi S, Jacques TS, et al. Mitochondrial dysfunction in a long-term rodent model of sepsis and organ failure. *Am J Physiol Regul Integr Comp Physiol* 2004;**286**:R491–7.

33. Levy RJ, Piel DA, Acton PD, et al. Evidence of myocardial hibernation in the septic heart. *Crit Care Med* 2005;**33**:2752–6.

34. Piel DA, Deutschman CS, Levy RJ. Exogenous cytochrome C restores myocardial cytochrome oxidase activity into the late phase of sepsis. *Shock* 2008;**29**:612–16.

35. Fredriksson K, Tjader I, Keller P, et al. Dysregulation of mitochondrial dynamics and the muscle transcriptome in ICU patients suffering from sepsis induced multiple organ failure. *PLoS One* 2008;**3**:e3686.

36. Fredriksson K, Hammarqvist F, Strigard K, et al. Derangements in mitochondrial metabolism in intercostal and leg muscle of critically ill patients with sepsis-induced multiple organ failure. *Am J Physiol Endocrinol Metab* 2006;**291**: E1044–50.

37. Brealey D, Brand M, Hargreaves I, et al. Association between mitochondrial dysfunction and severity and outcome of septic shock. *Lancet* 2002;**360**:219–23.

38. Smeding L, van der Laarse WJ, van Veelen TA, et al. Early myocardial dysfunction is not caused by mitochondrial abnormalities in a rat model of peritonitis. *J Surg Res* 2012;**176**:178–84.

39. Sjovall F, Morota S, Persson J, et al. Patients with sepsis exhibit increased mitochondrial respiratory capacity in peripheral blood immune cells. *Crit Care* 2013;**17**:R152.

40. Jeger V, Djafarzadeh S, Jakob SM, et al. Mitochondrial function in sepsis. *Eur J Clin Invest* 2013;**43**:532–42.

41. Fredriksson K, Flaring U, Guillet C, et al. Muscle mitochondrial activity increases rapidly after an endotoxin challenge in human volunteers. *Acta Anaesthesiol Scand* 2009;**53**:299–304.

42. Correa TD, Vuda M, Blaser AR, et al. Effect of treatment delay on disease severity and need for resuscitation in porcine fecal peritonitis. *Crit Care Med* 2012;**40**:2841–9.

43. Creteur J, De Backer D, Sakr Y, et al. Sublingual capnometry tracks microcirculatory changes in septic patients. *Intens Care Med* 2006;**32**:516–23.

44. Dubin A, Edul VS, Pozo MO, et al. Persistent villi hypoperfusion explains intramucosal acidosis in sheep endotoxemia. *Crit Care Med* 2008;**36**:535–42.

45. Rosengarten B, Hecht M, Auch D, et al. Microcirculatory dysfunction in the brain precedes changes in evoked potentials in endotoxin-induced sepsis syndrome in rats. *Cerebrovasc Dis* 2007;**23**:140–7.

46. Finfer S, Bellomo R, Lipman J, et al. Adult-population incidence of severe sepsis in Australian and New Zealand intensive care units. *Intens Care Med* 2004;**30**:589–96.

47. De Backer D, Dubois MJ, Schmartz D, et al. Microcirculatory alterations in cardiac surgery: effects of cardiopulmonary bypass and anesthesia. *Ann Thorac Surg* 2009;**88**:1396–403.

48. Atasever B, Boer C, Goedhart P, et al. Distinct alterations in sublingual microcirculatory blood flow and hemoglobin oxygenation in on-pump and off-pump coronary artery bypass graft surgery. *J Cardiothorac Vasc Anesth* 2010;**25**:784–90.

49. Jhanji S, Lee C, Watson D, et al. Microvascular flow and tissue oxygenation after major abdominal surgery: association with post-operative complications. *Intens Care Med* 2009;**35**:671–7.

50. Caldarone CA, Barner EW, Wang L, et al. Apoptosis-related mitochondrial dysfunction in the early postoperative neonatal lamb heart. *Ann Thorac Surg* 2004;**78**:948–55.

51. Oka N, Wang L, Mi W, et al. Cyclosporine A prevents apoptosis-related mitochondrial dysfunction after neonatal cardioplegic arrest. *J Thorac Cardiovasc Surg* 2008;**135**:123–30.

Chapter

9

Hemoglobin function and patient blood management

Aryeh Shander, Faraz Syed, and Mazyar Javidroozi

Introduction

With the stained safety and dubious efficacy of banked blood, in addition to past concerns with limited supply and increasing costs, a fundamental change in the clinicians' approach and attitude toward allogeneic blood transfusions have become necessary. Transfusion should no longer be considered a default decision, but should be a last resort to be used judiciously and sparingly and only when indicated. This shift is further fueled by the inherently complex and uncontrollable nature of allogeneic blood as a *de facto* "tissue allograft," which involves a complicated chain of procurement from live donors, processing, storage, and distribution. Any measures that can be used to reduce the use of allogeneic blood components without incurring harm to patients should be explored and adopted.[1–4]

When ordering any treatments, clinicians' primary goal is to provide the best care for their patients. By the same token, the goal in transfusion medicine should not be just limiting blood transfusion, but providing the best care for the patients. This is where Patient Blood Management (PBM) comes to play. PBM is defined as "the timely application of evidence-based medical and surgical concepts designed to maintain hemoglobin (Hb) concentration, optimize hemostasis and minimize blood loss in an effort to improve patient outcome."[5] In PBM, emphasis is placed on improving the clinical outcomes of the patients as opposed to simple reduction of blood transfusions; nonetheless, the latter is often achieved as a byproduct of implementing PBM strategies.[6] PBM strategies generally fall within one of the following approaches (Figure 9.1; visit www.sabm.org for more info):[7,8]

- Managing anemia
- Optimizing coagulation

- Interdisciplinary blood conservation modalities, and
- Patient-centered decision making.

PBM should be viewed as a comprehensive and multi-modality approach to be implemented throughout the course of care of patients. For example, in a surgical patient, this approach may span several weeks including prior to admission for an elective procedure into postdischarge follow-up visits and beyond. During this period, the patient should be assessed and reassessed for risk factors of both anemia and blood loss.[6] PBM and goal directed therapy (GDT) are complementary management strategies, and many of the PBM approaches can be implemented as part of a goal directed therapy strategy and vice versa.[9] PBM endorses GDT among the strategies to use to correct coagulation abnormalities, (Figure 9.1) and GDT often provides guidelines for transfusion of blood components based on objective and evidence-based criteria, which is also a key approach in PBM.[10] On the other hand, patients treated under GDT strategies can also benefit from PBM strategies by reducing their need and exposure to transfusions. For example, critically ill patients (who are often candidates for GDT) are at increased risk of receiving transfusions, and are possibly at increased risk of suffering unfavorable outcomes following transfusions,[11] and PBM measures can be highly beneficial to these patients by minimizing their need to receive allogeneic blood components.

Understanding the function of Hb, oxygen transportation by blood, and adaptations to anemia are the keys in applying PBM strategies in a goal directed fashion. These and other aspects of PBM that are more relevant to GDT are discussed here.

Perioperative Hemodynamic Monitoring and Goal Directed Therapy, ed. Maxime Cannesson and Rupert Pearse.
Published by Cambridge University Press. © Cambridge University Press 2014.

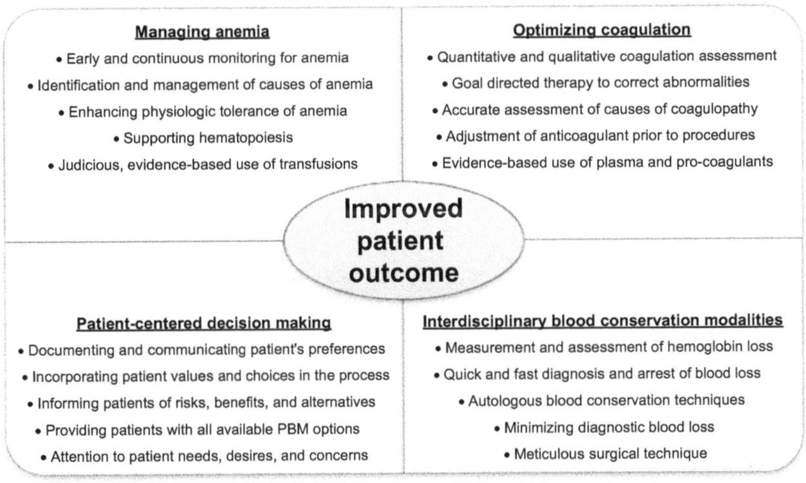

Managing anemia
- Early and continuous monitoring for anemia
- Identification and management of causes of anemia
- Enhancing physiologic tolerance of anemia
- Supporting hematopoiesis
- Judicious, evidence-based use of transfusions

Optimizing coagulation
- Quantitative and qualitative coagulation assessment
- Goal directed therapy to correct abnormalities
- Accurate assessment of causes of coagulopathy
- Adjustment of anticoagulant prior to procedures
- Evidence-based use of plasma and pro-coagulants

Improved patient outcome

Patient-centered decision making
- Documenting and communicating patient's preferences
- Incorporating patient values and choices in the process
- Informing patients of risks, benefits, and alternatives
- Providing patients with all available PBM options
- Attention to patient needs, desires, and concerns

Interdisciplinary blood conservation modalities
- Measurement and assessment of hemoglobin loss
- Quick and fast diagnosis and arrest of blood loss
- Autologous blood conservation techniques
- Minimizing diagnostic blood loss
- Meticulous surgical technique

Figure 9.1. Key strategies in patient blood management (PBM) with examples of each. These strategies are used in combination with the goal of improving patient outcomes (as opposed to mere reduction of allogeneic blood transfusions). Adapted from the Society for the Advancement of Blood Management; www.sabm.org.

Oxygen transportation – the pump, the vessels, and the medium

Evolution of single- to multi-cellular organisms necessitated development of elaborate mechanisms to deliver oxygen to cells lying far away from oxygen-rich environment in defiance of simple diffusion limitations. This task is achieved through the concerted function of three components – a medium capable of carrying oxygen, vessels for the medium to flow through, and a pump to circulate the medium through the vessels. The critical role of the cardiovascular system in maintaining oxygen delivery to the tissues throughout the body is discussed in detail in other chapters and here we focus on the role of the medium, blood.

Simply stated, blood (like most other aqueous fluids) is capable of loading oxygen when exposed to relatively high O_2 partial pressure (PO_2) and off-loading it when the PO_2 is relatively low. What makes blood particularly apt in doing this task is its ability to carry oxygen in two forms: dissolved (physically) in its aqueous phase and bound chemically to Hb molecules within the red blood cells (RBCs).

The Hb molecule is composed of four subunits, each capable of binding an oxygen molecule. Each Hb molecule can therefore bind with up to four oxygen molecules, which translates to up to 1.34 mL of oxygen per each gram of Hb or a total of 0.6–1 liter of oxygen in circulating blood of an average adult under physiologic conditions at sea level and 37 °C. Total Hb-bound oxygen content of each liter of blood can be calculated, based on the equation below:

Hb-bound oxygen (mL/Liter blood) = Hb concentration (g/L) × Hb oxygen saturation (SO_2)/100 × 1.34

In this equation, SO_2 is a value between 0 and 100%, representing the percentage of occupation (saturation) of oxygen-binding sites in Hb molecules. The complex tetrameric structure of Hb allows its affinity for oxygen molecules to be finely tuned. Binding of each oxygen molecule to a subunit induces conformational allosteric changes in the molecule that facilitates binding of the next oxygen molecule until all binding sites are occupied, and this cooperative binding of oxygen to Hb molecule is the reason why Hb–oxygen association (or dissociation) curve follows a sigmoidal shape. Other conditions such as increased levels of 2,3-diphosphoglycerate (2,3-DPG), which occurs in hypoxic conditions and acidic pH (due to increased CO_2 in peripheral tissues, in what is known as the Bohr effect) and increased temperature can affect the structure of the Hb molecule and facilitate dissociation and release of oxygen from the Hb–oxygen complex. As the result of these and other factors, Hb molecules are nearly completely saturated with oxygen at alveolar capillaries where PO_2 is high, and they can effectively release oxygen in other tissue where PO_2 is low and demand for oxygen is high (Figure 9.2).

Oxygen can also be dissolved in the aqueous phase of blood (namely plasma, but also the cytoplasm of all blood cells and platelets). Unlike the Hb-bound oxygen, the oxygen dissolved in the aqueous phase of blood behaves more simply, following Henry's law: the amount of oxygen dissolved in blood is directly related to PO_2 in a linear manner:

Blood-dissolved oxygen = PO_2 × Henry's law constant

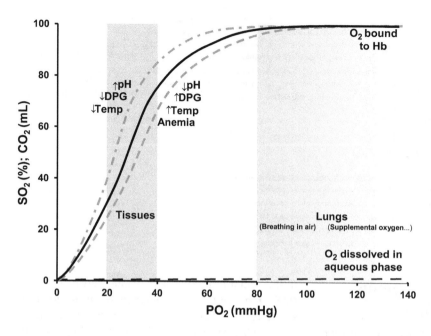

Figure 9.2. Relationship between partial pressure of oxygen (PO_2) and Hb oxygen saturation/content as well as dissolved oxygen in the aqueous phase (plasma and cytoplasm). To allow direct comparison of amounts of Hb-bound and dissolved oxygen, oxygen content (CO_2) based on an 150 mL aliquot of blood with hematocrit of 50% (total Hb content of 75 g) at 37 °C is provided. The solid black line represents normal Hb in RBC. The dashed gray lines represent the shift to left or right in Hb–oxygen dissociation curve as a result of changes in pH, 2,3-DPG, temperature, and anemia. Dashed black line represents the oxygen dissolved in the aqueous phase of blood, which normally represents just a small fraction of total oxygen content of blood. The gray areas represent the typical PO_2 levels in lung alveoli and the tissues throughout body.

Based on this equation, each liter of plasma is capable of dissolving about 0.03 mL oxygen per 1 mmHg PO_2 under normal physiologic conditions and temperature of 37 °C (Figure 9.2).

In order to calculate the total oxygen content of blood, the Hb-bound oxygen content and the blood-dissolved component should be added:

Total oxygen content of blood = Hb-bound oxygen + Blood-dissolved oxygen

This equation can be rewritten as follows for the oxygen content of arterial blood:

Total oxygen content of arterial blood (CaO_2; in mL) = (SaO_2/100 × Hb × 1.34) + (0.03 × PaO_2)

An important observation from this equation is that, under physiologic conditions, the bulk of oxygen content of blood (over 98%) is determined by the Hb-bound fraction. Assuming a Hb level of 150 g/L and near-complete (100%) SaO_2, the total oxygen content of each liter of blood will be approximately 204 mL: 201 mL bound to Hb and just 3 mL dissolved in blood.[12]

Understanding these two components of blood oxygen content (the Hb-bound and the dissolved part), and the way they behave in response to changes in other parameters, is critical to understanding the physiology and management of anemia and its most-dreaded consequences, hypoxia and ischemia. It must

be remembered that these equations only address oxygen content of blood. Nonetheless, "hypoxia" is a relative term, reflecting the ratio between the delivered oxygen and the oxygen needs (consumption) of the target tissues, which is determined and affected by a host of other factors.

While the equations so far focused on the oxygen content of blood, we can calculate the total arterial oxygen delivery (DO_2) to the organs using the equation below:

DO_2 = CaO_2 × Cardiac output (CO)

This equation incorporates the function of the heart (pump) in oxygen transportation throughout the body. CO provides another level of modulation and management in anemia: decreased CaO_2 can be compensated by increasing CO, and as discussed below, this is among the main mechanisms employed during physiologic adaptation to anemia.

It should be remembered that changes taking place in the body during anemia are substantially more complicated than the simplified examples provided here, which only focus on interactions between oxygen, Hb, and the aqueous phase of blood. Additionally, changes in rheological characteristics of blood during severe hemodilution can also interfere with oxygen delivery to the end-organ since a minimum level of blood viscosity and normal mechanical dynamics of RBCs are required to maintain microcirculation and avoid microhemodynamic aberrations.[13,14] We take a closer look at some of these issues in the next section.

Physiologic adaptation to anemia

Like many other systems in living organisms, the oxygen transportation system has a large reserve capacity and several redundant components, which allow maintenance of a stable oxygen supply to the tissues throughout the body despite changes in Hb level. Blood flow to the tissues is tightly regulated to maintain an adequate supply of oxygen. An important part of this regulation is the continuous monitoring of oxygen availability at organelle (e.g., mitochondrial), cellular, tissue, and organ levels.[3] Anemia results in decreased PO_2, which is detected by the renal cortex causing an increased production of erythropoietin, hematopoiesis, and eventually Hb level.[15] In the meantime, the peripheral chemoreceptors in the aortic arch and carotid arteries respond to arterial hypoxemia by modulating cardiovascular function.[16] These and other responses lead to the short-term physiologic adaptation to anemia which are hallmarked by increased heart rate (HR) and a combination of factors that increase the cardiac stroke volume (SV), including increased contractile force of heart, decreased after-load (reduced vascular resistance due to vasodilatation, reduced blood viscosity, and increased nitric oxide activity), and increased preload (increased venous return).[17] Increased HR and SV both directly increase CO:[18]

$$CO = \text{Stroke volume (SV)} \times \text{Heart rate (HR)}$$

In response to anemia, respiratory activity and ventilation are also increased, while improving the ventilation–perfusion matching to maximize the arterial oxygen pressure at alveolar sites. As a result, SaO_2 is usually maintained at near 100% during anemia, although as previously discussed, this should not be incorrectly interpreted as evidence of adequate oxygen delivery to the tissues since the total oxygen content of blood may still be too low.

Another important aspect of physiologic adaptation to anemia involves the regulation of oxygen extraction at various tissues. Generally speaking, not all oxygen molecules bound to Hb are off-loaded as the Hb molecules complete their journey through the tissue capillaries, leaving a reserve margin to allow higher extraction of oxygen from Hb depending on the demand and available Hb molecules. Considering the body as a whole, oxygen extraction from blood (EO_2) can be calculated by subtracting the oxygen content of blood leaving the tissues and returning to the heart (venous blood oxygen content; CvO_2) from the oxygen content of the arterial blood prior to entering the tissues (CaO_2):

$$EO_2 = CO \times (CaO_2 - CvO_2)$$

Similarly, oxygen consumption (VO_2) can be easily calculated, based on the oxygen content of blood and its extraction ratio as it passes through the tissues as follows:

$$VO_2 = EO_2 \times DO_2$$

Discussion of VO_2, DO_2, and EO_2 often leads to another important (and elusive) concept, critical DO_2 (DO_2 CRIT). As long as DO_2 is greater than VO_2/EO_2, the tissue in question is theoretically supplied with enough oxygen to keep up with the demand. As DO_2 drops, it reaches a level, denoted as DO_2 CRIT, where it can no longer match the oxygen demand (VO_2/EO_2), resulting in forced drop of VO_2 and occurrence of ischemia. While DO_2 CRIT is a very important threshold with important clinical implications (e.g., in determining the related "critical" Hb level as a "physiologic" transfusion trigger), it is obvious that DO_2 CRIT is a moving target, likely to change constantly depending on the VO_2 and EO_2 at each given tissue and at any given time. An extreme example is the case of "supply-dependency" encountered in critically ill septic patients, in which VO_2 keeps dropping with decreasing DO_2, even at DO_2 ranges that are expected to be substantially higher than what is normally needed to meet the metabolic needs.[19]

While an average systemic EO_2 can be calculated for the whole body based on the oxygen content of blood leaving the heart and oxygen content of blood returning to the heart (i.e., central venous blood oxygen content; $ScvO_2$), local EO_2 can vary significantly among different tissues and organs, with some tissues extracting a higher percentage of the blood oxygen content, leaving a narrower margin for compensation of decreased DO_2 in anemia by increasing EO_2. This is the case with heart muscle, which has a high baseline oxygen extraction ratio under normal conditions, making the oxygen delivery to heart largely flow dependent. In contrast, in brain capillaries under normal conditions, just about one-third of oxygen bound to Hb molecules is extracted, and the extraction ratio can be increased to 50% if needed.[15,20] This phenomenon is portrayed by a right shift in the oxygen-Hb dissociation curve during severe anemia (Figure 9.2), reducing the affinity of Hb for oxygen and facilitating its release in tissues facing hypoxia. This shift is caused by decreased pH, increased 2,3-DPG, and NO-mediated signaling pathways among others.[20] Other contributing factors include increased local blood flow and recruitment and redistribution of new capillaries at the tissue level.[21,22] Under normal conditions, the diffusion of oxygen from capillaries to the cells is effectively driven by a very small PO_2 difference between the capillaries to the interstitial space and into the cells, often just a few mmHg/μm.[23] Hence, it often only takes a very small change in the blood flow into the tissue to compensate for the negative impact of anemia and sustain stable oxygen delivery to the cells.[3]

As anemia progresses and tissue hypoxia develops, cells undergo further changes to adapt and protect themselves. Namely, increased expression (or more precisely, inhibition of degradation) of a group of transcription factors known collectively as hypoxia inducible factors (HIFs) in hypoxic conditions alters expression of various other genes that promote survival in hypoxic conditions and further improve cardiovascular adaption to anemia.[22,24] HIFs can promote hematopoiesis by increasing the expression of erythropoietin,[25] promote angiogenesis via up-regulating vascular endothelial growth factor (VEGF),[26] and can inhibit mitochondrial oxidative phosphorylation (aerobic) and promote glycolysis (anaerobic) to sustain ATP production with reduced dependency to oxygen availability.[27]

Interestingly, just as a "smart power grid" can regulate distribution of electricity during a shortage and divert it from non-critical users to more critical ones, oxygen transportation to critical organs such as heart can be selectively increased during anemia in context of stable or even reduced delivery to other organs. These active regulations are not just a result of circulatory changes, but involve metabolic changes including HIFs and other cellular mechanisms that take place during anemia.[28]

These are just some of the adaptations and compensatory mechanisms in play during anemia, and the responses will differ depending on the level of anemia and its acuity (acute vs. chronic). As a result of all these intricate and integrated processes, oxygen delivery to tissues remains relatively stable and commensurate to their critical needs despite reduced oxygen content of blood at systemic level.[3] These adaptive mechanisms can provide us with opportunities to better manage anemia, which is the basis for the third pillar of PBM, i.e., optimizing the physiologic adaptations to anemia to minimize its negative impacts.

PBM and adaptation to anemia – making the best out of a bad situation

As previously discussed, PBM strategies generally focus on one of these approaches: supporting hematopoiesis, minimizing blood loss, and optimizing the physiologic response to anemia, while using blood components appropriately and only when indicated.[5–7] Appropriate and timely management of anemia is a cornerstone of PBM, which often requires proactive planning and preparation to be most effective.[29] Nonetheless, when dealing with severely anemic and critically ill patients, the opportunity to be proactive and plan accordingly is often lost, as most approaches to manage anemia take some time to show clinical effects; a "time," which could define the line between survival and death (or ischemic sequels) in severely anemic patients.[30,31] Therefore, stop-gap measures to optimize and assist the physiologic adaptation mechanisms to severe anemia are essential while awaiting the results of longer-acting therapies.

Optimizing the physiologic response to anemia should never be regarded as a replacement for active management of anemia. Despite numerous adaptive and compensatory mechanisms discussed here and elsewhere, anemia remains an under-recognized and under-appreciated, yet potentially fatal condition. Therefore, every effort must be made to diagnose and manage it on a timely basis, throughout the course of clinical care.[32]

To summarize, tissue hypoxia and subsequent ischemia can be avoided by either increasing DO_2 (oxygen supply), increasing EO_2 (higher extraction of oxygen from Hb), or decreasing VO_2 (oxygen demand). DO_2 itself can be increased by increasing CaO_2 or increasing the CO. CO can be increased by increasing the SV or HR (although the high baseline EO_2 of heart and its high oxygen demand should be carefully considered to avoid cardiac ischemia). Finally, CaO_2 can be increased by increasing the Hb level or increasing the PaO_2. Each of these steps offers opportunities to intervene clinically and help an anemic patient avoid ischemia and its dire consequences.

Oxygen demand (VO_2) can be effectively controlled in severely anemic patients by some simple strategies. Conditions associated with increased metabolism

Table 9.1. Relationships between Hb level, PaO$_2$ and blood oxygen content. Note how SaO$_2$ remains unchanged as long as oxygen delivery to alveoli remains adequate, despite substantial changes in blood oxygen content. These cases are hypothetical illustrations only and they do not take other factors such as physiologic adaptations and changes in rheological characteristics of blood into account.

Scenarios	Variables			Blood O$_2$ content (mL)		
	Hb (g/L)	PO$_2$ (mmHg)	SaO$_2$	Hb-bound	Blood-dissolved	Total
A – Healthy adult breathing air	150	100	100%	201 (98.5%)	3 (1.5%)	204
B – Severely anemic patient breathing air (conditions otherwise similar)	75	100	100%	100.5 (97.1%)	3 (2.9%)	103.5
C – Severely anemic patient receiving supplemental oxygen in atmospheric pressure	75	600	100%	100.5 (84.8%)	18 (15.2%)	118.5
D – Moderately anemic patient breathing air	86.2	100	100%	115.5 (97.5%)	3 (2.5%)	118.5
E – Severely anemic patient undergoing hyperbaric oxygen therapy	75	1200	100%	100.5 (73.6%)	36 (26.4%)	136.5
F – Moderately anemic patient breathing air	99.6	100	100%	133.5 (97.8%)	3 (2.2%)	136.5

such as fever should be avoided and managed promptly and every effort should be made to keep the patient euthermic. Another source of oxygen consumption – muscle activity – should be kept at a minimum by confining patients to bed rest, and in severe cases (especially in patients who cannot be transfused), by using sedation or neuromuscular blockade.[33] Any unnecessary increases in cardiac workload should be avoided including hypovolemia, which can result in tachycardia thereby increasing cardiac work. Unless there is another clinical indication, patients should be kept euvolemic through appropriate and timely use of intravenous fluids.[34,35] As seen here, maintenance of normothermia (when clinically indicated) and avoiding increased oxygen consumption may help in management of severe anemia.[6,33,36]

As mentioned previously, raising the CaO$_2$ is another effective approach for increasing the oxygen delivery to the organs and avoiding ischemia. Table 9.1 depicts the effects of changing Hb levels (as seen in anemia) and PaO$_2$ (as seen in oxygen therapy) on blood oxygen content in a few hypothetical scenarios. Notice that, unlike the Hb-bound oxygen fraction that is saturated as PO$_2$ approaches ~100 mmHg (which is often achieved when breathing normally in atmospheric air),

the blood-dissolved oxygen fraction increases linearly with increasing PaO$_2$ as shown in Figure 9.2. SaO$_2$ is commonly found to be 100% in patients with severe anemia (indicating that all oxygen-binding sites on available Hb molecules are fully saturated with oxygen), but this is not necessarily indicative of adequate blood oxygen delivery since the total blood oxygen content is still reduced due to the reduced Hb level. In presence of severe anemia when the oxygen supply is unable to keep up with the demand at peripheral tissues, efforts should be made to increase the total oxygen content of blood. This can generally be achieved through these approaches:

- Increasing the Hb level (through blood transfusions or by stimulating hematopoiesis)
- Increasing the PaO$_2$ (through supplemental oxygen and hyperbaric oxygen therapy).

While blood transfusion can provide a quick increase of numerical Hb level, issues such as depleted 2,3-DPG and storage lesions are likely to hinder its effectiveness in boosting the blood oxygen content effectively.[37] This issue is avoided when hematopoiesis is stimulated (e.g., by using erythropoiesis-stimulating agents [ESAs]), but the time required for the response to reach clinically-significant levels means that this approach cannot be adequate in severely anemic patients at risk of impending tissue hypoxia and ischemia. In such cases, increasing the blood-dissolved oxygen fraction through supplying pure oxygen at atmospheric or hyperbaric pressure can be a life-saving acute measure to ensure adequate oxygen delivery to the tissues until Hb levels increase above the critical level.[38]

The use of artificial oxygen carriers is another option to increase the total oxygen content of blood in severe anemia. These agents are typically based on modified Hb molecules and can therefore provide additional oxygen-binding capacity. Some are based on inert fluids such as perfluorocarbons, which are capable of dissolving large amounts of oxygen.[39] Once pursued with much enthusiasm, development of these agents has faced hurdles related to safety issues in clinical trials.[40] Nonetheless, artificial oxygen carriers remain promising agents under active investigation with hope and a potential for revolutionizing the acute treatment of severe anemia.[41]

Other opportunities to improve the tolerance of anemia lie at the cellular level. ESAs are important pharmaceutical agents in management of anemia with therapeutic effects emerging within days. However, erythropoietin receptors have been detected on non-hematopoietic cells, and evidence suggests their role in protecting cells against ischemia and reperfusion injury.[42] Another potential candidate is estrogen and its derivatives, which have been shown to offer protection against ischemia and ischemia-reperfusion injury in various organs in a number of animal models.[43–45] While still under investigation to determine clinical implications, these agents open exciting new horizons in managing severe anemia and mitigating the detrimental effects of hypoxemia. Finally, the early use of tranexamic acid in bleeding trauma patients has been shown to be associated with improved survival.[46] While the main mode of action of tranexamic acid is believed to be through its anti-fibrinolytic and hemostatic effects, other evidence points toward the potential beneficial effects on inflammatory pathways and ischemic-reperfusion injury.[47]

PBM and transfusion indications

There are times that, despite all efforts, Hb level should be raised quickly and urgently to avoid impending ischemia or to mitigate its consequences. Appropriate use of allogeneic blood transfusions when indicated as supported by evidence-based criteria is an important aspect of PBM. Numerous guidelines have been developed to aid clinicians in making transfusion decisions in various settings. While these guidelines usually acknowledge the importance of considering factors such as risk of ischemia, extent and rate of blood loss, hemodynamic status, and other co-morbidities when deciding on transfusion, they invariably rely on Hb levels to define the main transfusion criteria.[48] This is partly due to the simplicity and availability of Hb measurement and the unavailability of other practical measures of ischemia, or oxygen delivery and consumption at a tissue level. Use of Hb-based transfusion triggers should never divert the focus of management from treating the patients and achieving clinical endpoints to correcting a number.[49]

Ever since the Transfusion Requirements in Critical Care (TRICC) randomized controlled trial demonstrated the safety and feasibility of a "restrictive" versus "liberal" transfusion strategy in critically ill patients,[50] there have been a number of other trials supporting the same notion in other patient populations.[51–53] Subsequently, the Hb triggers for transfusion have been dropping from the now-outdated 100 g/l to 60–80 g/l in non-symptomatic patients. Other factors that are commonly considered alongside Hb levels in making transfusion decisions include older age and co-morbidities.[48,54]

Use of Hb as a transfusion trigger comes with other complexities. Hb is commonly determined as part of complete blood count performed on a blood sample obtained for a patient. Nonetheless, the Hb measurement can be affected by a host of other factors including the type of device and method used to measure Hb, source and site of blood sample and whether it was obtained using a tourniquet or not, body position at time of blood draw, and even the time of day.[55] Additionally, Hb and hematocrit are known to be sluggish to change and be reflective of actual levels during acute changes in blood volume.

Recently developed continuous Hb monitoring technologies provide certain advantages, given their lack of dependence on blood sampling and their provision of continuous, real-time data at the point-of-care. The measure – called Total Hb (SpHb) – is derived along with other parameters such as blood oxygen content, carboxyhemoglobin, methemoglobin, SpO_2, perfusion index (PI), and Pleth variability index (PVI). This is based on analysis of lights with various wavelengths that are emitted and detected by a non-invasive sensor placed on the finger (Masimo Corp,

Irvine, CA). The accuracy of SpHb compared with standard methods remains controversial, with some studies indicating limited accuracy in comparison with established laboratory measurement methods. The reported difference between SpHb and directly measured Hb may exceed 20 g/L in some patients, while some other reports support the usefulness of incorporation of SpHb as part of transfusion decision making process.[56–62] Ability to monitor the Hb changes non-invasively in real time (with some margin of error) is certainly highly desirable in clinical settings, and more advances in this field are expected to improve the quality of care. Until availability of more evidence and further refinement of the technology, use of SpHb particularly to monitor the Hb and other trends seems to be reasonable and can add value when used in combination with other measures and as an ancillary device, but given the accuracy concerns, reliance on SpHb measures alone in making transfusion decisions cannot be recommended yet.[63]

Currently available functional coagulation tests are mainly based on characterizing the viscoelastic properties of blood during coagulation tests. These so-called viscoelastic hemostatic assays (VHAs) include thromboelastography (TEG) and thromboelastometry. There are other platforms that analyze platelet function. These are powerful tools to provide clinicians with accurate and readily-available information on the status of coagulation system at point of care. Their usage as part of a GDT approach to guide transfusion of blood components has been under clinical investigation. These devices can be useful in assisting the clinicians in choosing blood components (and other coagulation factors and hemostatic agents) more carefully and appropriately to better address the specific deficits in the coagulation system.[64] Studies support effectiveness of these measures as part of a GDT approach and to better manage coagulation and hemostasis, reduce blood loss and possibly the RBC transfusions, and improve the outcomes of the patients, particularly those at high risk of significant blood loss.[65–67]

The future in transfusion indications is likely to revolve around efforts toward replacing Hb and hematocrit levels as transfusion triggers with other more meaningful physiologic indicators of tissue oxygen levels. While there are currently no universally accepted physiologic triggers, some proposed candidates include plasma lactate level, venous O_2 saturation (SvO$_2$), ScvO2, EO$_2$, and electrodiagnostic changes indicative of impaired tissue oxygenation (e.g., ST-segment changes in electrocardiography), and abnormalities in vital signs (e.g., relative hypotension or tachycardia) not explained by other probable causes.[68–70] ScvO2 is among the parameters used in GDT and it is discussed in more detail in other chapters.

The field of physiologic transfusion triggers is understandably a technology-driven field, and its ultimate widespread clinical application will depend on availability of devices to measure and monitor tissue oxygenation status, preferably in real time and in non- or minimally invasive manner. Brain tissue oxygen monitoring using probes that are placed into the white matter has been clinically available for years and studies support its usefulness in management of patients with brain injury (e.g., as part of a GDT protocol),[71] but the invasive nature of this approach limits its usage beyond neuro-critical care units. Alternatively, non-invasive devices are available that can measure regional tissue oxygen saturation using near infrared spectroscopy (e.g., INVOS, Covidien, Mansfield, MA, USA). In a recent randomized controlled trial, use of such a device to guide blood transfusion, based on the brain tissue oxygen saturation, achieved some levels of success in patients undergoing cardiac surgery,[72] but more studies are needed to define the role of these devices as part of transfusion decision making process. Establishment and validation of physiologic transfusion triggers are expected to allow true goal directed transfusion therapy as opposed to reliance on arbitrary Hb or hematocrit values.

PBM, the new standard of care

Regardless of the triggers defined to prescribe transfusion, one should never forget that every transfusion decision (no matter how sound and appropriate *per se*) can be viewed as failure in appropriate management of the patient according to the principles of PBM. Many transfusions in the surgical setting are direct results of low baseline Hb levels and excessive surgical blood loss,[73] both preventable, manageable, and modifiable risk factors. Rather than being trapped in the quest for the "ultimate" transfusion triggers, another sensible and readily available approach could be to tweak the risk factors leading to transfusion in order to avoid the transfusion triggers altogether.[36,74] Unfortunately, the preventive strategy is often lost in the midst of all the debates over transfusion, ignoring the fact that allogeneic blood is, after all, merely a temporary fix with limitations of its own.

The lost opportunities and their significant health consequences can be illustrated with the case of hospital-acquired anemia (HAA). In a recent multi-center study, which included one academic and nine community hospitals, three out of every four hospitalized adult patients developed HAA, with 30% of cases ending up being severely anemic. HAA was also associated with increased risk of mortality and length of stay.[75] Most of the patients with moderate to severe HAA might have been considered to be candidates for transfusion, and many were eventually transfused during their hospital stay, while they could have avoided HAA (or its more severe forms) by some simple measures, such as limiting diagnostic blood draws,[76] and proactive screening for and management of anemia before it turns into a major problem.

PBM offers a clear pathway toward improving patient outcomes through evidence-based and appropriate use of various modalities and interventions. The evidence supporting feasibility, safety, and efficacy of PBM and its positive impact on clinical outcomes of patients in various clinical settings is emerging,[77] and PBM is increasingly being endorsed and adopted as a standard of care in management of various patient populations.[78–80]

Conflicts of interest

Aryeh Shander has been a consultant or speaker with an honorarium for, or has received research support from, Bayer, Luitpold, Masimo, Novartis, Novo Nordisk, OrthoBiotech, Pfizer, and Zymogenetics; He is a founding member of SABM. Mazyar Javidroozi has been a contractor for SABM.

References

1. Shander A, Fink A, Javidroozi M, et al. Appropriateness of allogeneic red blood cell transfusion: the international consensus conference on transfusion outcomes. *Transfus Med Rev* 2011;**25**:232–46.

2. Acheson AG, Brookes MJ, Spahn DR. Effects of allogeneic red blood cell transfusions on clinical outcomes in patients undergoing colorectal cancer surgery: a systematic review and meta-analysis. *Ann Surg* 2012;**256**:235–44.

3. Shander A, Javidroozi M, Ozawa S, Hare GM. What is really dangerous: anaemia or transfusion? *Br J Anaesth* 2011;**107 Suppl 1**:i41–i59.

4. Shander A, Puzio T, Javidroozi M. Variability in transfusion practice and effectiveness of strategies to improve it. *J Cardiothorac Vasc Anesth* 2012;**26**:541–4.

5. Shander A, Hofmann A, Isbister J, Van AH. Patient blood management – the new frontier. *Best Pract Res Clin Anaesthesiol* 2013;**27**:5–10.

6. Goodnough LT, Shander A. Patient blood management. *Anesthesiology* 2012;**116**:1367–76.

7. Isbister JP. The three-pillar matrix of patient blood management – an overview. *Best Pract Res Clin Anaesthesiol* 2013;**27**:69–84.

8. Gombotz H, Hofman A, Rehak P, Kurz J. [Patient blood management (part 2). Practice: the 3 pillars]. *Anasthesiol Intensivmed Notfallmed Schmerzther* 2011;**46**:466–74.

9. Reuben AD, Appelboam AV, Higginson I, Lloyd JG, Shapiro NI. Early goal-directed therapy: a UK perspective. *Emerg Med J* 2006;**23**:828–32.

10. Kocian R, Spahn DR. Haemoglobin, oxygen carriers and perioperative organ perfusion. *Best Pract Res Clin Anaesthesiol* 2008;**22**:63–80.

11. Fuller BM, Gajera M, Schorr C, et al. The impact of packed red blood cell transfusion on clinical outcomes in patients with septic shock treated with early goal directed therapy. *Indian J Crit Care Med* 2010;**14**:165–9.

12. Astrup P, Severinghaus J. *The History of Blood Gases, Acids and Bases.* Copenhagen: Munksgaard, 1986.

13. Salazar Vazquez BY, Wettstein R, Cabrales P, Tsai AG, Intaglietta M. Microvascular experimental evidence on the relative significance of restoring oxygen carrying capacity vs. blood viscosity in shock resuscitation. *Biochim Biophys Acta* 2008;**1784**:1421–7.

14. Yalcin O, Ortiz D, Tsai AG, Johnson PC, Cabrales P. Microhemodynamic aberrations created by transfusion of stored blood. *Transfusion* 2013.

15. Halperin ML, Cheema-Dhadli S, Lin SH, Kamel KS. Properties permitting the renal cortex to be the oxygen sensor for the release of erythropoietin: clinical implications. *Clin J Am Soc Nephrol* 2006;**1**:1049–53.

16. Pittman RN. *Regulation of Tissue Oxygenation.* San Rafael, CA: Morgan & Claypool Life Sciences, 2011.

17. Hare GM, Tsui AK, Ozawa S, Shander A. Anaemia: can we define haemoglobin thresholds for impaired oxygen homeostasis and suggest new strategies for treatment? *Best Pract Res Clin Anaesthesiol* 2013;**27**:85–98.

18. Metivier F, Marchais SJ, Guerin AP, Pannier B, London GM. Pathophysiology of anaemia: focus on the heart and blood

vessels. *Nephrol Dial Transpl* 2000;**15 Suppl 3**:14–18.

19. Madjdpour C, Spahn DR. Allogeneic red blood cell transfusion: physiology of oxygen transport. *Best Pract Res Clin Anaesthesiol* 2007;**21**:163–71.

20. El Hasnaoui-Saadani R, Pichon A, Marchant D, et al. Cerebral adaptations to chronic anemia in a model of erythropoietin-deficient mice exposed to hypoxia. *Am J Physiol Regul Integr Comp Physiol* 2009;**296**: R801–11.

21. Wilson DF, Lee WM, Makonnen S, et al. Oxygen pressures in the interstitial space and their relationship to those in the blood plasma in resting skeletal muscle. *J Appl Physiol* 2006;**101**:1648–56.

22. Tsui AK, Dattani ND, Marsden PA, et al. Reassessing the risk of hemodilutional anemia: some new pieces to an old puzzle. *Can J Anaesth* 2010;**57**:779–91.

23. Sakadzic S, Roussakis E, Yaseen MA, et al. Two-photon high-resolution measurement of partial pressure of oxygen in cerebral vasculature and tissue. *Nat Methods* 2010;**7**:755–9.

24. Myllyharju J, Koivunen P. Hypoxia-inducible factor prolyl 4-hydroxylases: common and specific roles. *Biol Chem* 2013;**394**: 435–48.

25. Lee FS, Percy MJ. The HIF pathway and erythrocytosis. *Annu Rev Pathol* 2011;**6**:165–92.

26. Wagner PD. The critical role of VEGF in skeletal muscle angiogenesis and blood flow. *Biochem Soc Trans* 2011;**39**:1556–9.

27. Goda N, Kanai M. Hypoxia-inducible factors and their roles in energy metabolism. *Int J Hematol* 2012;**95**:457–63.

28. Semenza GL. Oxygen-dependent regulation of mitochondrial respiration by hypoxia-inducible factor 1. *Biochem J* 2007;**405**:1–9.

29. Goodnough LT, Maniatis A, Earnshaw P, et al. Detection, evaluation, and management of preoperative anaemia in the elective orthopaedic surgical patient: NATA guidelines. *Br J Anaesth* 2011;**106**:13–22.

30. Mackenzie CF, Moon-Massat PF, Shander A, Javidroozi M, Greenburg AG. When blood is not an option: factors affecting survival after the use of a hemoglobin-based oxygen carrier in 54 patients with life-threatening anemia. *Anesth Analg* 2010;**110**:685–93.

31. Tobian AA, Ness PM, Noveck H, Carson JL. Time course and etiology of death in patients with severe anemia. *Transfusion* 2009;**49**:1395–9.

32. Shander A, Javidroozi M, Goodnough LT. Anemia screening in elective surgery: definition, significance and patients' interests. *Anesth Analg* 2006;**103**:778–9.

33. Shander A, Javidroozi M. The approach to patients with bleeding disorders who do not accept blood-derived products. *Semin Thromb Hemost* 2013;**39**:182–90.

34. Goodnough LT, Shander A, Spence R. Bloodless medicine: clinical care without allogeneic blood transfusion. *Transfusion* 2003;**43**:668–76.

35. Shander A, Goodnough LT. Objectives and limitations of bloodless medical care. *Curr Opin Hematol* 2006;**13**:462–70.

36. Shander A, Moskowitz DM, Javidroozi M. Blood conservation in practice: an overview. *Br J Hosp Med (Lond)* 2009;**70**:16–21.

37. van de Watering L. Red cell storage and prognosis. *Vox Sang* 2011;**100**:36–45.

38. Van Meter KW. A systematic review of the application of hyperbaric oxygen in the treatment of severe anemia: an evidence-based approach.

Undersea Hyperb Med 2005;**32**:61–83.

39. Goodnough LT, Shander A. Current status of pharmacologic therapies in patient blood management. *Anesth Analg* 2013;**116**:15–34.

40. Natanson C, Kern SJ, Lurie P, Banks SM, Wolfe SM. Cell-free hemoglobin-based blood substitutes and risk of myocardial infarction and death: a meta-analysis. *JAMA* 2008;**299**:2304–12.

41. Galvagno SM, Jr., Mackenzie CF. New and future resuscitation fluids for trauma patients using hemoglobin and hypertonic saline. *Anesthesiol Clin* 2013;**31**:1–19.

42. Kagaya Y, Asaumi Y, Wang W, et al. Current perspectives on protective roles of erythropoietin in cardiovascular system: erythropoietin receptor as a novel therapeutic target. *Tohoku J Exp Med* 2012; **227**:83–91.

43. Inagaki T, Kaneko N, Zukin RS, Castillo PE, Etgen AM. Estradiol attenuates ischemia-induced death of hippocampal neurons and enhances synaptic transmission in aged, long-term hormone-deprived female rats. *PLoS One* 2012;**7**:e38018.

44. Kawasaki T, Chaudry IH. The effects of estrogen on various organs: therapeutic approach for sepsis, trauma, and reperfusion injury. Part 2: liver, intestine, spleen, and kidney. *J Anesth* 2012;**26**:892–9.

45. Kawasaki T, Chaudry IH. The effects of estrogen on various organs: therapeutic approach for sepsis, trauma, and reperfusion injury. Part 1: central nervous system, lung, and heart. *J Anesth* 2012;**26**:883–91.

46. Shakur H, Roberts I, Bautista R, et al. Effects of tranexamic acid on death, vascular occlusive events, and blood transfusion in trauma patients with significant haemorrhage (CRASH-2): a

randomised, placebo-controlled trial. *Lancet* 2010;**376**:23–32.

47. Pusateri AE, Weiskopf RB, Bebarta V, et al. Tranexamic acid and trauma: current status and knowledge gaps with recommended research priorities. *Shock* 2013;**39**:121–6.

48. Shander A, Gross I, Hill S, Javidroozi M, Sledge S. A new perspective on best transfusion practices. *Blood Transfus* 2013;**11**:193–202.

49. Shander A, Javidroozi M. Strategies to reduce the use of blood products: a US perspective. *Curr Opin Anaesthesiol* 2012;**25**:50–8.

50. Hebert PC, Wells G, Blajchman MA, et al. A multicenter, randomized, controlled clinical trial of transfusion requirements in critical care. Transfusion Requirements in Critical Care Investigators, Canadian Critical Care Trials Group. *N Engl J Med* 1999;**340**:409–17.

51. Carson JL, Terrin ML, Noveck H, et al. Liberal or restrictive transfusion in high-risk patients after hip surgery. *N Engl J Med* 2011;**365**:2453–62.

52. Hajjar LA, Vincent JL, Galas FR, et al. Transfusion requirements after cardiac surgery: the TRACS randomized controlled trial. *JAMA* 2010;**304**:1559–67.

53. Lacroix J, Hebert PC, Hutchison JS, et al. Transfusion strategies for patients in pediatric intensive care units. *N Engl J Med* 2007;**356**:1609–19.

54. Carson JL, Kuriyan M. What should trigger a transfusion? *Transfusion* 2010;**50**:2073–5.

55. Berkow L. Factors affecting hemoglobin measurement. *J Clin Monit Comput* 2013; **27** (5):499–508.

56. Dewhirst E, Naguib A, Winch P, et al. Accuracy of noninvasive and continuous hemoglobin measurement by pulse co-oximetry during preoperative phlebotomy. *J Intens Care Med* 2013; Apr 22[epub ahead of print].

57. Giraud B, Frasca D, Debaene B, Mimoz O. Comparison of haemoglobin measurement methods in the operating theatre. *Br J Anaesth* 2013; **111**(6): 946–54.

58. Joseph B, Hadjizacharia P, Aziz H, et al. Continuous noninvasive hemoglobin monitor from pulse ox: ready for prime time? *World J Surg* 2013;**37**:525–9.

59. Knutson T, la-Giustina D, Tomich E, et al. Evaluation of a new nonnvasive device in determining hemoglobin levels in emergency department patients. *West J Emerg Med* 2013;**14**:283–6.

60. Skelton VA, Wijayasinghe N, Sharafudeen S, et al. Evaluation of point-of-care haemoglobin measuring devices: a comparison of Radical-7 pulse co-oximetry, HemoCue((R)) and laboratory haemoglobin measurements in obstetric patients. *Anaesthesia* 2013;**68**:40–5.

61. Shah N, Osea EA, Martinez GJ. Accuracy of noninvasive hemoglobin and invasive point-of-care hemoglobin testing compared with a laboratory analyzer. *Int J Lab Hematol* 2013; Jun 27.doi:10.1111/ijlh.12118 [epub ahead of print]

62. Miller RD, Ward TA, Shiboski SC, Cohen NH. A comparison of three methods of hemoglobin monitoring in patients undergoing spine surgery. *Anesth Analg* 2011;**112**:858–63.

63. Park YH, Lee JH, Song HG, et al. The accuracy of noninvasive hemoglobin monitoring using the radical-7 pulse CO-oximeter in children undergoing neurosurgery. *Anesth Analg* 2012;**115**:1302–7.

64. Gorlinger K, Shore-Lesserson L, Dirkmann D, et al. Management of hemorrhage in cardiothoracic surgery. *J Cardiothorac Vasc Anesth* 2013;**27**:S20–S34.

65. Theusinger OM, Levy JH. Point of care devices for assessing bleeding and coagulation in the trauma patient. *Anesthesiol Clin* 2013;**31**:55–65.

66. Johansson PI, Ostrowski SR, Secher NH. Management of major blood loss: an update. *Acta Anaesthesiol Scand* 2010;**54**:1039–49.

67. Walsh M, Thomas SG, Howard JC, et al. Blood component therapy in trauma guided with the utilization of the perfusionist and thromboelastography. *J Extra Corpor Technol* 2011;**43**:162–7.

68. Vallet B, Adamczyk S, Barreau O, Lebuffe G. Physiologic transfusion triggers. *Best Pract Res Clin Anaesthesiol* 2007;**21**:173–81.

69. Orlov D, O'Farrell R, McCluskey SA, et al. The clinical utility of an index of global oxygenation for guiding red blood cell transfusion in cardiac surgery. *Transfusion* 2009;**49**:682–8.

70. Madjdpour C, Spahn DR, Weiskopf RB. Anemia and perioperative red blood cell transfusion: a matter of tolerance. *Crit Care Med* 2006;**34**: S102–S108.

71. Narotam PK, Morrison JF, Nathoo N. Brain tissue oxygen monitoring in traumatic brain injury and major trauma: outcome analysis of a brain tissue oxygen-directed therapy. *J Neurosurg* 2009;**111**:672–82.

72. Vretzakis G, Georgopoulou S, Stamoulis K, et al. Monitoring of brain oxygen saturation (INVOS) in a protocol to direct blood transfusions during cardiac surgery: a prospective randomized clinical trial. *J Cardiothorac Surg* 2013;**8**:145.

73. Gombotz H, Rehak PH, Shander A, Hofmann A. Blood use in elective surgery: the Austrian

benchmark study. *Transfusion* 2007;**47**:1468–80.

74. Spahn DR, Shander A, Hofmann A. The chiasm: transfusion practice versus patient blood management. *Best Pract Res Clin Anaesthesiol* 2013;**27**:37–42.

75. Koch CG, Li L, Sun Z, et al. Hospital-acquired anemia: prevalence, outcomes, and healthcare implications. *J Hosp Med* 2013; **8(9)**: 506–12.

76. Salisbury AC, Reid KJ, Alexander KP, et al. Diagnostic blood loss from phlebotomy and hospital-acquired anemia during acute myocardial infarction. *Arch Intern Med* 2011;**171**:1646–53.

77. Gross I, Shander A, Sweeney J. Patient blood management and outcome, too early or not? *Best Pract Res Clin Anaesthesiol* 2013;**27**:161–72.

78. Bruce W, Campbell D, Daly D, Isbister J. Practical recommendations for patient blood management and the reduction of perioperative transfusion in joint replacement surgery. *ANZ J Surg* 2013;**83**:222–9.

79. De Leon EM, Szallasi A. "Transfusion indication RBC (PBM-02)": gap analysis of a Joint Commission Patient Blood Management Performance Measure at a community hospital. *Blood Transfus* 2012;1–5.

80. Shander A, Van AH, Colomina MJ, et al. Patient blood management in Europe. *Br J Anaesth* 2012;**109**:55–68.

Chapter

10

A rational approach to fluid and volume management

Daniel Chappell and Matthias Jacob

Introduction

Fluid and volume application remains a frequently discussed issue in anesthesia and intensive care. After the more drug-centered discussions of the last decade around the ideal composition and total amount of intravenous fluids in general,[1] the focus is now moving on to distinguish between different patient groups. Fluid handling should obviously be done "procedure-specifically" in the perioperative setting, and the old, originally transatlantic "crystalloid versus colloid" debate was revitalized with the help of very recent data focusing on patients with severe sepsis.[2] And this appears quite justified: cardiopulmonary healthy patients going into elective surgery are supposed to be primarily normovolemic, having a functioning vascular barrier and intact fluid compartments. Therefore, they are endangered by acute perioperative bleeding. Critically ill patients, by contrast, are often systemically inflamed, suffering from imbalances affecting not only cardiac preload. This might impact markedly on their pathophysiology. In the non-inflamed patient it might be reasonable to distinguish between a crystalloid for maintenance and the care for cardiac preload with a combination of vasopressors and iso-oncotic colloids in order to maintain steady state for as long as possible.[1] In the septic patient with a presumably impaired vascular barrier, functioning things seem to be completely different. Unfortunately, experts around the world are discordant on this issue, especially concerning the use of colloids in general, but also concerning timing, amount, and situation when using this class of drugs. One important fact, however, is often ignored: the only rational pathway to success is a careful analysis of all the available information, concentrating on facts while excluding extrapolation and expert opinion as far as possible.

Outcome-based evidence in fluid handling – what is the problem?

Evidence-based medicine was initiated in the early 1990s as a new and promising approach for looking at clinical problems. It was a consequential reaction to the observation that, despite analyzing problems quite rationally, theoretical considerations often do not lead to the central target of an enhanced medical treatment: a measurable improvement in patient outcome. The idea behind it was the assumption that the superiority of a new therapeutic idea can only be reliably proven if it has been shown by a prospectively performed randomized comparison to the current standard, focusing on outcome. This led to great success in many schematically performed causal therapies, e.g., in chemotherapy of cancer patients. In this case, it is quite easy to define "good" or "bad" outcome parameters, and the relation of the treatment result to the drug is obvious. It was only logical to transfer this modern way of making science to fluid and volume handling in critically ill patients. Importantly, however, in fluid management there are major differences: (i) it is not a causal therapy, but a supportive measure, therefore, (ii) ideal outcome values are difficult to determine, and, perhaps most importantly, (iii) there is still no clear "standard," making each comparison to a "new" approach difficult. Generally, it appears impossible to heal patients with IV fluids. Rather, the intention behind the approach is to optimize the hemodynamic situation and to keep the patient alive as long as it takes causal therapies and nature to cure the primary problem. Beyond that, the influence of infusion therapy on the overall outcome might strongly depend on the quality of the rest of the supportive treatment. Choosing the right antibiotic, nutrition, vasopressor,

Perioperative Hemodynamic Monitoring and Goal Directed Therapy, ed. Maxime Cannesson and Rupert Pearse.
Published by Cambridge University Press. © Cambridge University Press 2014.

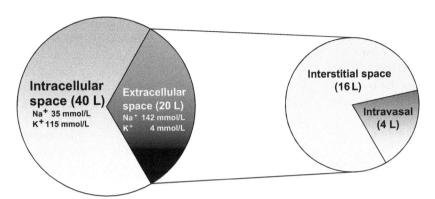

Figure 10.1. Distribution of total body water.

inotrope, diuretic, pain medication, sedative, and anti-coagulant; optimizing ventilation, hemodynamics, kidney function, and coagulation; deciding on the necessity of blood and plasma products, organ replacement therapies, X-rays, CT scans, ultrasound, laboratory values; and picking the adequate monitoring of all these aspects as early and precisely as possible shows how difficult and multi-factorial the treatment of critically ill patients actually is. It appears justified to at least ask the question whether we actually can measurably reduce mortality by improving infusion therapy. It is very likely that any success here is strongly related to the individual therapeutic context in which the data have been produced and even more to the quality of the control treatment, which is, due to the lack of a generally accepted standard, normally not reflecting the reader's approach. Accordingly, a major prerequisite of an outcome-study in the field of fluid and volume handling is to carefully report what actually happened to the patients in detail, allowing the readers to weigh up whether the data are applicable to their practice.

A rational approach to fluid and volume handling

When stabilizing macrohemodynamics of a patient, we are presuming maintenance of cardiac output to be a good idea. Beyond that it appears reasonable to avoid interstitial edema for as long as possible. A good basis for that might be to carefully maintain steady state of all compartments and to protect the vascular barrier.[1]

Concerning compartments and barriers

The human body water amounts to 60% of the total body mass and is stored under steady state conditions by two-thirds within the cells, while one-third is distributed extracellulary. The cellular membrane, despite being extremely frail versus hydrostatic gradients, functionally separates the large intracellular compartment almost completely from the rest. The vascular barrier, by contrast, separates two extracellular subcompartments from each other and prevents blood components from being driven toward the interstitial space, despite an outwards-directed gradient generated by the blood pressure. The reason is the biology of the endothelial surface layer (ESL), a small structure consisting of the endothelial glycocalyx and bound plasma constituents attached to the endothelial surface.[3] In general, inserting IV lines only provides direct access to the minor part of the fluid compartments (Figure 10.1).

Normovolemia – the ultimate goal

The principal goal in perioperative fluid management is to maintain normovolemia of all compartments, presuming that this might be beneficial to the patient. This means to maintain fluid compartments and sustain vascular barrier functioning to avoid fluid accumulations within the body while upholding an optimized cardiac preload. However, the attending anesthesiologist is faced with several principal and practical problems: the individual patients' hydration state before surgery is unknown and the compartments cannot be assessed in clinical routine. The most important and desirable target is the total body blood volume, which presumably should be kept at least within individual normal ranges even in the face of acute blood losses. However, double-label blood volume measurement, the current standard to assess total body blood volume, is invasive, complex, personnel-intensive, and currently not available in daily routine. A technically easier possible alternative, hematocrit dilution, is often based on estimated basic values and can only assess changes in the *circulating part* of the blood volume, ignoring a considerable non-circulating part of the plasma situated within the ESL. As the thickness of the latter normally decreases due to intravascular volume exchanges, indirectly measured blood volumes using this hematocrit method, and therefore also volume effects of fluids in literature, are often markedly overestimated and should be interpreted with great caution (see below). Measures such as pulmonary catheters are invasive and are also not capable of determining blood volume. Therefore, physicians are currently relying on short-term patient history, clinical impressions, and monitoring surrogates with low predictive value to estimate the current state and changes of blood volume. A further problem is that exact measurement of perioperative losses is difficult. In the context of surgery, clinicians are mainly relying on estimations. Therefore, it is necessary to base them on the best available data. This requirement is crucial.

Fluid or volume – what losses, when and why?

It has been increasingly established that it might be rational to differentiate between fluid losses and volume deficits.[1] Fluid loss is an on-going issue the body knows from daily life, comprising insensible perspiration and urinary output, i.e., net losses out of the body primarily affecting the extracellular compartment. Beyond that, volume deficits exclusively concern the circulatory space, normally being related to acute bleeding. But also a shift of protein-rich fluid from the vasculature toward the tissues is frequently observed when the vascular barrier is altered in critical illness. Various recommendations exist in the literature and in textbooks on how, why, when, and with what perioperative losses should be replaced.

Fluid losses – a clear indication for crystalloids

Traditional recommendations concerning the preoperative volume state act on the assumption that preoperative fasting causes distinct intravascular hypovolemia. A prospective trial, however, directly measuring blood volume in cardiopulmonary healthy patients scheduled for elective surgery revealed intravascular normovolemia even after a fasting period of 10 hours.[4] The reason for what appears illogical at first sight might be the recruitment of interstitially stored fluid in the periphery due to the horizontal position during the night. Applying current fasting guidelines with a recommendation for the ingestion of clear water up to 2 hours prior to surgery[5] should clearly avoid a relevant impact of preoperative fasting on the body compartments in the vast majority of patients. In rare cases of prolonged fasting or preoperative bowel preparation, which can cause an extracellular fluid deficit, a continuous crystalloidal infusion already during this period, before surgery, seems to be rational.

Perioperative insensible perspiration is traditionally believed to dramatically increase during major surgery and trauma, requiring large amounts of fluid. However, Lamke and co-workers who designed a specific evaporation measuring chamber detected an average evaporation rate of $0.5 \ \mathrm{mL/kg \ h^{-1}}$, which is, even in the surgical worst case of opening the abdominal cavity and exposing the entire bowel to environment, at most doubled.[6,7] This means that perspiration, which affects the entire extracellular space, should be sufficiently replaced with around $1 \ \mathrm{mL/kg \ h^{-1}}$ of crystalloids in healthy, normothermic surgical patients if the target is maintaining steady state and avoiding interstitial edema.

Urine output is often believed to be a crucial rapid alert system for acute renal failure. However, surgery and trauma *per se* cause a hormone-driven reduction of urine output as the body tries to preserve its fluid compartments. Short-term reductions below $0.5 \ \mathrm{mL/kg \ h^{-1}}$ have been shown to have no influence on the incidence of acute renal failure in previously healthy kidneys. Urine output is normally protein-free, affects the extracellular compartment, and a 1:1 loss replacement with crystalloids during the entire perioperative period should be sufficient to maintain the integrity of the compartments.

Volume losses – are crystalloids a suitable alternative?

Blood losses do not occur in every surgical patient to a relevant extent. Even in major surgery, modern techniques have reduced blood losses dramatically. Nevertheless, as these kinds of losses only affect the intravascular space, a replacement with iso-oncotic colloids seems rational as they target this compartment, require lower amounts, and avoid interstitial fluid accumulation.[1] In the recent past, however, crystalloids have been suggested to be a suitable and well-tolerated alternative, especially when considering the potential harm related to colloid use increasingly reported in the literature.[8]

When contemplating the type of fluid for a specific situation and presuming that maintenance of the compartments might be a good idea, we first have to check whether the distribution spaces match our expectations. For blood replacement this means knowing to what extent the respective solution contributes to the filling state of the circulatory compartment. This extent is called the "volume-effect."

Shift or stay? Volume effects of crystalloids and colloids

Many things have been written in literature concerning volume effects of crystalloids and colloids, and many of them are inaccurate. In fact, most data around this pharmacokinetic property of these drugs in literature are suffering from an easy, but insufficient methodology called "hematocrit dilution." It is important to know the limitations of this frequently applied technique using the extent of hematocrit dilution to estimate the capacity of a volume preparation to expand blood volume. First, an apparent initial blood volume is not measured but estimated from height, weight, and/or body surface area. By measuring venous hematocrit, an apparent plasma volume is calculated. After an intravenous infusion, the hematocrit is reassessed, from which the apparent new plasma volume and the volume effect of the chosen solution are calculated. In simple words, the hematocrit dilution technique for assesing volume effects is based on the belief that the more a certain amount of fluid is able to dilute the circulating red blood cells, the higher the intravascular persistence/volume effect. And this is certainly true. However, this theoretically brilliant principle is severely limited by the existence of the already mentioned ESL, which contains and harbors up to 1 liter of plasma as an exclusion zone for the red cells.[3] The hematocrit is exclusively assessed within the circulating part of the blood volume, ignoring the amount of plasma bound within the ESL. Unfortunately, the volume of the ESL is not constant and its degradation (i.e., by a hypervolemic fluid infusion) releases plasma from the non-circulating to the circulating plasma volume.[9] This indirectly increases the distribution

space of red blood cells, causing false-high and overestimated volume effects. The only reliable and timely scientific method for assessing changes in blood volume is to directly and simultaneously measure red cell and plasma volumes before and after a volume challenge by tracer dilution. The following unquestioned data are the result of such an approach, labeling red cells with sodium fluorescein and plasma with indocyanine green.[9–11]

Situation I: the bleeding patient

The only appropriate indication for the substitution of "volume" is a deficit in the intravascular state versus normal. Therefore, the model to test this indication-based use of volume preparations is the bleeding patient. In a clinical trial this was simulated by acute normovolemic hemodilution in preoperative patients (ASA I-II), withdrawing 1–1.5 liters of blood in 30 min and simultaneously replacing these losses by (i) the threefold amount of Ringer's lactate or (ii) a comparable amount of iso-oncotic colloids (Figure 10.2). The observations confirmed the physiological expectation that crystalloids are not retained by the vascular barrier, even if the circulation is in need of preload to maintain normal conditions. They were distributed evenly across the whole extracellular compartment, the volume effect was 17±10%, meaning that over 80% were shifted toward the interstitial space.[12] Iso-oncotic colloids, however, used with an adequate indication in the bleeding patient, were able to maintain blood volume; their mean volume effects were between 85% and 98%, depending on the substance.[10,11] Obviously, the intact vascular barrier is able to retain artificial and natural large molecules, together with the accompanying water load.

Situation II: artificial hypervolemia

Things are completely different if a primarily normovolemic circulation is challenged with an additional intravenous bolus. The study setup for hypervolemia was the same as above, except that the patients in steady state received an intravenous bolus of more than 1 liter of iso-oncotic colloid without simultaneous blood withdrawal (Figure 10.2). This led, in fact, to an expansion of blood volume, but much lower than the infused amount. The volume effects were down to around 40% and were accompanied by a severe reduction of the total volume of the ESL.[9] It seems likely that the hypervolemia-related release of

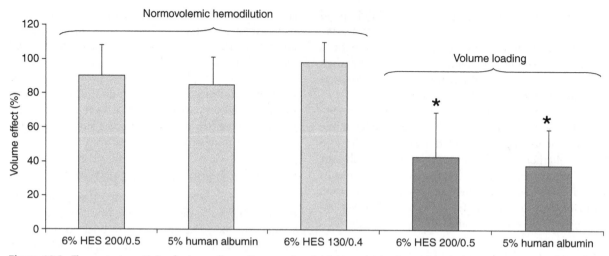

Figure 10.2. The context-sensitivity of volume effects of iso-oncotic colloids (the volume effect is that part of the colloid that remains within the circulation and does not primarily shift outwards). As a substitute during acute bleeding, carefully maintaining normovolemia throughout the procedure, 6% HES 200/0.5, 5% human albumin, and 6% HES 130/0.4 (left-hand columns) had volume effects of more than 90%. Volume loading of the normovolemic, by contrast, led to volume effects of 6% HES 200/0.5 and 5% human albumin (right-hand columns) of about 40%. Blood volumes were assessed before and after intervention via double-label-technique.[9–11]
$n = 10$ each. Values are mean ± SD. * $P<0.05$ vs. normovolemic hemodilution. HES = hydroxyethyl starch. Reproduced from Chappell et al.[1] with permission.

atrial natriuretic peptide (ANP) activates metalloproteases, which digest the endothelial glycocalyx within a very short period of time.[13] Obviously, using the highly potent drug "colloid" without a good indication severely affects a core structure of vascular barrier competence. This can cause pronounced and lasting interstitial edema, actively inducing biological problems to compartments and barriers that the patient has to deal with throughout the perioperative period.

Volume effects of crystalloids and colloids: what lesson do we have to learn?

There are two types of fluid shifting:[1] Type I-shifting is not a pathophysiological surprise, it is the inevitable, constant, and reproducible consequence of the therapeutic concept to use crystalloids to also stabilize cardiac preload in the face of acute bleeding. Type I-shifting is not related to a compromised vascular barrier competence, but is the consequence of crystalloidal fluid overload. Type II-shifting, by contrast, is related to a breakdown of the vascular barrier. First of all, this might be caused by surgical trauma or inflammation during major surgery, but also hypervolemia should be avoided as far as possible if

maintaining the steady state is considered to be an important aspect in the anesthesiological strategy.

From theory to bedside: fluid management in clinical practice
The surgical patient

Normovolemia of all compartments appears to be a current and reasonable goal in perioperative treatment, at least in major surgery. To target this goal, crystalloids should be infused to replace on-going fluid losses such as urine output and insensible perspiration and colloids if the patient is in need of volume.[1] Guidelines recommend measuring volume responsiveness using algorithm-based fluid boluses in order to optimize tissue perfusion on the basis of a maximized cardiac output.[14] The underlying assumption is that, concerning cardiac output, maximization is the same as optimization. This might be true, but we should consider that, at the current stage, it remains unclear if this accounts for every patient in every situation.

Guiding fluid therapy

Guiding fluid therapy by measuring volume responsiveness has repeatedly been recommended in high-risk surgical populations. This concept, occasionally referred to as a "goal directed" approach, is, at first sight, an interesting alternative to directly measuring blood volume because it also functionally considers systemic vasotension. Formerly, the most commonly applied measures in this context were the pulmonary artery and central venous catheter. The pulmonary catheter measures left ventricular preload, systemic vascular resistance, and cardiac output, but not blood volume or fluid responsiveness. A drawback is that such measurements are not provided in real time and are static rather than dynamic. In most clinical circumstances, however, a clinical prediction of pre-load responsiveness is required.[15] Moreover, the pulmonary catheter is invasive, can cause severe complications such as ventricular fibrillation or valve perforation, and has not been shown to reduce mortality in critically ill patients. This has resulted in a decreased use of this device.[16] Consequently, the pulmonary catheter should only be used in selected patient collectives such as cardiac surgery or acute heart failure, e.g., where information on pressures in the small circulation is necessary. Many surgical high-risk patients will have a central venous catheter to infuse vasopressors, fluids, and to calibrate thermo-dilution devices. Despite frequently being used to guide fluid therapy, the central venous pressure (CVP) is a poor indicator of cardiac preload and does not predict the effect of a fluid bolus, making therapeutic decisions on fluid responsiveness very difficult. Although being part of the current Surviving Sepsis Campaign recommendations, a recent meta-analysis showed that CVP actually cannot guide fluid therapy. The authors even recommended that using CVP for fluid therapy should be "abandoned."[17] However, in our opinion the trend of CVP can be used as an indicator for pathological changes and initiate further investigations.

Current outcome data in surgery

Other methods such as systolic pressure and pulse pressure variation have been shown to predict fluid responsiveness, but not that they improve patient outcome. Stroke volume maximization via esophageal Doppler guided fluid boluses in contrast appears to improve outcome, especially in elderly and frail patients. Even though this method cannot be performed in every institution and in every patient for practical and financial reasons and is difficult to apply in awake patients, it is currently the best investigated measure for perioperative GDT.[14]

Above that, outcome data in surgery are difficult to determine. Mortality in elective patients is meanwhile so low that several ten-thousands of patients would be necessary to detect any clinically relevant difference. Nevertheless, the results of trials on goal directed therapy, using a basal crystalloidal maintenance infusion to replace on-going losses and indication-triggered colloidal boluses beyond, are actually relatively homogenous. Recently, Feldheiser et al. compared the esophageal Doppler-guided use of a balanced 6% HES 130/0.4 with that of a balanced crystalloid in a double-blinded manner.[18] HES led to a significantly improved stroke volume, corrected flow time, cardiac index, and hemodynamic stability despite requiring 35% less intravenous fluids. Patients in the crystalloid group required fresh frozen plasma more frequently (92% vs. 62%) and in higher amounts (6 vs. 3.5 units). Several other trials with comparable settings have shown that colloids improve the micro-circulation, tissue oxygen tension, gut mucosal perfusion, and hemodynamic stability and reduce lactate levels whilst requiring less fluid and causing less tissue edema. In a meta-analysis from 2011, Hamilton and colleagues analyzed 48 trials on over 4800 patients, concluding that early GDT using colloids reduces complications and morbidity.[19] The importance of reducing perioperative complications was shown by Khuri and co-workers, who evaluated over 100 000 patients after surgery.[20] They showed that, independent of the preoperative patient risk, the occurrence of only one complication (from a list of 22), e.g., delayed weaning, ileus, or wound infection in the first 30 postoperative days reduced median patient survival by 69%.

Moreover, clinical trials in major abdominal surgery have repeatedly shown that large amounts of crystalloids cause complications such as impaired wound healing, postoperative weight increase, increased cardiac and pulmonary complication rates, as well as disturbed bowel mobility and prolonged hospital stay.[21–23] Despite difficulties in comparing these trials among each other – as each protocol and study group definition differed significantly – the main conclusion was quite clear: fluid overload is not beneficial for patient outcome. In minor surgical procedures such as laparoscopy, the infusion of large amounts of crystalloids (e.g., 40 mL/kg) seemed to reduce the incidence of PONV.[24]

Obviously, most surgical patients will not require a colloid and will do fine with a pure crystalloid fluid regime. However, acute bleeding or hypovolemia-associated decrease in cardiac output initiates the infusion of iso-oncotic colloids to the benefit of the perioperative patient outcome. But are the data from healthy elective patients transferable to the critically ill on the ICU?

The ICU patient

While the surgical patient presents with mortality rates of about 1%–2%, up to 50% of those patients entering the ICU with septic shock will die. One important aspect of critically ill patients is a change in vascular integrity, which clinically displays with the contradictory impressions of interstitial hypervolemia (tissue edema) and intravascular hypovolemia, which responds inadequately to fluid boluses. One reason for this leakiness of the vessels is, next to a separation of the endothelial cell line, an impaired integrity of the endothelial glycocalyx, which means an impairment of vascular barrier functioning. The glycocalyx is severely degraded in septic patients, and this destruction itself is associated with an increased mortality.[25] In this situation colloids are not retained completely by the vascular wall. Rather, they are partly shifted toward the tissues after intravenous infusion, leading to a dramatic reduction of their volume effect. Beyond that, colloids in tissue are suspected to have negative side effects. Hydroxyethyl starch is stored in cells for prolonged periods and can cause renal impairment or itching.[8] Apart from anaphylaxis, gelatins seem to be well tolerated. However, large trials evaluating this product are missing and the exact volume effect of this small bovine protein remains unknown. At least in Europe, dextrans almost completely disappeared from the market, due to severe anaphylactic reactions and renal affection. Albumin, a human colloid, seems to have no severe negative effects in this situation, but large trials and meta-analyses have also shown no benefit to overall outcome compared with crystalloids.[26] Fresh frozen plasma is a (natural) blood product, but is currently not recommended as a first-line treatment for general volume therapy. Therefore, the high price of these non-artificial products makes it difficult to argue for their use.

Another important aspect in these patients is fluid overload. While many still believe that this is a trivial aspect, several studies have shown that positive fluid balances, which is nothing other than fluid accumulations inside the body, are associated with an increased mortality, especially in septic patients.[27,28] Therefore, the most important goal should be to resuscitate the patient as quickly as possible, while keeping the unavoidable positive fluid balance as small as feasible. In uncomplicated sepsis, defined as two of five SIRS criteria plus infection,[29] patients are hemodynamically stable and are often able to drink orally. They do not depend on large amounts of IV fluids, especially not colloids. This might change during development of severe sepsis or septic shock. In these patients it is extremely challenging to choose the optimal type, amount, and timing for fluid resuscitation. Emanuel Rivers and colleagues did not evaluate the type of fluid, but showed that the most crucial aspect seems to be the time point of fluid infusion.[30] Rivers performed an early goal directed approach and clearly demonstrated that the initial resuscitation phase following a strict protocol, in his trial the first 6 hours, was crucial for patient outcome and mortality.

When discussing trials comparing colloids versus crystalloids on ICU it is crucial (i) to try to constitute a control group that reflects daily practice and (ii) strictly abide to study groups, i.e., not infusing colloids in a "crystalloid" study group.

Outcome data in sepsis

Preliminary results of the RaFTinG (Rational Fluid Therapy in Germany, ClinicalTrials.gov Identifier: NCT01122277) trial, a prospectively performed, non-interventional registry including 4500 patients in 61 German ICUs and relating fluid handling to outcome, revealed that, in practice, artificial colloids are applied to patients within the very first period of their ICU stay at a mean daily amount of around 800 mL. Obviously, colloid use today is already the result of carefully outweighing risk and benefit in the individual situation. This is important when discussing the recent randomized trials, which demonstrated that large daily amounts of HES might negatively impact outcome, especially when infused over several days in septic patients. Discussions among experts concerning this collective are on-going. Meanwhile, even political authorities have been involved, despite the story being quite simple: the community agrees unanimously that long-term use of HES in patients with sepsis has no benefits for patients, but increases the risk. This is reflected by the main result of two recent trials, VISEP[31] and 6S.[32]

In VISEP, patients were randomized up to 24 h after diagnosis of severe sepsis.[31] During the initial resuscitation phase, which was documented observationally as it was not part of the interventional trial, the vast majority of patients even in the crystalloid group were pretreated with HES. How many received albumin, fresh frozen plasma, or gelatine later is not reported. Therefore, it is not surprising that the majority of patients were hemodynamically stabilized at study onset, lacking a proper indication for colloids. Nevertheless, the HES group received large amounts of this artificial colloid over days. What, in fact, caused the observed increased need for renal replacement therapy related to HES use in these studies obviously was the treatment with this highly potent drug *outside* a proper indication. Beyond that, it is remarkable that a further 33% in the "crystalloid" group received colloids *during* the trial. Therefore, the VISEP "crystalloid" group actually appears to be a "low amount of colloid in the early phase and indication-based thereafter" group. The study "colloid" group was receiving large amounts of HES (partly beyond daily recommended amounts) over several days. This clearly does not reflect daily practice. In summary, any conclusion on a theoretically possible approach stabilizing patients in shock exclusively with crystalloids is not possible from this trial.

Similar aspects account for the 6S trial.[32] In their "crystalloid" group over 60% had already received up to 1000 mL of colloid for initial resuscitation before the trial started, which was up to 24 hours after diagnosis. A remarkable further 32% in this "crystalloid" group received a colloid *during* the trial. This means that practically all patients in the "crystalloid" group received a colloid at some time point. Therefore, the "crystalloid" group of 6S was also more of a "low amounts of colloids" group. The "colloid" group, by contrast, once again received large amounts of HES every day throughout the trial (theoretically for up to 90 days). As this trial had no protocol, no criteria for RRT, and with the vast majority of patients being, once again, hemodynamically stabilized at study onset, it is difficult to comprehend the clinical relevance of what actually happened to the patients. Therefore, the conclusion again is to use colloids in low amounts in the initial resuscitation phase and to refrain from their use in maintenance, especially in high dosages over longer time periods. Any recommendations concerning a purely crystalloidal treatment is not based on the data and, therefore, is pure speculation.

The CHEST trial included 7000 patients, presenting a heterogeneous ICU collective, which was randomized into receiving HES or saline.[33] It is not understood whether there was a clear indication for the study fluid, as the single indications stated in the protocol (e.g., mean arterial pressure <70 mmHg, heart rate >90 bpm or CVP < 10 mmHg) are, by no means, a trigger for fluid resuscitation with colloids in clinical practice. As there were no relevant differences in outcome in this trial, it seems that HES in hemodynamically stable ICU patients has no relevant benefits, so that crystalloids should be used preferably for maintenance. Any discussion around the data beyond that, is, once again, speculative.

All these three trials did not include the initial stabilization phase, but were initiated *after* pretreatment during the outcome-sensitive phase of fluid resuscitation. In October 2013 the first prospective trial including this crucial initial phase into the observation period was published in written form. Despite being an open-label trial, CRISTAL randomized patients in severe sepsis, septic, or hypovolemic shock into a colloid or a crystalloid group, resuscitating the respective groups accordingly.[34] All patients received additional on-going basal crystalloid replacement therapy. With 2 L of colloids infused practically only within the first 48 h after diagnosis, the total amount was much lower and the time point much earlier than in 6S and VISEP. Not very surprisingly, the results were the complete opposite: in the colloid group of CRISTAL mortality, mechanical ventilation and need for vasopressors were lower, showing no sign of organ failure or need for RRT. Moreover, the most effective colloid was HES. These results are in line with RaFTinG, which also showed advantages for HES in comparison to crystalloids when used in limited amounts at an early time point. Moreover, RaFTinG showed a clear advantage of modern third-generation starches (HES 130/0.4) compared with second-generation large molecule starches (HES 200/0.5). From all available trials, it seems as though small amounts of colloids individually targeting the intravascular compartment at an early time point seem to improve patient outcome. Continuing with large dosages of a no longer indicated drug after having reached the target should obviously be avoided, and also avoided in volume therapy.

Science meets politics – what will the future bring?

The Pharmacovigilance Risk Assessment Committee (PRAC) European Medicines Agency (EMA) concluded on June 13, 2013, that the "benefits of infusion solutions containing hydroxyethyl starch (HES) no longer outweigh their risks," and therefore it recommended suspension of the marketing authorizations for these drugs. The decision was based on the above-mentioned trials VISEP, 6S, and CHEST. Despite the marketing, authorization holders requested an immediate re-examination, arguing together with many international experts that the available studies do not reflect the core indication of these drugs and therefore cannot justify such an invasive recommendation. Some member states (UK and Italy) decided to suspend the use of HES products in their countries. This triggered a further review of HES solutions under Article 107i of Directive 2001/83/EC, running in parallel with the re-examination of the previous PRAC recommendation from June 2013. An invitation of all stakeholders to provide comments and new data to the PRAC to facilitate a decision on the future of HES products revealed that the vast majority of those who are working at the bedside are not willing to lose this, in their view, important therapeutic option. Beyond that, new data from CRISTAL, BASES, and RaFTinG were introduced and markedly influenced the final recommendation the PRAC forwarded to the so-called Coordination Group for Mutual Recognition and Decentralized Procedures – Human (CMDh) after having finalized both procedures on October 10, 2013. This led to the recommendation that HES solutions must no longer be used in patients with sepsis, burn injuries, renal failure, severe coagulopathy, or in critically ill patients. Moreover, HES solutions should only be used for the treatment of hypovolemia, due to acute blood loss at the lowest effective dose for the shortest period of time.

From a political point of view, the procedure was conducted satisfactorily. From an emotional point of view, many colleagues are happy that this drug will most likely remain a therapeutic option. From a scientific point of view, the decision is disappointing. It remains questionable whether this recommendation will increase patient safety, as neither VISEP nor 6S or CHEST evaluated a strategy completely denying colloids during initial stabilization in shock. Beyond that, there is new evidence that it might even be harmful. The listed contraindications for HES are sensible and comprehensible. However, they are neither new nor sensational and most clinicians would have agreed to them, even without the decision of an authority, as it reflects current European clinical practice. At the end of the day there remains a bad feeling as, under great external pressure, an official authority exceeded its competence, trying to end an on-going medical expert discussion and limiting the freedom of action of those who want to treat their patients the best way they can.

Conclusions

The on-going debate on optimal fluid management is still not over. The primary goal should be to maintain steady state in all patients, maintaining fluid compartments including intravascular normovolemia. Both hypo- and hypervolemia should be avoided as far as possible. In surgical patients with intact vascular barrier, using a rational approach with isotonic balanced crystalloids to replace on-going losses, combined with goal directed indication-triggered boluses of balanced iso-oncotic colloids seems rational. In patients requiring fluid resuscitation, the indication for a colloid is limited to the early initial stabilization phase. Patients with renal impairment or an impaired vascular barrier function should be primarily treated with crystalloids supplemented with small amounts of human albumin if indicated to limit fluid overload.

References

1. Chappell D, Jacob M, Hofmann-Kiefer K, Conzen P, Rehm M. A rational approach to perioperative fluid management. *Anesthesiology* 2008;**109**:723–40.

2. Chappell D, Jacob M. Hydroxyethyl starch – the importance of being earnest. *Scand J Trauma Resusc Emerg Med* 2013;**21**:61.

3. Becker BF, Chappell D, Jacob M. Endothelial glycocalyx and coronary vascular permeability: the fringe benefit. *Basic Res Cardiol* 2010;**105**:687–701.

4. Jacob M, Chappell D, Conzen P, Finsterer U, Rehm M. Blood volume is normal after pre-operative overnight fasting. *Acta Anaesth Scand* 2008;**52**:522–9.

5. Smith I, Kranke P, Murat I, et al. Perioperative fasting in adults and children: guidelines from the European Society of Anaesthesiology. *Eur J Anaes* 2011;**28**:556–69.

6. Lamke LO, Nilsson GE, Reithner HL. Water loss by evaporation from the abdominal cavity during surgery. *Acta Chir Scand* 1977;**143**:279–84.

7. Lamke LO, Nilsson GE, Reithner HL. Insensible perspiration from the skin under standardized environmental conditions. *Scand J Clin Lab Invest* 1977;**37**:325–31.

8. Reinhart K, Perner A, Sprung CL, et al. Consensus statement of the ESICM task force on colloid volume therapy in critically ill patients. *Intens Care Med* 2012;**38**:368–83.

9. Rehm M, Haller M, Orth V, et al. Changes in blood volume and hematocrit during acute preoperative volume loading with 5% albumin or 6% hetastarch solutions in patients before radical hysterectomy. *Anesthesiology* 2001;**95**:849–56.

10. Rehm M, Orth V, Kreimeier U, et al. Changes in intravascular volume during acute normovolemic hemodilution and intraoperative retransfusion in patients with radical hysterectomy. *Anesthesiology* 2000;**92**:657–64.

11. Jacob M, Rehm M, Orth V, et al. [Exact measurement of the volume effect of 6% hydoxyethyl starch 130/0.4 (Voluven) during acute preoperative normovolemic hemodilution]. *Der Anaesthesist* 2003;**52**:896–904.

12. Jacob M, Chappell D, Hofmann-Kiefer K, et al. The intravascular volume effect of Ringer's lactate is below 20%: a prospective study in humans. *Crit Care* 2012;**16**:R86.

13. Mulivor AW, Lipowsky HH. Inhibition of glycan shedding and leukocyte-endothelial adhesion in postcapillary venules by suppression of matrixmetalloprotease activity with doxycycline. *Microcirculation* 2009;**16**:657–66.

14. Powell-Tuck JG, Lobo DN, Allison SP, et al. British Consensus guidelines on intravenous fluid therapy for adult surgical patients, 2011.

15. Benington S, Ferris P, Nirmalan M. Emerging trends in minimally invasive haemodynamic monitoring and optimization of fluid therapy. *Eur J Anaesthesiol* 2009;**26**:893–905.

16. Wiener RS, Welch HG. Trends in the use of the pulmonary artery catheter in the United States, 1993-2004. *JAMA* 2007;**298**:423–9.

17. Marik PE, Cavallazzi R. Does the central venous pressure predict fluid responsiveness? An updated meta-analysis and a plea for some common sense. *Crit Care Med* 2013;**41**:1774–81.

18. Feldheiser A, Pavlova V, Bonomo T, et al. Balanced crystalloid compared with balanced colloid solution using a goal-directed haemodynamic algorithm. *Br J Anaesth* 2013;**110**:231–40.

19. Hamilton MA, Cecconi M, Rhodes A. A systematic review and meta-analysis on the use of preemptive hemodynamic intervention to improve postoperative outcomes in moderate and high-risk surgical patients. *Anesth Analg* 2011;**112**:1392–402.

20. Khuri SF, Henderson WG, DePalma RG, et al. Determinants of long-term survival after major surgery and the adverse effect of postoperative complications. *Ann Surg* 2005;**242**:326–41; discussion 41–3.

21. Brandstrup B, Tonnesen H, Beier-Holgersen R, et al. Effects of intravenous fluid restriction on postoperative complications: comparison of two perioperative fluid regimens: a randomized assessor-blinded multicenter trial. *Ann Surg* 2003;**238**:641–8.

22. Lobo DN, Bostock KA, Neal KR, et al. Effect of salt and water balance on recovery of gastrointestinal function after elective colonic resection: a randomised controlled trial. *Lancet* 2002;**359**:1812–18.

23. Nisanevich V, Felsenstein I, Almogy G, et al. Effect of intraoperative fluid management on outcome after intraabdominal surgery. *Anesthesiology* 2005;**103**:25–32.

24. Holte K, Klarskov B, Christensen DS, et al. Liberal versus restrictive fluid administration to improve recovery after laparoscopic cholecystectomy: a randomized, double-blind study. *Ann Surg* 2004;**240**:892–9.

25. Nelson A, Berkestedt I, Schmidtchen A, Ljunggren L, Bodelsson M. Increased levels of glycosaminoglycans during septic shock: relation to mortality and the antibacterial actions of plasma. *Shock* 2008;**30**:623–7.

26. Finfer S, Bellomo R, Boyce N, et al. A comparison of albumin and saline for fluid resuscitation in the intensive care unit. *N Engl J Med* 2004;**350**:2247–56.

27. Micek ST, McEvoy C, McKenzie M, et al. Fluid balance and cardiac function in septic shock as predictors of hospital mortality. *Crit Care* 2013; **17**:R246.

28. Boyd JH, Forbes J, Nakada TA, Walley KR, Russell JA. Fluid resuscitation in septic shock: a positive fluid balance and elevated central venous pressure are associated with increased mortality. *Crit Care Med* 2011;**39**:259–65.

29. Dellinger RP, Levy MM, Rhodes A, et al. Surviving Sepsis Campaign: international guidelines for management of severe sepsis

and septic shock, 2012. *Intens Care Med* 2013;**39**:165–228.

30. Rivers E, Nguyen B, Havstad S, et al. Early goal-directed therapy in the treatment of severe sepsis and septic shock. *N Engl J Med* 2001;**345**:1368–77.

31. Brunkhorst FM, Engel C, Bloos F, et al. Intensive insulin therapy and pentastarch resuscitation in severe

sepsis. *N Engl J Med* 2008;**358**:125–39.

32. Perner A, Haase N, Guttormsen AB, et al. Hydroxyethyl starch 130/0.42 versus Ringer's acetate in severe sepsis. *N Engl J Med* 2012;**367**:124–34.

33. Myburgh JA, Finfer S, Bellomo R, et al. Hydroxyethyl starch or saline for fluid resuscitation in

intensive care. *N Engl J Med* 2012;**367**:1901–11.

34. Annane D, Siami S, Jaber S, et al. Effects of fluid resuscitation with colloids vs crystalloids on mortality in critically ill patients presenting with hypovolemic shock: the CRISTAL randomized trial. *JAMA* 2013;**310**:1809–17.

Vasopressors and inotropes

Robert H. Thiele and James M. Isbell

Introduction

Goal directed therapy algorithms can be classified by a variety of means, most commonly either by the trigger for intervention (e.g., cardiac output, stroke volume variation) or by the intervention itself (fluid administration, pharmacotherapy, or both). For algorithms that utilize pharmacotherapy to achieve a physiologic goal, it is critical for the practitioner to understand the global physiologic as well as organ-specific effects of the various pharmacologic agents available. The purpose of this chapter is to review the relevant physiology and pharmacology related to agents commonly implemented as part of goal directed therapy algorithms. Phosphodiesterase inhibitors and calcium sensitizers, while important to the intensivist, are not commonly employed in structured hemodynamic management algorithms and will not be reviewed here.

Receptors

Alpha adrenergic receptors

There are two subtypes of α-adrenergic receptors (AR) in humans, $\alpha_1 AR$ and $\alpha_2 AR$.[1] Stimulation of $\alpha_1 AR$, an excitatory G protein-coupled receptor (G_s), leads to an increase in intracellular Ca^{2+} via activation of phospholipase C (PLC).[2] Stimulation of $\alpha_2 AR$, an inhibitor G protein-coupled receptor (G_i), leads to inactivation of adenyl cyclase (AC), and ultimately decreases the production of cAMP.[2] $\alpha_1 AR$ have been demonstrated in the vasculature of myocardial, cerebral, renal, muscular, and cutaneous tissue in animals,[3] and in the central arteries, gastrointestinal tract, kidneys, lungs, and coronary arteries in humans.[1]

Beta adrenergic receptors

There are at least three beta-adrenergic receptors (βARs) in humans, β_1, β_2, and β_3.[4] Stimulation of β_1 and β_2 receptors leads to the activation of adenylate cyclase (AC) and subsequent increase in cyclic AMP (cAMP) through excitatory G-protein (G_s) mediated mechanisms.[2] β_1 receptors have been identified in myocardial,[4] cerebral,[5] renal,[2] and adipose tissue,[6,7] and agonism primarily leads to an increase in cardiac contractility and peripheral lipolysis. In healthy humans, the majority of ventricular βARs are of the β_1 subtype, although in chronic heart failure this may not be the case.[2] βARs appear to be down-regulated in the setting of chronic heart failure.[8] β_2 receptors have been identified in cardiac,[2] pulmonary,[9,10] vascular smooth muscle,[11–14] and uterine tissue,[2] and primarily lead to broncho-dilation[9,10] and peripheral vasodilation,[11–14] and in parturients, uterine relaxation.[2] Agonism of β_3 receptors leads to decreases in contractility,[4] but the importance of this βAR subtype is not well understood.

Dopamine receptors

Two dopamine receptors are present in human tissue, DA_1 and DA_2.[2] Stimulation of DA_1 receptors leads to the activation of adenylate cyclase (AC) and subsequent increase in cyclic AMP (cAMP) through G-protein mediated mechanisms, whereas DA_2 receptors lead to the inhibition of adenylate cyclase (AC).[2] DA_1 receptors are located in renal, mesenteric, cerebral, and coronary vascular beds and lead to direct vasodilation.[2] DA_2 receptors are located in renal and larger vascular beds and lead to indirect vasodilation, and are also located on sympathetic nerve endings

Perioperative Hemodynamic Monitoring and Goal Directed Therapy, ed. Maxime Cannesson and Rupert Pearse.
Published by Cambridge University Press. © Cambridge University Press 2014.

and autonomic ganglia, where they lead to the inhibition of endogenous norepinephrine release.[2]

Vasopressin receptors

There are at least three distinct vasopressin receptors, V_{1a}, V_{1b}, and V_2, all of which are G-protein coupled receptors and all of which are related to the oxytocin (OT) receptor.[15] V_{1a} (V_1) receptors are present in both the arterial and venous vasculature, activate phospholipase C (which leads to phosphotidylinositol hydrolysis), and ultimately lead to intracellular Ca^{2+} release and vascular smooth muscle contraction.[15–17] V_2 receptors are exclusively present in the kidneys. They activate adenylate cyclase thus enhancing the cyclic AMP (cAMP)-mediated incorporation of aquaporins into the distal tubules and collecting ducts, leading to increased retention of free water.[15,18,19] The V_{1b} (V_3) receptor is primarily located in the anterior pituitary and affects adrenocorticotropic hormone (ACTH) release.[15,17] V_{1a} is also present on platelets[17] and leads to increased platelet aggregation.[20–22] V_2-agonism leads to the release of factor VIII.[23]

Pharmacology
Vasoconstrictors
Phenylephrine

Phenylephrine is an $\alpha_1 AR$ agonist that is structurally related to epinephrine (the only difference is the lack of a hydroxyl on position 4 of the benzene ring).[24] The peak onset of phenylephrine occurs approximately 40 seconds after bolus administration[25] and loses its effect within 20 minutes.[26]

Vasopressin and terlipressin

Vasopressin is a nonapeptide produced by the hypothalamus and is also referred to as antidiuretic hormone (ADH). The human version of vasopressin contains arginine, thus it is referred to as *arginine vasopressin* (AVP) to distinguish it from synthetic analogs (e.g., terlipressin, desmopressin).[27] AVP is a mixed V_{1a}/V_2 agonist with approximately 1:1 selectivity for both receptors.[28]

Onset occurs within minutes after intravenous administration of AVP and the plasma half-life ranges from 4 to 24 minutes,[27,29] thus it is typically infused when not being used in the context of advanced cardiac life support (ACLS).[27] Doses of 0.01–0.04 U/min

lead to plasma concentrations of approximately 20–30 pg/mL in humans, which enhances the action of endogenous catecholamines without producing overt deleterious effects on vital organ systems.[30] Doses above 0.04 U/min lead to plasma concentrations in excess of 100 pg/mL and may lead to vasoconstriction of coronary, pulmonary, mesenteric, and renal vasculature.[30]

Terlipressin is an AVP analog which is longer-acting than AVP. Its duration of action and lower incidence of side effects have made it the favored agent for the treatment of acute esophageal variceal bleeding.

Inoconstrictors
Dopamine

Dopamine is a naturally occurring catecholamine found in sympathetic nervous tissue as well as in the adrenal glands. It is the immediate precursor to norepinephrine in the catecholamine synthesis pathway.[31] It is both a direct acting agent (with activity at dopamine receptors, αARs, and βARs) as well as an indirect-acting agent (leading to release of endogenous norepinephrine from catecholamine storage sites).[31] The activity of dopamine on various receptors is dependent on the dose administered, with large doses leading to predominant αAR activity, thus leading to systemic vasoconstriction.[32,33] Epinene (the N-methyl derivative of dopamine) can directly bind and activate both β_1 and β_2 receptors.[2]

Norepinephrine

Norepinephrine is a naturally occurring catecholamine that is synthesized from dopamine.[31] It is active at $\alpha_1 AR$, $\beta_1 AR$, and $\beta_2 AR$ in a dose-dependent manner and differs from epinephrine primarily by exhibiting less $\beta_2 AR$ activity.

Epinephrine

Epinephrine is a naturally occurring catecholamine that is synthesized from norepinephrine (which is synthesized from dopamine).[31] It is active at $\alpha_1 AR$, $\beta_1 AR$, and $\beta_2 AR$ in a dose-dependent manner and differs from norepinephrine primarily by exhibiting more $\beta_2 AR$ activity. It is rapidly metabolized by catecholamine o-methyl-transferase (COMT) and monoamine oxidase (MOA) in the liver.

Inodilators

Dobutamine

Dobutamine is a synthetic catecholamine that primarily activates β_1ARs and β_2ARs (approximately 3:1 relative activity[34]), with mild activity at α_1ARs.[35–39]

Isoproterenol

Isoproterenol is a synthetic catecholamine that primarily activates β_1ARs and β_2ARs (with approximately equal activity at both) and has very little activity at α_1ARs.[34]

Physiologic effects

Vasoconstrictors

Phenylephrine

In addition to causing systemic arterial vasoconstriction, phenylephrine causes systemic *venous* constriction,[33,40–43] pulmonary artery vasoconstriction,[44] and, in high doses, may increase myocardial contractility.[45] Administration of methoxamine (a longer-acting α_1AR agonist) increases left ventricular wall stress and decreases left ventricular function in animals[46] and presumably phenylephrine, which has an identical mechanism of action, would do the same.

The effects of α_1AR agonists on myocardial supply and demand are complex. Clearly, α_1AR agonists increase oxygen demand, both by increasing afterload (through vasoconstriction) and, at high doses, by increasing contractility.[45] Methoxamine (a longer-acting α_1AR agonist) has been demonstrated to decrease coronary artery blood flow in dogs.[47] Animal studies utilizing phenylephrine have demonstrated no change[48] or even an increase[49] in coronary artery blood flow, as have some human studies using methoxamine.[50]

Human studies have demonstrated decreased left ventricular function, increased wall motion abnormalities, and increased left ventricular end-systolic wall stress when phenylephrine is utilized to maintain normal blood pressure in the setting of deep anesthetic levels.[51] The effect of α_1AR-agonists on cardiac output is dependent upon the balance of both arterial and venous effects (in the pulmonic and systemic vasculatures). Twenty five percent of total blood volume is present in splanchnic organs and α_1AR-agonists may initially increase venous return due to venoconstriction,[52] potentially leading to increased cardiac output at low doses (as has been demonstrated with methoxamine [in animals],[53] but not phenylephrine). At doses commonly used, human studies

consistently demonstrate decreased cardiac output with the administration of phenylephrine.[54,55]

α_1AR are present in human kidneys in relatively high densities and while human physiologic studies are rare, animal studies suggest that α_1AR-agonists reduce renal blood flow and urine output.[3,47,56]

Vasopressin and terlipressin

Administration of exogenous vasopressin to achieve supranormal levels has been demonstrated to produce vasoconstriction in multiple vascular beds, including muscle,[57–59] coronary vasculature,[47,57,60,61] renal vasculature,[47] mesentery,[47,57,58,62–64] and skin[57] in animals and the muscle,[65] mesentery,[66] and subcutaneous tissue[65] in humans.

Vasopressin has also been demonstrated to produce *vasodilation* in some vascular beds.[67–69] The relative amount of vasoconstriction or vasodilation in each particular vascular bed has not been firmly established and is likely both species and concentration dependent.

Based on animal studies, it appears that vasopressin primarily causes vasoconstriction in the splanchnic, hepatic, cardiac, and muscular beds. Animal studies that compare pure α_1AR agonists (methoxamine) to vasopressin suggest that vasopressin has a more profound effect on heart rate (leading to substantial bradycardia), left ventricular function (reduced dP/dt), and coronary artery flow.[47]

While clearly present in the brain,[70–72] vasopressin produces relatively little effect on the cerebral vasculature.[57,58,68,69,73] Vasopressin also has a relatively mild effect on the renal[47,57,59,63] and pulmonary[74,75] vasculature based on animal studies and, while it does appear to increase pulmonary vascular resistance (PVR) in humans, the increase in PVR is significantly less than that produced by alpha-agonists.[76] Vasodilation due to vasopressin[67–69] occurs only at low doses, and the receptor responsible has not been identified, although it is likely that the phenomenon is mediated by nitric oxide release.[30]

Low doses of vasopressin lead to a diuretic effect in humans,[77–79] possibly due to vasoconstriction of the efferent arterioles.[80] At higher doses, vasopressin leads to renal vasoconstriction[81,82] and decreased urine output, likely due to a combination of both free water retention (V_2-mediated) and V_1-mediated reductions in renal blood flow.[30]

While administration of vasopressin universally increases systemic vascular resistance and produces reflex bradycardia, its effect on cardiac output can be variable. In human patients with myocardium capable of handling an increase in afterload, exogenous vasopressin may increase blood pressure without affecting cardiac output.[83,84] Intact and denervated animal models have both demonstrated decreases in cardiac output following vasopressin administration.[85] Animal studies, which directly compare pure α_1AR agonists (methoxamine) to vasopressin, suggest that vasopressin has a more profound effect on cardiac output as compared to α_1AR agonists.[47]

Additionally, vasopressin may act as a myocardial depressant either through direct actions on the myocardium (although this may only occur at high concentrations) or via coronary artery vasoconstriction and a reduction in myocardial blood flow.[3,47] Vasopressin also potentiates the actions of endogenous catecholamines.[3]

Normal vasopressin levels in humans are not sufficient to activate the vasoactive response of the V_{1a} receptors,[15,86] and endogenous vasopressin administration does not reliably increase blood pressure when autonomic systems are intact.[87] Furthermore, blockade of vasopressin receptors in healthy humans does not result in hypotension,[88] nor does mild lower body negative pressure lead to an increase in vasopressin release.[89] These data suggest that the primary role of AVP in maintaining cardiovascular hemostasis is related to maintenance of intravascular volume, not peripheral vascular tone. Indeed, the primary trigger for vasopressin release in healthy humans is increased osmolarity, not hypotension.[90]

Endogenous vasopressin levels are decreased in the setting of septic shock,[30,76] but are increased in the settings of cardiogenic shock, cardiac arrest, and hemorrhagic shock[76] (hypovolemia has been shown to cause AVP release in both animal and human models[86]). Vasopressin levels have also been shown to rise in the setting of impaired autonomic function,[87,91,92] orthostatic hypotension,[93] and extreme lower body negative pressure (-40 mmHg).[94] Thus several authors have hypothesized that endogenous vasopressin may function as a "back-up" mechanism to preserve blood pressure in a variety of pathologic states.[27,91]

Inoconstrictors
Dopamine

Administration of dopamine in low doses leads to hypotension in animal models – this discovery, and the realization that this response could not be blocked with traditional adrenergic blocking agents,[32] led to the search for an additional adrenergic receptor, since identified as the dopamine receptor(s).[2] More recent animal studies (canine heart failure model) suggest that dopamine increases cardiac output and renal blood flow over the range of 5–20 μcg/kg min^{-1}.[95] At large doses (~50 μcg/kg/min) dopamine begins to resemble norepinephrine in animal models, leading to increases in both mean arterial pressure and systemic vascular resistance.[32]

In humans given dopamine at 3–12 μcg/kg min^{-1}, dopamine leads to an increase in cardiac output due to a fall in systemic vascular resistance (mean arterial pressure is not affected).[96,97] In critically ill humans, dopamine at 10–12 μcg/kg min^{-1} increases cardiac output by approximately 50%[98] and in humans post-cardiopulmonary bypass (CPB), doses of up to 2.5 μcg/kg min^{-1} increase renal blood flow without affecting cardiac output.[99] At 4 μcg/kg min^{-1}, cardiac output begins to increase in the post-CPB patient population.[99] In humans with heart failure, a linear relationship between dose and cardiac output has been observed, with boluses ranging from 2 to 6 μcg.[100] Dopamine simultaneously decreases left ventricular end-systolic volume and lowers early diastolic pressure, leading to a leftward shift in the diastolic pressure–dimension relationship.[100]

Administration of dopamine to patients undergoing CPB leads to a significant increase in venous reservoir volumes (implying venoconstriction) at both low (0.2 mg bolus) and high (4 mg bolus) doses. Perfusion pressure only increased with high dose dopamine, suggesting a dose-dependent effect of this drug on afterload (presumably by binding to α_1ARs).[33]

Overall, it is assumed that dopamine has primarily dopaminergic effects at doses less than 3 μcg/kg min^{-1}, stimulates βARs at 3–10 μcg/kg min^{-1}, and stimulates α_1ARs at doses greater than 10 μcg/kg min^{-1}, although the interindividual variation in the response to dopamine may exceed that of other vasopressors.[101]

In addition to peripheral vascular effects, dopamine administration leads to natriuresis (due to DA_1 activation), although it is not clear whether this is due to an increase in renal perfusion or to a direct tubular effect.[2] Dopamine doses of up to 7 μcg/kg min^{-1} have been demonstrated to increase renal blood flow.[32]

Norepinephrine

In dogs, administration of norepinephrine from 0 to 0.5 μcg/kg min^{-1} leads to a linear increase in mean arterial pressure, with no change in cardiac output[36] and coronary arterial vasoconstriction.[102] Interestingly, administration of norepinephrine in animals increases left ventricular function and *decreases* left ventricular wall stress, most likely by increasing contractility (which reduces the radius of the ventricular cavity and hence wall stress in accordance with Lame's equation, which states that wall stress is equal to pressure times radius divided by wall thickness).[46]

In humans, norepinephrine boluses of 0.05 – 0.1 µcg/kg can restore mean arterial pressure in hypotensive subjects without affecting ventricular function, in contrast to phenylephrine which, at bolus doses of 2 µcg/kg, leads to decreased ventricular function.[103,104] Norepinephrine also increases pulmonary vascular resistance in humans, presumably due to its effect on α_1ARs,[105] and appears to decrease cerebral blood flow despite causing an increase in mean arterial pressure, also due to its effect on α_1ARs.[106,107]

Epinephrine

In humans post-CPB, epinephrine doses of 0.02–0.08 µcg/kg min^{-1} increase cardiac output without affecting renal blood flow.[99] In humans undergoing epidural anesthesia, epinephrine infusions (1 to 5 µcg/min) have been shown to preserve cardiac output when compared with phenylephrine at equipotent doses (2 to 20 µcg/min, which significantly decreases cardiac output).[108] Similar results were demonstrated in a cross-over comparison of these two drugs in patients undergoing spinal anesthesia, with epinephrine increasing cardiac output by 38% and phenylephrine decreasing it by 28%.[109]

Inodilators

Isoproterenol

Isoproterenol increases cardiac output, decreases SVR, and has no effect on renal blood flow over the range of 0.01–0.05 µcg/kg min^{-1} in a canine model of heart failure.[95] In animal myocardial infarction models, isoproterenol increases myocardial oxygen consumption significantly and can lead to infarct extension.

In humans, isoproterenol consistently increases cardiac output and heart rate while lowering mean arterial pressure.[110] Renal blood flow is either unaffected or decreased.[110] Administration of isoproterenol in patients undergoing cardiopulmonary bypass leads to a significant decrease in venous reservoir volumes (implying venodilation) and a decrease in perfusion pressure, suggesting peripheral vasodilation (likely due to β_2AR agonism).[33]

Dobutamine

Dobutamine increases cardiac output with relatively little effect on SVR and renal blood flow over the range of 1–5 µcg/kg min^{-1} in a canine model of heart failure.[95] Administration of dobutamine in animals increases left ventricular function and decreases left ventricular wall stress, probably due to a combination of reduced systemic vascular resistance and increased contractility (which reduces the radius of the ventricular cavity and thus wall stress).[46]

In a variety of human models, dobutamine has been shown to increase cardiac output over a range of approximately 2 to 15 µcg/kg min^{-1} [35,99,111–113] or with boluses ranging from 2 to 10 µcg.[100] Dobutamine simultaneously decreases left ventricular end-systolic volume and lowers early diastolic pressure, leading to a leftward shift in the diastolic pressure–dimension relationship.[100] Central venous pressure and pulmonary capillary wedge pressure typically decrease,[114,115] as does end-diastolic volume and thus left ventricular wall stress.[115] As compared with isoproterenol, dobutamine leads to less tachycardia and less decrease in blood pressure at equivalent cardiac outputs.[115] Dobutamine increases myocardial oxygen consumption by as much as 58%.[116]

Conclusions

Only with thorough knowledge of physiology (particularly with regard to the autonomic nervous system) and pharmacology can practitioners develop a pharmacologic strategy designed to achieve a specific physiologic goal. The myriad of available vasoactive agents are best thought of in terms of the distribution and end-organ effects of the receptors on which they act.

References

1. Rudner XL, Berkowitz DE, Booth JV, et al. Subtype specific regulation of human vascular alpha(1)-adrenergic receptors by vessel bed and age. *Circulation* 1999;**100(23)**: 2336–43.

2. Brodde OE. Physiology and pharmacology of cardiovascular catecholamine receptors: implications for treatment of chronic heart failure. *Am Heart J* 1990;**120 (6 Pt 2)**:1565–72.

3. Hoffbrand BI, Forsyth RP. Regional blood flow changes during norepinephrine, tyramine and methoxamine infusions in the unanesthetized rhesus monkey. *J Pharmacol Exp Ther* 1973;**184**(3):656–61.

4. Kaumann AJ, Molenaar P. Modulation of human cardiac function through 4 beta-adrenoceptor populations. *Naunyn Schmiedebergs Arch Pharmacol* 1997;**355**(6):667–81.

5. Bylund DB, Snyder SH. Beta adrenergic receptor binding in membrane preparations from mammalian brain. *Mol Pharmacol* 1976;**12**(4):568–80.

6. Molinoff PB. Alpha- and beta-adrenergic receptor subtypes properties, distribution and regulation. *Drugs* 1984;**28 Suppl** 2:1–15.

7. Harms HH, Van der Meer J. Isoprenaline antagonism of cardioselective beta-adrenergic receptor blocking agents on human and rat adipocytes. *Br J Clin Pharmacol* 1975;**2**(4):311–15.

8. White M, Yanowitz F, Gilbert EM, et al. Role of beta-adrenergic receptor downregulation in the peak exercise response in patients with heart failure due to idiopathic dilated cardiomyopathy. *Am J Cardiol* 1995;**76**(17):1271–6.

9. Davis C, Conolly ME, Greenacre JK. Beta-adrenoceptors in human lung, bronchus and lymphocytes. *Br J Clin Pharmacol* 1980;**10**(5):425–432.

10. Harms HH. Isoproterenol antagonism of cardioselective beta adrenergic receptor blocking agents: a comparative study of human and guinea-pig cardiac and bronchial beta adrenergic receptors. *J Pharmacol Exp Ther* 1976;**199**(2):329–35.

11. Koch-Weser J, Frishman WH. beta-Adrenoceptor antagonists: new drugs and new indications. *N Engl J Med* 1981;**305**(9):500–6.

12. Lands AM, Arnold A, McAuliff JP, Luduena FP, Brown TG, Jr. Differentiation of receptor systems activated by sympathomimetic amines. *Nature* 1967;**214**(5088):597–8.

13. Dunlop D, Shanks RG. Selective blockade of adrenoceptive beta receptors in the heart. *Br J Pharmacol Chemother* 1968;**32**(1):201–18.

14. Michel MC, Brodde OE, Insel PA. Peripheral adrenergic receptors in hypertension. *Hypertension* 1990;**16**(2):107–20.

15. Koshimizu TA, Nakamura K, Egashira N, et al. Vasopressin V1a and V1b receptors: from molecules to physiological systems. *Physiol Rev* 2012;**92**(4):1813–64.

16. Morel A, O'Carroll AM, Brownstein MJ, Lolait SJ. Molecular cloning and expression of a rat V1a arginine vasopressin receptor. *Nature* 1992;**356**(6369):523–6.

17. Sugimoto T, Saito M, Mochizuki S, et al. Molecular cloning and functional expression of a cDNA encoding the human V1b vasopressin receptor. *J Biol Chem* 1994;**269**(43):27088–92.

18. Lolait SJ, O'Carroll AM, McBride OW, et al. Cloning and characterization of a vasopressin V2 receptor and possible link to nephrogenic diabetes insipidus. *Nature* 1992;**357**(6376):336–9.

19. Birnbaumer M, Seibold A, Gilbert S, et al. Molecular cloning of the receptor for human antidiuretic hormone. *Nature* 1992;**357**(6376):333–5.

20. Bichet DG, Razi M, Lonergan M, et al. Hemodynamic and coagulation responses to 1-desamino[8-D-arginine]vasopressin in patients with congenital nephrogenic diabetes insipidus. *N Engl J Med* 1988;**318**(14):881–7.

21. Haslam RJ, Rosson GM. Effect of vasopressin on human blood platelets. *J Physiol* 1971;**219**(2):36P–8P.

22. Haslam RJ, Rosson GM. Aggregation of human blood platelets by vasopressin. *Am J Physiol* 1972;**223**(4):958–67.

23. Mannucci PM, Canciani MT, Rota L, Donovan BS. Response of factor VIII/von Willebrand factor to DDAVP in healthy subjects and patients with haemophilia A and von Willebrand's disease. *Br J Haematol* 1981;**47**(2):283–93.

24. Hardman JG. *Goodman and Gilman's: The Pharmacological Basis of Therapeutics.* 9th edn. New York: McGraw-Hill, 1996.

25. Schwinn DA, Reves JG. Time course and hemodynamic effects of alpha-1-adrenergic bolus administration in anesthetized patients with myocardial disease. *Anesth Analg* 1989;**68**(5):571–8.

26. Craig CR, Stitzel RE. *Modern Pharmacology With Clinical Applications.* Vol 6th: Lippincott Williams & Wilkins, 2003.

27. Treschan TA, Peters J. The vasopressin system: physiology and clinical strategies. *Anesthesiology.* 2006;**105**(3):599–612; quiz 639–40.

28. Rehberg S, Ertmer C, Lange M, et al. Role of selective V2-receptor-antagonism in septic shock: a randomized, controlled, experimental study. *Crit Care* 2010;**14**(6):R200.

29. Baumann G, Dingman JF. Distribution, blood transport, and degradation of antidiuretic hormone in man. *J Clin Invest* 1976;**57**(5):1109–16.

30. Holmes CL, Patel BM, Russell JA, Walley KR. Physiology of vasopressin relevant to management of septic shock. *Chest* 2001;**120**(3):989–1002.

31. Goldberg LI. Dopamine – clinical uses of an endogenous

catecholamine. *N Engl J Med* 1974;**291**(14):707–10.

32. Goldberg LI. Cardiovascular and renal actions of dopamine: potential clinical applications. *Pharmacol Rev* 1972;**24**(1):1–29.

33. Marino RJ, Romagnoli A, Keats AS. Selective venoconstriction by dopamine in comparison with isoproterenol and phenylephrine. *Anesthesiology* 1975;**43**(5):570–2.

34. Overgaard CB, Dzavik V. Inotropes and vasopressors: review of physiology and clinical use in cardiovascular disease. *Circulation* 2008;**118** (10):1047–56.

35. Gillespie TA, Ambos HD, Sobel BE, Roberts R. Effects of dobutamine in patients with acute myocardial infarction. *Am J Cardiol* 1977;**39**(4):588–94.

36. Robie NW, Nutter DO, Moody C, McNay JL. In vivo analysis of adrenergic receptor activity of dobutamine. *Circ Res* 1974;**34** (5):663–71.

37. De Backer D, Zhang H, Manikis P, Vincent JL. Regional effects of dobutamine in endotoxic shock. *J Surg Res* 1996;**65**(2):93–100.

38. Tuttle RR, Mills J. Dobutamine: development of a new catecholamine to selectively increase cardiac contractility. *Circ Res* 1975;**36**(1):185–96.

39. Ruffolo RR, Jr., Yaden EL. Vascular effects of the stereoisomers of dobutamine. *J Pharmacol Exp Ther* 1983;**224** (1):46–50.

40. Appleton C, Olajos M, Morkin E, Goldman S. Alpha-1 adrenergic control of the venous circulation in intact dogs. *J Pharmacol Exp Ther* 1985;**233** (3):729–34.

41. Eichler HG, Ford GA, Blaschke TF, Swislocki A, Hoffman BB. Responsiveness of superficial hand veins to phenylephrine in essential hypertension. Alpha adrenergic blockade during prazosin therapy. *J Clin Invest* 1989;**83**(1):108–12.

42. Hirakawa S, Itoh H, Kotoo Y, et al. The role of alpha and beta adrenergic receptors in constriction and dilation of the systemic capacitance vessels: a study with measurements of the mean circulatory pressure in dogs. *Jpn Circ J* 1984;**48**(7):620–32.

43. Pang CC. Autonomic control of the venous system in health and disease: effects of drugs. *Pharmacol Ther* 2001;**90** (2–3):179–230.

44. Tuman KJ, McCarthy RJ, March RJ, Guynn TP, Ivankovich AD. Effects of phenylephrine or volume loading on right ventricular function in patients undergoing myocardial revascularization. *J Cardiothorac Vasc Anesth* 1995;**9** (1):2–8.

45. Landzberg JS, Parker JD, Gauthier DF, Colucci WS. Effects of myocardial alpha 1-adrenergic receptor stimulation and blockade on contractility in humans. *Circulation* 1991;**84** (4):1608–14.

46. Lang RM, Borow KM, Neumann A, Janzen D. Systemic vascular resistance: an unreliable index of left ventricular afterload. *Circulation* 1986;**74**(5):1114–23.

47. Heyndrickx GR, Boettcher DH, Vatner SF. Effects of angiotensin, vasopressin, and methoxamine on cardiac function and blood flow distribution in conscious dogs. *Am J Physiol* 1976;**231** (5 Pt. 1):1579–87.

48. Woodman OL, Vatner SF. Coronary vasoconstriction mediated by alpha 1- and alpha 2-adrenoceptors in conscious dogs. *Am J Physiol* 1987;**253** (2 Pt 2):H388–93.

49. Crystal GJ, Kim SJ, Salem MM, Abdel-Latif M. Myocardial oxygen supply/demand relations during phenylephrine infusions in dogs. *Anesth Analg* 1991;**73**(3):283–8.

50. Loeb HS, Saudye A, Croke RP, et al. Effects of pharmacologically-induced hypertension on myocardial ischemia and coronary hemodynamics in patients with fixed coronary obstruction. *Circulation* 1978;**57** (1):41–6.

51. Smith JS, Roizen MF, Cahalan MK, et al. Does anesthetic technique make a difference? Augmentation of systolic blood pressure during carotid endarterectomy: effects of phenylephrine versus light anesthesia and of isoflurane versus halothane on the incidence of myocardial ischemia. *Anesthesiology* 1988;**69**(6):846–53.

52. Gelman S, Mushlin PS. Catecholamine-induced changes in the splanchnic circulation affecting systemic hemodynamics. *Anesthesiology* 2004;**100**(2):434–9.

53. Zandberg P, Timmermans PB, van Zwieten PA. Hemodynamic profiles of methoxamine and B-HT 933 in spinalized ganglion-blocked dogs. *J Cardiovasc Pharmacol* 1984;**6**(2):256–62.

54. Langesaeter E, Rosseland LA, Stubhaug A. Continuous invasive blood pressure and cardiac output monitoring during cesarean delivery: a randomized, double-blind comparison of low-dose versus high-dose spinal anesthesia with intravenous phenylephrine or placebo infusion. *Anesthesiology* 2008;**109**(5):856–63.

55. Stewart A, Fernando R, McDonald S, et al. The dose-dependent effects of phenylephrine for elective cesarean delivery under spinal anesthesia. *Anesth Analg* 2010;**111** (5):1230–7.

56. Grangsjo G, Persson E. Influence of some vaso-active substances on regional blood flow in the dog kidney. A study on normovolaemic and hypovolaemic dogs. *Acta*

Anaesthesiol Scand 1971;**15** (2):71–95.

57. Liard JF, Deriaz O, Schelling P, Thibonnier M. Cardiac output distribution during vasopressin infusion or dehydration in conscious dogs. *Am J Physiol* 1982;**243**(5):H663–9.

58. Ericsson BF. Effect of vasopressin on the distribution of cardiac output and organ blood flow in the anesthetized dog. *Acta Chir Scand* 1971;**137**(8):729–38.

59. Schmid PG, Abboud FM, Wendling MG, et al. Regional vascular effects of vasopressin: plasma levels and circulatory responses. *Am J Physiol* 1974;**227** (5):998–1004.

60. Michel JB, Tedgui A, Bardou A, Levy B. Effect of vasopressin on phasic coronary blood flow. *Basic Res Cardiol.* 1985;**80**(3):221–30.

61. Pantely GA, Ladley HD, Anselone CG, Bristow JD. Vasopressin-induced coronary constriction at low perfusion pressures. *Cardiovasc Res* 1985;**19** (7):433–41.

62. Martin DS, McNeill JR. Sensitivity of intestinal resistance vessels to vasopressin after ganglionic blockade in the conscious cat. *J Cardiovasc Pharmacol* 1987;**9** (3):368–74.

63. Hofbauer KG, Studer W, Mah SC, et al. The significance of vasopressin as a pressor agent. *J Cardiovasc Pharmacol* 1984;**6** Suppl 2:S429–38.

64. Kerr JC, Hobson RW, 2nd, Seelig RF, Swan KG. Influence of vasopressin on colon blood flow in monkeys. *Gastroenterology* 1977;**72**(3):474–8.

65. Hammer M, Skagen K. Effects of small changes of plasma vasopressin on subcutaneous and skeletal muscle blood flow in man. *Acta Physiol Scand* 1986;**127** (1):67–73.

66. Erwald R, Wiechel KL, Strandell T. Effect of vasopressin on regional splanchnic blood flows in conscious man. *Acta Chir Scand* 1976;**142**(1):36–42.

67. Okamura T, Ayajiki K, Fujioka H, Toda N. Mechanisms underlying arginine vasopressin-induced relaxation in monkey isolated coronary arteries. *J Hypertens* 1999;**17**(5):673–8.

68. Katusic ZS, Shepherd JT, Vanhoutte PM. Vasopressin causes endothelium-dependent relaxations of the canine basilar artery. *Circ Res* 1984;**55**(5):575–9.

69. Vanhoutte PM, Katusic ZS, Shepherd JT. Vasopressin induces endothelium-dependent relaxations of cerebral and coronary, but not of systemic arteries. *J Hypertens Suppl* 1984;**2** (3):S421–2.

70. Tribollet E, Barberis C, Jard S, Dubois-Dauphin M, Dreifuss JJ. Localization and pharmacological characterization of high affinity binding sites for vasopressin and oxytocin in the rat brain by light microscopic autoradiography. *Brain Res* 1988;**442**(1):105–18.

71. Phillips PA, Abrahams JM, Kelly J, et al. Localization of vasopressin binding sites in rat brain by in vitro autoradiography using a radioiodinated V1 receptor antagonist. *Neuroscience* 1988;**27** (3):749–61.

72. Ostrowski NL, Lolait SJ, Bradley DJ, et al. Distribution of V1a and V2 vasopressin receptor messenger ribonucleic acids in rat liver, kidney, pituitary and brain. *Endocrinology* 1992;**131**(1):533–5.

73. Lassoff S, Altura BM. Do pial terminal arterioles respond to local perivascular application of the neurohypophyseal peptide hormones, vasopressin and oxytocin? *Brain Res* 1980;**196** (1):266–9.

74. Walker BR, Haynes J, Jr., Wang HL, Voelkel NF. Vasopressin-induced pulmonary vasodilation in rats. *Am J Physiol* 1989;**257** (2 Pt 2):H415–22.

75. Wallace AW, Tunin CM, Shoukas AA. Effects of vasopressin on pulmonary and systemic vascular mechanics. *Am J Physiol* 1989;**257** (4 Pt 2):H1228–34.

76. Jeon Y, Ryu JH, Lim YJ, et al. Comparative hemodynamic effects of vasopressin and norepinephrine after milrinone-induced hypotension in off-pump coronary artery bypass surgical patients. *Eur J Cardiothorac Surg* 2006;**29**(6):952–6.

77. Landry DW, Levin HR, Gallant EM, et al. Vasopressin pressor hypersensitivity in vasodilatory septic shock. *Crit Care Med* 1997;**25**(8):1279–82.

78. Eisenman A, Armali Z, Enat R, Bankir L, Baruch Y. Low-dose vasopressin restores diuresis both in patients with hepatorenal syndrome and in anuric patients with end-stage heart failure. *J Intern Med* 1999;**246**(2):183–90.

79. Gold J, Cullinane S, Chen J, et al. Vasopressin in the treatment of milrinone-induced hypotension in severe heart failure. *Am J Cardiol* 2000;**85**(4):506–8.

80. Edwards RM, Trizna W, Kinter LB. Renal microvascular effects of vasopressin and vasopressin antagonists. *Am J Physiol* 1989;**256**(2 Pt 2):F274–8.

81. McVicar AJ. Dose–response effects of pressor doses of arginine vasopressin on renal haemodynamics in the rat. *J Physiol* 1988;**404**:535–46.

82. Harrison-Bernard LM, Carmines PK. Juxtamedullary microvascular responses to arginine vasopressin in rat kidney. *Am J Physiol* 1994;**267**(2 Pt 2):F249–56.

83. Braunwald E, Wagner HN, Jr. The pressor effect of the antidiuretic principle of the posterior pituitary in orthostatic hypotension. *J Clin Invest* 1956;**35**(12):1412–18.

84. Tsuneyoshi I, Yamada H, Kakihana Y, et al. Hemodynamic and metabolic effects of low-dose

vasopressin infusions in vasodilatory septic shock. *Crit Care Med* 2001;**29**(3):487–93.

85. Cowley AW, Jr., Monos E, Guyton AC. Interaction of vasopressin and the baroreceptor reflex system in the regulation of arterial blood pressure in the dog. *Circ Res* 1974;**34**(4):505–14.

86. Share L. Role of vasopressin in cardiovascular regulation. *Physiol Rev* 1988;**68**(4):1248–84.

87. Williams TD, Da Costa D, Mathias CJ, Bannister R, Lightman SL. Pressor effect of arginine vasopressin in progressive autonomic failure. *Clin Sci (Lond)* 1986;**71**(2):173–8.

88. Bussien JP, Waeber B, Nussberger J, et al. Does vasopressin sustain blood pressure of normally hydrated healthy volunteers? *Am J Physiol* 1984;**246**(1 Pt 2): H143–7.

89. Goldsmith SR, Francis GS, Cowley AW, Cohn JN. Response of vasopressin and norepinephrine to lower body negative pressure in humans. *Am J Physiol* 1982;**243**(6):H970–3.

90. Goldsmith SR. Baroreceptor-mediated suppression of osmotically stimulated vasopressin in normal humans. *J Appl Physiol* 1988;**65**(3):1226–30.

91. Jordan J, Tank J, Diedrich A, Robertson D, Shannon JR. Vasopressin and blood pressure in humans. *Hypertension* 2000;**36**(6): E3–4.

92. Kaufmann H, Oribe E, Miller M, et al. Hypotension-induced vasopressin release distinguishes between pure autonomic failure and multiple system atrophy with autonomic failure. *Neurology* 1992;**42**(3 Pt 1):590–3.

93. Zerbe RL, Henry DP, Robertson GL. Vasopressin response to orthostatic hypotension. Etiologic and clinical implications. *Am J Med* 1983;**74**(2):265–71.

94. Leimbach WN, Jr., Schmid PG, Mark AL. Baroreflex control of plasma arginine vasopressin in humans. *Am J Physiol* 1984;**247** (4 Pt 2):H638–44.

95. Argenta LC, Kirsh MM, Bove EL, et al. A comparison of the hemodynamic effects of inotropic agents. *Ann Thorac Surg* 1976;**22** (1):50–7.

96. Horwitz D, Fox Sm D, Goldberg LI. Effects of dopamine in man. *Circ Res* 1962;**10**:237–43.

97. McDonald RH, Jr., Goldberg LI, McNay JL, Tuttle EP, Jr. Effect of dopamine in man: augmentation of sodium excretion, glomerular filtration rate, and renal plasma flow. *J Clin Invest* 1964;**43**:1116–24.

98. Maestracci P, Grimaud D, Livrelli N, Philip F, Dolisi C. Increase in hepatic blood flow and cardiac output during dopamine infusion in man. *Crit Care Med* 1981;**9** (1):14–16.

99. Sato Y, Matsuzawa H, Eguchi S. Comparative study of effects of adrenaline, dobutamine and dopamine on systemic hemodynamics and renal blood flow in patients following open heart surgery. *Jpn Circ J* 1982;**46** (10):1059–72.

100. Carroll JD, Lang RM, Neumann AL, Borow KM, Rajfer SI. The differential effects of positive inotropic and vasodilator therapy on diastolic properties in patients with congestive cardiomyopathy. *Circulation* 1986;**74**(4):815–25.

101. Johnston AJ, Steiner LA, O'Connell M, et al. Pharmacokinetics and pharmacodynamics of dopamine and norepinephrine in critically ill head-injured patients. *Intens Care Med* 2004;**30**(1):45–50.

102. Vatner SF, Higgins CB, Braunwald E. Effects of norepinephrine on coronary circulation and left ventricular dynamics in the conscious dog. *Circ Res* 1974;**34**(6):812–23.

103. Goertz AW, Lindner KH, Seefelder C, et al. Effect of phenylephrine bolus administration on global left ventricular function in patients with coronary artery disease and patients with valvular aortic stenosis. *Anesthesiology* 1993;**78** (5):834–41.

104. Goertz AW, Schmidt M, Seefelder C, Lindner KH, Georgieff M. The effect of phenylephrine bolus administration on left ventricular function during isoflurane-induced hypotension. *Anesth Analg* 1993;**77**(2):227–31.

105. Fowler NO, Westcott RN, Scott RC, Mc GJ. The effect of norepinephrine upon pulmonary arteriolar resistance in man. *J Clin Invest* 1951;**30**(5):517–24.

106. King BD, Sokoloff L, Wechsler RL. The effects of l-epinephrine and l-norepinephrine upon cerebral circulation and metabolism in man. *J Clin Invest* 1952;**31**(3):273–9.

107. Sensenbach W, Madison L, Ochs L. A comparison of the effects of l-norepinephrine, synthetic l-epinephrine, and U.S.P. epinephrine upon cerebral blood flow and metabolism in man. *J Clin Invest* 1953;**32**(3):226–32.

108. Sharrock NE, Go G, Mineo R, Harpel PC. The hemodynamic and fibrinolytic response to low dose epinephrine and phenylephrine infusions during total hip replacement under epidural anesthesia. *Thromb Haemost* 1992;**68**(4):436–41.

109. Brooker RF, Butterworth JF, 4th, Kitzman DW, et al. Treatment of hypotension after hyperbaric tetracaine spinal anesthesia. A randomized, double-blind, cross-over comparison of phenylephrine and epinephrine. *Anesthesiology* 1997;**86** (4):797–805.

110. Rosenblum R, Berkowitz WD, Lawson D. Effect of acute intravenous administration of

isoproterenol on cardiorenal hemodynamics in man. *Circulation* 1968;**38(1)**: 158–68.

111. Renard M, Bernard R. Clinical and hemodynamic effects of dobutamine in acute myocardial infarction with left heart failure. *J Cardiovasc Pharmacol* 1980;**2** **(5)**:543–52.

112. Ruffolo RR, Jr. The pharmacology of dobutamine. *Am J Med Sci* 1987;**294(4)**:244–8.

113. Akhtar N, Mikulic E, Cohn JN, Chaudhry MH. Hemodynamic effect of dobutamine in patients with severe heart failure. *Am J Cardiol* 1975;**36(2)**:202–5.

114. Leier CV, Webel J, Bush CA. The cardiovascular effects of the continuous infusion of dobutamine in patients with severe cardiac failure. *Circulation* 1977;**56(3)**:468–72.

115. Sonnenblick EH, Frishman WH, LeJemtel TH. Dobutamine: a new synthetic cardioactive sympathetic amine. *N Engl J Med* 1979;**300** **(1)**:17–22.

116. Ukkonen H, Saraste M, Akkila J, et al. Myocardial efficiency during calcium sensitization with levosimendan: a noninvasive study with positron emission tomography and echocardiography in healthy volunteers. *Clin Pharmacol Ther* 1997;**61** **(5)**:596–607.

Chapter

12

Cardiovascular physiology applied to critical care and anesthesia

Nils Siegenthaler and Karim Bendjelid

Introduction

Hemodynamic management of the patient in a perioperative setting and especially in intensive care is considered a cornerstone of patient treatment.[1,2] Guidelines and protocols provide a standard basis for the management of such patients. However, mastering the cardiovascular physiology, and identifying the pathophysiological mechanisms and archetypes involved, allow the clinician to manage each situation according to the specific characteristics of the state of the patient. Moreover, implementation of hemodynamic monitoring at the bedside faces many challenges.

Monitoring devices and hemodynamic markers assessed at the bedside have evolved significantly over the last 30 years, resulting in the availability of a large variety of methods and procedures with specific features and limitations. In the present setting, adequate use of these devices and machines requires a full knowledge of the concepts used to obtain the measured parameters. Thus, in order to guide therapy, physician skills should be based on physiological concepts rather than on simple guidelines.[3,4] Indeed, no hemodynamic monitoring, *per se*, has been associated with an improvement in patient survival[5–9] unless integrated in an early and clinically relevant therapy.[1] Finally, the habitually measured macrohemodynamic parameters may not always allow assessment of tissue perfusion. Indeed, in some circumstances, macrocirculatory perfusion may be decoupled from microcirculation perfusion, resulting in situations where, even if macrocirculatory parameters are adequate, tissue hypoperfusion may persist.[10,11]

The objective of the present chapter is to describe the essential physiological mechanisms involved in the hemodynamic management of patients in a perioperative setting and in intensive care. The chapter was conceived primarily to provide up-to-date information to anesthesiologists and intensivists in order to be able to understand adequately measured hemodynamic parameters and to adapt the therapy according to the pathophysiological state of patients.

Hemodynamics and oxygenation

The "Pathway of oxygen," described previously by the Swiss biologist ER Weibel, successively combines a system able to extract oxygen from the atmosphere and eliminate CO_2 produced by the cells, i.e., the respiratory system. Then, the cardiovascular system is charged to transport oxygen from the lungs to the tissues. Within the cells, cellular respiration will use the oxygen to produce adenosine triphosphate and other high-energy compounds through aerobic metabolism. The cardiovascular system can be separated into two circulations, with specific characteristics, arranged in series. Macrocirculation, which includes the heart, arteries and veins, is responsible for the transport of oxygen to the organs and for the transport of metabolic wastes to their elimination sites. Microcirculation includes arterioles, capillaries, and venules and ensures adequate and homogeneous perfusion of tissues. Even if these two systems are arranged in series, the specificity of each system means there may be a situation where, despite one part seeming to operate correctly, the other one may be altered. This particular state, called macro-microcirculatory decoupling, explains why in specific situations, signs of tissue hypoperfusion may persist despite normalization and optimization of macrohemodynamic parameters.[11]

The hemodynamic goal of macrocirculation is to generate an oxygenated blood flow (DO_2). DO_2 is

Perioperative Hemodynamic Monitoring and Goal Directed Therapy, ed. Maxime Cannesson and Rupert Pearse.
Published by Cambridge University Press. © Cambridge University Press 2014.

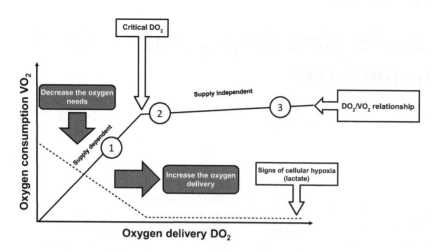

Figure 12.1. The relationship between total cellular consumption of oxygen (VO$_2$) and the O$_2$ delivery (DO$_2$). In the supply independent zone, a decrease in DO$_2$ is compensated by an increase in O$_2$ extraction, which preserves O$_2$ cellular need without change in O$_2$ consumption. A further decrease in DO$_2$, under the critical point of DO$_2$, could not be compensated by an increase in O$_2$ extraction, and thus will result in a decrease in O$_2$ cellular consumption. Two therapeutic strategies can allow the re-equilibration of DO$_2$/VO$_2$ relationship: a decrease in O$_2$ needs or an increase in DO$_2$. (1) Low DO$_2$/VO$_2$ relationship indicating shock state. (2) adequate DO$_2$/VO$_2$ relationship. (3) high DO$_2$/VO$_2$ relationship representing supra-physiologic resuscitation.

defined as the quantity of oxygen per unit of volume of blood (CaO$_2$ = [1.39 × Hb (g.liter^{-1})] × [SaO$_2$ (%)] + [(0.23 × PaO$_2$ k Pa^{-1})]) debited at a rate equivalent to the cardiac output (CO) in liters per minute (DO$_2$ = CO × CaO$_2$). DO$_2$ is adequate when the present value is equivalent to the metabolic oxygen requirement (oxygen consumption: VO$_2$). The relationship linking DO$_2$ to VO$_2$ presents with two zones (Figure 12.1). Initially, a decrease in DO$_2$ is compensated by an increase in extraction of oxygen in order to maintain the aerobic metabolism (zone of supply independency). However, when DO$_2$ decreases further, oxygen extraction may not be able to compensate for the decrease in delivery (critical DO$_2$ point) and cells suffer from a lack of oxygen, limiting their aerobic metabolism, which may result in cellular hypoxia, ischemia, lactate production, and lastly death (zone of supply dependency) (Figure 12.1). Therefore, the goal of tissue resuscitation is to use any method possible to balance the relationship between DO$_2$ and VO$_2$. A therapeutic management that allows achievement of a high DO$_2$ value (far above VO$_2$) may also result in the situation of supraphysiologic oxygenation that has been demonstrated to be associated with an excess of morbidity and mortality (Figure 12.1).[12] The present concept of DO$_2$/VO$_2$ balance applies not only in a global shock state, but also in a situation where local perfusion is altered (intracranial hypertension, cerebral vasospasm, mesenteric ischemia, intra-abdominal compartment syndrome). Imbalance between DO$_2$/VO$_2$ can be identified by the occurrence of signs of cellular hypoxia (Figure 12.1): organ dysfunction (oliguria, confusion),

elevation in the plasmatic concentration of lactate, or signs of excessive extraction of oxygen (low venous blood saturation).

Equilibration of DO$_2$/VO$_2$ can be obtained by two methods (Figure 12.1): a decrease in the oxygen requirement (VO$_2$) or an increase in the oxygen delivery (DO$_2$). First, VO$_2$ depends mainly on cellular metabolism, which may be increased by a rise in cellular metabolism (temperature or muscular activity). In a critically ill patient, the respiratory cost of spontaneous breathing may be important. Field et al. estimated the cost of breathing in a patient with cardiorespiratory disease to be about 24% of the VO$_2$ total, but it may be higher in specific patients.[13] Therefore, respiratory support to decrease VO$_2$ may allow re-equilibration of the DO$_2$/VO$_2$ relationship until DO$_2$ improves. This concept is especially important in a patient where a refractory low cardiac output limits the DO$_2$. For example, after a cardiopulmonary bypass, myocardial function may be transitorily decreased, limiting DO$_2$. In this case, the increased cost of breathing during an early weaning of positive pressure ventilation can be associated with a DO$_2$/VO$_2$ imbalance, resulting in cellular hypoxia.

The second way to re-equilibrate DO$_2$/VO$_2$ is to increase DO$_2$ (Figure 12.2). The arterial oxygen content, CaO$_2$, can be optimized by increasing the hemoglobin content or by raising the SaO$_2$. The usual goal is to achieve a hemoglobin concentration between 7.0 and 9.0 g/dL. SaO$_2$ could be increased by raising FiO$_2$ or by improving the pulmonary gas exchange (decreasing the pulmonary shunt [zones with low ventilation/perfusion ratio]).

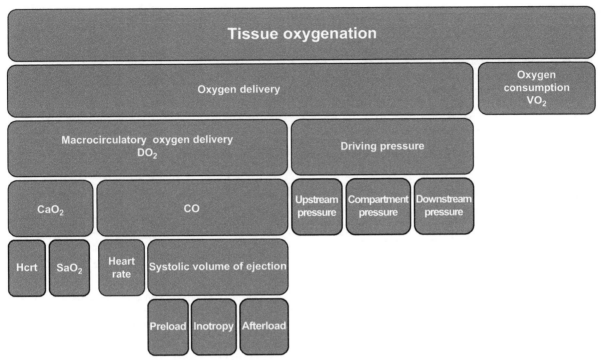

Figure 12.2. Hemodynamic determinants of tissue oxygenation. Tissue oxygenation is adequate when O_2 delivery is equilibrated with O_2 needs. O_2 delivery is determined by the arterial content in oxygen (CaO_2 × cardiac output (CO)). The main determinants of CaO_2 are the arterial mass in red cells (Hematocrit: Hcrt) and the O_2 arterial hemoglobin saturation (SaO_2). CO is determined by the stroke volume multiplied by the heart rate. The value of preload, inotropy, and afterload influence stroke volume. A sufficient driving pressure across the tissue is mandatory in order to maintain tissue perfusion. Driving pressure is determined by the upstream pressure (arterial pressure), the downstream pressure (venous pressure), and the pressure around the tissue.

As optimization of DO_2 by SaO_2 and hemoglobin concentration is limited, CO is thus the main determinant of DO_2 in a shock state. CO is defined as the systolic volume (SV) of ejection (stroke volume: SV) multiplied by the heart rate ($CO \text{ (liter min}^{-1}) = SV \text{ (liter)} \times HR \text{ (beat min}^{-1})$) (Figure 12.2). The three main determinants of SV are ventricular preload, ventricular inotropy, and ventricular afterload (or aortic impedance in a pulsatile system). Each of these determinants will be discussed separately in the next part of the chapter. The second determinant of CO is heart rate. Heart rate must be high enough to ensure CO; however, an increase in heart rate is at the expense of a decreased duration of diastole, necessary to generate enough preload, and is associated with an increase in myocardial work. Finally, even if a macrocirculatory oxygenated blood flow is generated (optimal DO_2), it must be transmitted to arterial and tissue circulation. Therefore, arterial pressure must be enough to overcome vascular resistance and downstream pressure, maintaining an adequate perfusion pressure (blood flow = perfusion pressure/resistance).

Perfusion pressure, often called driving pressure, depends on upstream pressure (aortic or postarteriolar pressure for the capillary circulation) and on downstream pressure (venous pressure) (Figure 12.3A). In some cases (intracranial hypertension, abdominal compartment syndrome, limb compartment syndrome), pressure surrounding the tissue is higher than downstream vascular pressure. In this situation, similarly to a Starling resistor, the external pressure will determine driving pressure and thus the flow across the tissue (Figure 12.3B). Flow can be maintained by increasing the arterial pressure (therapeutic hypertension) or by lowering the extramural tissue pressure (decompressive craniectomy, opening of the abdominal wall, draining excessive abdominal fluid, fasciotomy). An increase in downstream vascular pressure (high central venous pressure) may also limit perfusion pressure and may

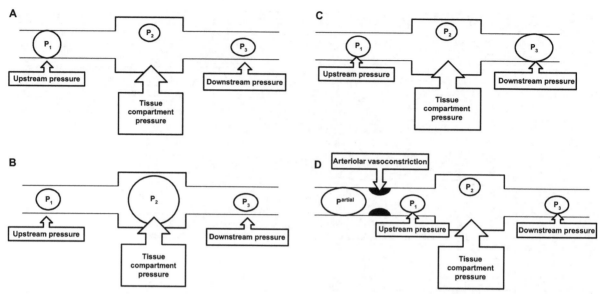

Figure 12.3. The main hemodynamic determinant of the driving pressure (i.e., pressure allowing perfusion of tissue). Upstream pressure represents input arterial pressure and downstream pressure represents the outlet venous pressure. The tissue compartment pressure represents the pressure around the tissue. In a normal situation (A) upstream pressure is higher than downstream pressure, that is higher than the tissue compartment pressure resulting in a positive, driving pressure allowing tissue perfusion. When the tissue compartment pressure increases (intracranial hypertension, abdominal compartment, etc.) at a value higher than downstream pressure, the pressure surrounding the organ determines the flow across the tissue. In the case where the present pressure increases more than the upstream pressure, blood flow across the tissue ceases. In various situations, such as venous congestion, increasing downstream pressure may also limit the blood flow across the tissue, even if upstream pressure seems adequate (C). The upstream pressure of the capillaries lies next to the arteriolar site of vasoconstriction. Therefore, when arteriolar vasoconstriction is excessive, even if arterial pressure may be high, upstream pressure determining the driving pressure across capillaries may be low, resulting in a decreased tissue blood flow.

contribute to organ dysfunction (venous congestion), as in the cardio-renal syndrome, for example (Figure 12.3C).[14,15] Finally, even if the arterial pressure seems adequate, increasing arteriolar vasoconstriction induced by the use of vasopressors, for example, may be responsible for significant perfusion pressure loss (Figure 12.3D). Consequently, postarteriolar pressure decreases, leading to a decrease in capillary perfusion pressure, inducing tissue hypoperfusion. This mechanism (peripheral resistance-induced macro-microcirculatory decoupling) can be observed in the distal limb of hypovolemic patients under high doses of norepinephrine.

Preload and venous return

To improve SV, preload must be adequate. Excessive preload, especially in cases of decreased ventricular compliance, however, may be associated with the high ventricular pressure responsible for pulmonary and/or systemic congestion. Preload is defined as the degree of tension of the cardiac muscle (stretching of cardiomyocyte) before contraction. As this cannot be measured directly, clinicians may estimate preload either by volumetric indices or by ventricular filling pressure measurements. Since volumetric indices may be better related with the degree of stretch of the myocardium than with pressure, preload can be defined as the ventricular end-diastolic volume.[16]

The volume–pressure relationship depends on the compliance of the cavity. Any change in ventricular compliance may change the measured pressure for the same volume. Therefore, a preload state may be the same for different measured pressures. Moreover, measured pressures reflect intra-cavitary pressures and not the physiologically relevant transmural pressures (transmural pressure = intra-cavitary Pr –extra-mural Pr). As a result, no static parameters (central venous pressure, pulmonary artery occlusion pressure) allow accurate preload estimations.

The preload has two roles: to provide enough fluid to be ejected and to recruit the force of contraction through the Frank–Starling mechanism.

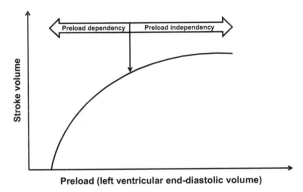

Figure 12.4. Starling's law of the heart. The relationship between ventricular preload and stroke volume determines the heart function curve. The heart function curve can be separated in to two zones, depending on the effect of change in preload on the stroke volume. In the preload-dependent zone, an increase in preload will result in a significant increase in stroke volume and thus in cardiac output. In the preload independent zone, a further increase in preload will no longer result in a significant increase in stroke volume.

The Frank–Starling law of the heart states that, over a specific range of preload, an increase in preload will result in an increase in ejection volume defining a situation of preload dependency (Figure 12.4). Above a certain preload, the force of contraction cannot be increased. Over this range of preload, any increase in preload will be associated with an increase in ventricular pressure, with no increase in SV, defining a situation of preload independency. In clinical practice, fluid infusion may improve the hemodynamic state only if the specific function of the heart is in a preload-dependent state. Otherwise, fluid infusion will result in fluid overload. For the left heart, fluid overload and associated high ventricular pressure can induce a rise in pulmonary capillary pressure, resulting in pulmonary edema. The amplitude of the increase in pressure depends on left ventricular compliance, therefore in a situation where the left ventricular (LV) compliance is low, as in LV diastolic dysfunction (acute ischemia, ventricular hypertrophy) a rise in LV end-diastolic pressure could be significant. Therefore, with low LV compliance, the optimal range of ventricular volume is also narrow.

Ventricular preload is generated by the venous return to the heart.[17–19] The venous compartment contains a large fraction of the total systemic blood volume (70%). The part of this volume that did not contribute to pressure generation is called the unstressed blood volume (i.e., venous blood volume at a venous transmural pressure near zero).

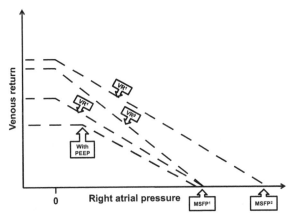

Figure 12.5. The relationship between venous return and right atrial pressure (i.e., the downstream pressure or back pressure of venous return) at different values of mean systemic filling pressure (MSFP; representing the upstream pressure of venous return) and venous resistance (VR). At a fixed MSFP, venous return increases when the right atrial pressure decreases until a negative venous transmural pressure results in a venous collapse, limiting a further increase in the venous return. At a constant resistance to the venous return (VR[1]), an increase in MSFP (MSFP[1] to MSFP[2]) will result, at any fixed value of right atrial pressure, in an increase in venous return. On the other hand, at a fixed value of MSFP (MSFP[1]), a decrease in venous resistance will result in a higher venous return for any fixed value of right atrial pressure. Positive pressure ventilation with PEEP will result in a right-ward shift in the venous return curve, limiting the return of blood to the heart.

This volume keeps the venous system open, but without pressure. Then, as the venous blood volume increases, the venous pressure will increase and determine the stressed blood volume (i.e., venous blood volume above the unstressed blood volume that is responsible for the generation of a positive venous transmural pressure). Magder et al. suggested that the stressed blood volume represents only a quarter of the total blood volume, providing a large reserve of unstressed blood volume.[20] As soon as the stressed blood volume generates a pressure above the downward pressure (right atrial pressure), the positive pressure gradient generates a flow: the venous return. The venous return is thus determined by the pressure difference (driving pressure of the venous return) between upstream pressure (mean systemic filling pressure: MSFP) and downstream pressure (right atrial pressure [RAP]) and can be described by the equation: Venous return = (MSFP – RAP) / Venous resistance (Figure 12.5). Venous return will then increase if MSFP increases for a constant RAP and venous resistance, or if RAP decreases with a constant MSFP and venous resistance. However, if RAP decreases under a critical pressure (close to the extramural pressure), the transmural pressure becomes negative, leading to the collapse of the vein, limiting the flow of the venous return. This phenomenon of flow limitation may protect the heart from excessive venous return (excessive ventricular preload) when the patient generates very low pleural pressure, for example, during high inspiratory effort.

As pressure and volume are linked by compliance, MSFP pressure may increase as a consequence of two interventions: an increase in volume, such as during fluid expansion, for a constant venous compliance, or by a decrease in venous compliance with a constant volume, such as following venoconstriction.[21] Fluid loading increases the stressed blood volume without impacting on the unstressed blood volume, while venoconstriction contributes unstressed blood toward the stressed blood volume. At the bedside, clinicians may thus increase venous return, and consequently ventricular preload, by infusing fluid or by inducing venoconstriction (phenylephrine, norepinephrine). Fluid infusion may be more efficient, as the second determinant of venous return, apart from the driving pressure, is the venous resistance (Figure 12.5).

For any driving pressure, venous return decreases when venous resistance increases. Fluid infusion increases the diameter of the vein and thus reduces the venous resistance, while the impact of venoconstriction on venous resistance is difficult to predict (there are different effects on large veins from those on venules). Various situations may increase the venous resistance to flow. For instance, an increased intra-abdominal pressure (abdominal compartment syndrome, pregnancy) may limit venous return, despite an insufficient increase in MSFP. This situation may result in a preload-dependent decrease in cardiac output that would not necessarily respond to fluid infusion or venoconstriction, but that would dramatically improve after freeing up the abdominal constraint (opening the abdominal wall or draining the cavity).

Generation of the ventricular preload is mainly determined by the diastolic phase of the heart cycle (relaxation phase), and a normal heart filling is almost completed at early diastole. However, in situations characterized by an alteration of the relaxation phase (diastolic failure), filling needs time, and occurs during the entire diastole. Therefore, any factor that would decrease the capacity of the ventricle to fill may be associated with a limitation in preload generation. This situation may occur when ventricular compliance is decreased by intrinsic change of the ventricle

(hypertrophic cardiomyopathy) or by extrinsic factors (pericardial restriction, cardiac tamponade, or lung hyperinflation). Duration of the diastole and the contribution of the atrial contraction (30%–40% of the filling) to ventricular filling may then limit generation of the preload.[22]

Assessment of the preload and especially the preload dependency–independency state is difficult. The static preload parameters (central venous pressure or pulmonary artery occlusion pressure) that are influenced by various physiological parameters (volume, compliance, heart function, or extramural pressure), do not allow adequate prediction of fluid responsiveness.[23,24] The dynamic parameters (pulse pressure variation [PPV] or stroke volume variation) are better indices as they are based on the influence of cardiopulmonary interactions, which are amplified in a state of preload dependency (see heart–lung interactions).

Inotropy (contractility)

The second determinant of stroke volume, cardiac inotropy, refers to the intrinsic ability of the myocardial muscle to change its generation of force independently of the preload. Inotropy can be described in various terms: in terms of a length–tension relationship (Frank–Starling curves: as an increase in tension for a determined length [preload]); as the maximal force generated at any ventricular volume (end-systolic pressure–volume relationship); in terms of a force (afterload)–velocity (of muscle shortening) relationship; as an increase in velocity of shortening at zero force (Vmax); or as an increase in the rate of pressure generation that can be estimated by the ratio of pressure change (dP) over a period of time (dt) : dP/dt.

With a constant value of preload and afterload, the consequence of a variation in inotropy is a change in stroke volume. When inotropy decreases, the Frank–Starling curve is shifted downward and to the right, resulting in decreased stroke volume, increased end-diastolic volume, and increased end-diastolic pressure (Figure 12.6). The amplitude of the increase in end-diastolic pressure depends on the ventricular compliance. In terms of preload, a decrease in inotropy may thus transform a state of preload dependency into a state of preload independency. Conversely, an increase in inotropy will results in increased stroke volume, decreased end-diastolic volume, and decreased pressure. Usually, this change in preload can be observed at the bedside after initiation of

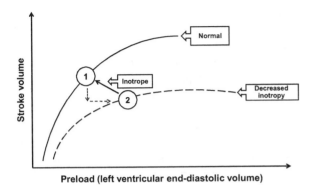

Figure 12.6. Relationship between ventricular preload and stroke volume whatever the contractility. As ventricular contractility (inotropy) decreases, the heart function curve is shifted right and downwards (1 to 2) resulting in a decrease in stroke volume and an increase in left ventricular end-diastolic volume. Inotropic drugs may improve stoke volume, while decreasing left ventricular end-diastolic volume and thus ventricular pressure as the heart function curve returns toward the baseline.

inotropes that induces a decrease in central venous pressure or pulmonary artery occlusion pressure. The present paradigm explains why a fixed static value of central venous pressure or pulmonary artery occlusion pressure is not able to accurately estimate fluid responsiveness.

Myocardial contraction is related to actin–myosin interaction, facilitated by calcium (Ca^{2+}) binding to troponin C and ATP. To maintain or improve inotropy, first, oxygen delivery must be adapted to the cellular needs. Unlike other organs, the myocardium has a low reserve of oxygen extraction that can compensate for a decrease in oxygen supply. (Oxygen extraction of the left ventricular myocardium is close to 75% at rest.) The myocardium must thus depend on an increase in coronary blood flow to meet increased metabolic demand. Coronary perfusion must then be maintained and the coronary flow reserve (the difference between resting and maximal coronary blood flow) must be adequate, otherwise the force of contraction may be limited. If hypoxia persists, cellular ischemia will ensue, inducing transitory or definitive loss of cardiac cells and myocardial function.[25,26]

Before stimulating the myocardium with inotropes, it is therefore essential that the coronary flow reserve can meet the increased demand in oxygen by the myocardium. Once myocardial oxygen delivery has been confirmed, inotropic stimulation may be used. Inotropes increase contractility by different pathways: by stimulation of beta-adrenergic receptors – subtype 1 (dopamine, dobutamine, isoprenaline, adrenalin),

inhibition of intracellular cAMP corrosion by the inhibition of phosphodiesterase III (Milrinone), or by an improvement in the efficiency of myofilament contraction (calcium sensitizers). Although they allow an acute increase in the force of contraction, catecholamines may also lead, in excess, to stress cardiomyopathy, resulting in a decrease in heart function. Increased sensibility to circulating catecholamines at the apex of the heart may explain the geometric characteristics of takotsubo cardiomyopathy.[27,28]

Afterload

The afterload is the tension developed by the ventricle during ejection and can be considered as the load (impedance in a pulsatile system) against which the heart must contract in order to open the aortic valve and promote forward flow (blood ejection). The end-systolic ventricular pressure defines this parameter.[16] Afterload can be described, according to Laplace's law, as the repeated instantaneous wall stress of the ventricles, ventricular wall stress being wall tension (ventricular pressure × ventricular radius, during ejection) divided by wall thickness. Thus, afterload integrates various parameters: ventricular structure, ventricular function, impedance, and resistance to the ejection. This last component, when aortic or pulmonary valve or outflow tract are normal, is mainly determined by the characteristics of the arteries (systemic or pulmonary arterial load). To maintain the same ejection, an increase in afterload will be associated with an increase in the myocardial work. If the ventricle is unable to generate enough work, the volume of ejection will decrease, resulting in a reduction of the cardiac output and an increase in ventricular volume (Figure 12.7).

Afterload must then be maintained as low as possible, especially in situations with a decreased contractility and for the right ventricle. However, a certain amount of aortic pressure is mandatory for maintaining coronary perfusion and the driving pressure of organ perfusion. Therefore, in cases where an afterload value cannot be tolerated, mechanical assistance (intra-aortic balloon counterpulsation, ventricular assistance, etc...) may be required.

Specificity of the right ventricle

The right ventricle (RV) differs from the left ventricle (LV) in various ways and can be considered to be a high-volume-low-pressure pump (volume primed but

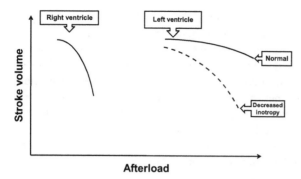

Figure 12.7. Influence of afterload on right- and left-ventricular stroke volume. On the left side of the heart, the stroke volume of a normal left ventricle is influenced only at high afterload, as ventricular work reserve is high. However, at decreased left ventricular contractility (decreased inotropy), stroke work reserve may not allow compensation for an increase in afterload and may result in a decrease in stroke volume. Unlike the left ventricle, due to anatomical structural and geometrical factors the right ventricle does not tolerate any further increases in afterload.

pressure unprepared). The RV is thinner (one-sixth of the LV), decreasing its capacity of force generation. Its geometry is crescent-shaped, lying on the LV and it contracts inward, longitudinally, and by traction on the free wall, resulting in greater longitudinal than radial shortening. As the RV lies on, and is bound to, the LV through the septum, its contractility is partly generated by the LV.[29] Unlike the LV, the RV is highly sensitive to afterload, relying on preload and force of contraction (Figure 12.7). Moreover, the RV is excessively preload sensitive allowing it to recruit a force of contraction through the Frank–Starling mechanism. However, volume overload of the RV may result in right–left ventricular interaction, impairing left ventricular diastolic function.[30,31]

Heart–lung interactions

It is essential to understand heart–lung interactions in order to understand hemodynamic interactions in patients under mechanical ventilation and during the assessment of dynamic parameters of preload.[32,33]

Influence of static heart–lung interactions on preload

A stable increase in intrathoracic pressure (PEEP) has multiple influences. First, pressure may be transmitted to the right atrium, resulting in a decrease in the pressure gradient of venous return. Second, the influence of intrathoracic pressure on venous return may be amplified through an increase in venous

resistance.[34] Both of these effects result in a decrease in venous return, ventricular preload, and thus right ventricular stroke volume,[32,35] but can be limited by a simultaneous increase in mean systemic filling pressure (the input pressure of the venous return), maintaining the venous return. This adaptation to increased intrathoracic pressure (PEEP) is mediated through neurohumoral[36] and mechanical factors,[37] but may be blunted during hypovolemia. This explains why PEEP may induce a significant decrease in cardiac output in hypovolemic patients that generally improves after fluid replacement. It must be noted that severe lung inflation may induce a progressive compression of the heart, resulting in a restriction of ventricular diastolic filling.[38]

Influence of static heart–lung interactions on afterload

During the inspiration phase of positive pressure ventilation, the aortic transmural pressure decreases (increase in pleural pressure), reducing the left ventricular afterload and favoring ejection. This effect can be especially beneficial in the presence of left ventricular heart failure. Conversely, during spontaneous respiration, the decrease in pleural pressure will result in an increase in left ventricular afterload (increase in aortic transmural pressure), imposing a greater load on the LV.

The effect of heart–lung interaction on the right ventricle is different. As the lung volume increases above its functional residual capacity, in spontaneous or positive pressure ventilation, the pulmonary arterial resistance increases due to the compression of the vascular bed (capillaries) by the expanding lung (increase in lung West zones I and II at the expense of zone III).[39]

Cyclic influence of mechanical ventilation on the hemodynamic state

First, as already stated, on the right side, a positive intrathoracic pressure is responsible for an increase in right atrial pressure and an increase in venous resistance to the venous flow, resulting in a decrease in venous return. Second, as the expanding lung volume increases the right ventricular afterload, right ventricular ejection decreases, resulting in a decrease in transpulmonary blood flow. This limits the left ventricular preload, which may decrease further in the case of right ventricular volume or pressure overload (septal shift to the left compresses the LV and limits its diastolic expansion, decreasing LV compliance). After a few heartbeats, corresponding to the pulmonary vascular transit time, the left ventricular preload decreases, with a concomitant decrease in LV stroke volume.

The relative increase in venous return on the right side during expiration results in an increase in left ventricular preload and SV a few heartbeats later, during the mechanical breath. Moreover, at inspiration, the increase in transpulmonary pressure ($P_{alv} > P_{pl}$) expands lung volume and may "squeeze" the capillaries, recruiting lung blood and resulting in an early and transitory increase in the left ventricular preload.[40] At the same time, due to the increase in pleural pressure, the left ventricular afterload decreases, resulting in an increase in LV stroke volume.

Various factors may affect these heart–lung interactions during positive pressure ventilation. In hypovolemia, resulting in a state of preload dependency, the amplitude of the variation of left ventricular ejection increases with ventilation. When there is spontaneous respiration during positive pressure ventilation, as pleural pressure and alveolar pressure are influenced by movable respiratory rate and spontaneous effort, cardiopulmonary interactions described may be unpredictable. The tidal volume also influences the importance of cardiopulmonary interaction, particularly because of the influence of lung volume on transpulmonary pressure.

Cardiopulmonary interactions may be used to treat patients. For example, the physiological management of pulmonary edema is determined by the relation between the left ventricular volume and compliance. An elevated left ventricular pressure induces a postcapillary pulmonary vascular hypertension responsible for initial interstitial edema. Left ventricular pressure rises as ventricular volume increases and/or as ventricular compliance decreases. Therefore, in clinical practice, the treatment of pulmonary edema consists of reducing ventricular pressure essentially by a decrease in the end-diastolic volume (preload). This can be achieved by decreasing venous return through increasing venous compliance with venodilatators, a decrease in blood volume (diuretics), or by positive pressure ventilation (decreasing venous return to the LV). Moreover, the left ventricular volume can be decreased by increasing left ventricular ejection through decreasing afterload.[41]

Considering the weaning of positive pressure ventilation, two factors therefore seem important: heart function must be recovered and fluid overload avoided. Positive pressure ventilation decreases the oxygen requirement from the respiratory muscles and supports the heart, assisting systolic function and limiting venous return. Thus weaning failure may be due to the inability of the hemodynamic system to support the new physiology and maintain oxygen supply to the organs. First, heart function must have recovered sufficiently to support the decreased assistance of the LV by positive intrathoracic pressure. An apparent imbalance DO_2/VO_2 during weaning, representing an inability of the heart to ensure the increased oxygen demand, can be assessed by various means, for example, by the trend of central venous blood saturation.[42] Second, as positive pressure limits the venous return and thus protects the heart (Figure 12.5), any excess circulating blood volume must be avoided before weaning of positive pressure ventilation. An increase in ventricular pressure (pulmonary artery occlusion pressure, for example) during weaning may indicate an inadequacy between the increase in venous return and the heart function.[43]

Dynamic cardiopulmonary interactions may also be used to determine the physiologic state of the hemodynamic system. Dynamic indices of preload, used to predict a state of preload dependency, originate from these interactions. Among the dynamic indices, pulse pressure variation is widely used (Figure 12.8). The origin of pulse pressure variation is related to cyclic perturbation of the cardiovascular system by the respiratory system. The perturbator (respiratory system) increases or decreases the LV volume of ejection as discussed previously. However, to be clinically relevant, the present perturbation must be sufficient (enough tidal volume [> 6 mL/kg], stable chest compliance, stable transmission of pressure), unperturbed with constant respiratory cycles (no spontaneous respiration), and a stable cardiovascular system (regular cardiac rhythm).

From macrocirculation to microcirculation

Microcirculation is the "vital" part of the cardiovascular system, consisting of a network of small vessels (5–200 μm) including arterioles, capillaries, and

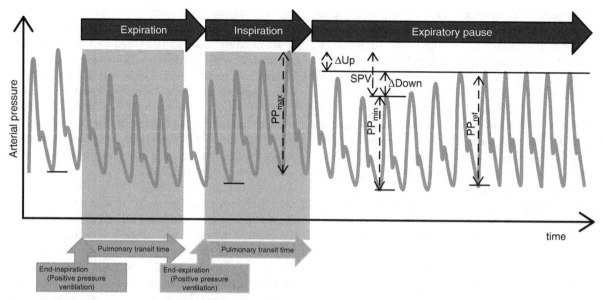

Figure 12.8. Arterial pressure variations during positive pressure ventilation without spontaneous effort. Due to cardiopulmonary interactions, inspiration induces a decrease in right ventricular stroke volume, due to a decrease in venous return and an increase in right ventricular afterload. After a few heart beats (pulmonary transit time), the present decrease affects the left ventricular filling and stroke volume. The pulse pressure (PP) represents the difference between systolic and diastolic arterial pressure. Pulse pressure is maximal (PP_{max}) a few heart beats after the end of expiration and lower (PP_{min}) a few heart beats after inspiration. The difference between maximal and minimal pulse pressure determines the pulse pressure variation (PP_v). The difference between maximal and minimal systolic pressure define the systolic pressure variation (SPV) that comprises two values (ΔUp and ΔDown), according to the reference value of systolic arterial pressure (PP_{ref}) obtained after an expiratory pause.

venules.[11] Its function resides in the regulation of exchanges between blood flow and tissue. Therefore, its anatomical and functional integrity is essential to assure cellular oxygenation.

Microcirculatory perfusion is determined by macrocirculatory parameters (arterial blood pressure, viscosity, DO_2) and by specific microcirculatory parameters. In various situations, microcirculatory perfusion may be decoupled from macrocirculatory parameters. During septic shock, for example, tissue hypoperfusion may persist, despite normal macrocirculatory parameters. Consequently, in some cases, commonly measured macrocirulatory parameters may not allow prediction of tissue perfusion. Various mechanisms contribute to changes in microvascular perfusion: perfusion pressure, rheological factors, and alteration of the microcirculation autoregulation. Considering capillary perfusion pressure, the input pressure of the capillary bed resides in the vascular pressure next to the arteriole, which is the main site of vasoconstriction and resistance (capillaries are devoid of muscular tissue). Therefore, an increased arteriolar vasoconstriction results in an increase in

macrocirculatory pressure, but it may also be associated with a paradoxical reduction in the capillary bed perfusion pressure, due to the loss of pressure in the highly resistant arteriolar vascular network.[44]

Conclusions

In summary, the key to treating the changes that occur in a patient's cardiovascular status is understanding the underlying physiology and how this has been disturbed. When applied to anesthesia and critical care, cardiovascular physiology provides paradigms and knowledge that could be used to treat patients and to improve their critical state on a daily basis. Recently, great progress was made in perioperative hemodynamic monitoring and goal directed therapy for these kinds of patients, with a primary focus on concepts and algorithms able to assess cardiovascular integration and tissue resuscitation. At the beginning of the new millennium, this evolution is an important indicator, highlighting the major shift of hemodynamic monitoring toward a pragmatic approach.

References

1. Rivers E, Nguyen B, Havstad S, et al. Early goal directed therapy in the treatment of severe sepsis and septic shock. *N Engl J Med* 2001;**345**(19):1368–77.

2. Lees N, Hamilton M, Rhodes A. Clinical review: goal-directed therapy in high risk surgical patients. *Crit Care* 2009;**13**(5):231.

3. Gnaegi A, Feihl F, Perret C. Intensive care physicians' insufficient knowledge of rightheart catheterization at the bedside: time to act? *Crit Care Med* 1997;**25**(2):213–20.

4. Jain M, Canham M, Upadhyay D, Corbridge T. Variability in interventions with pulmonary artery catheter data. *Intensive Care Med* 2003;**29**(11):2059–62.

5. Connors AF, Jr., Speroff T, Dawson NV, et al. The effectiveness of right heart catheterization in the initial care of critically ill patients. SUPPORT Investigators. *JAMA* 1996;**276**(11):889–97.

6. Shah MR, Hasselblad V, Stevenson LW, et al. Impact of the pulmonary artery catheter in critically ill patients: meta-analysis of randomized clinical trials. *JAMA* 2005;**294**(13):1664–70.

7. Harvey S, Young D, Brampton W, et al. Pulmonary artery catheters for adult patients in intensive care. *Cochrane Database Syst Rev* 2006;**19**(3):CD003408.

8. Binanay C, Califf RM, Hasselblad V, et al. Evaluation study of congestive heart failure and pulmonary artery catheterization effectiveness: the ESCAPE trial. *JAMA* 2005;**294**(13):1625–33.

9. Harvey S, Stevens K, Harrison D, et al. An evaluation of the clinical and cost effectiveness of pulmonary artery catheters in patient management in intensive care: a systematic review and a randomised controlled trial. *Health Technol Assess* 2006;**10**(29):1–133.

10. De Backer D, Creteur J, Preiser JC, Dubois MJ, Vincent JL. Microvascular blood flow is altered in patients with sepsis. *Am J Respir Crit Care Med* 2002;**166**(1):98–104.

11. Siegenthaler N, Giraud R, Piriou V, Romand JA, Bendjelid K. Microcirculatory alterations in critically ill patients: pathophysiology, monitoring and treatments. *Ann Fr Anesth Reanim* 2010;**29**(2):135–44.

12. Hayes MA, Timmins AC, Yau EH, et al. Elevation of systemic oxygen delivery in the treatment of critically ill patients. *N Engl J Med* 1994;**330**(24):1717–22.

13. Field S, Kelly SM, Macklem PT. The oxygen cost of breathing in patients with cardiorespiratory disease. *Am Rev Respir Dis* 1982;**126**(1):9–13.

14. Mullens W, Abrahams Z, Francis GS, et al. Importance of venous congestion for worsening of renal function in advanced decompensated heart failure. *J Am Coll Cardiol* 2009;**53**(7):589–96.

15. Tang WH, Mullens W. Cardiorenal syndrome in decompensated heart failure. *Heart* 2010;**96**(4):255–60.

16. Rothe C. Toward consistent definitions for preload and afterload–revisited. *Adv Physiol Educ* 2003;**27**(1–4):44–45.

17. Funk DJ, Jacobsohn E, Kumar A. The role of venous return in critical illness and shock-part I: physiology. *Crit Care Med* 2013;**41**(1):255–62.

18. Funk DJ, Jacobsohn E, Kumar A. Role of the venous return in critical illness and shock: part II-shock and mechanical ventilation. *Crit Care Med* 2013;**41**(2):573–9.

19. Gelman S. Venous function and central venous pressure: a physiologic story. *Anesthesiology* 2008;**108**(4):735–48.

20. Magder S, De Varennes B. Clinical death and the measurement of stressed vascular volume. *Crit Care Med* 1998;**26**(6):1061–4.

21. Monnet X, Jabot J, Maizel J, Richard C, Teboul JL. Norepinephrine increases cardiac preload and reduces preload dependency assessed by passive leg raising in septic shock patients. *Crit Care Med* 2011;**39**(4):689–94.

22. Cohen-Solal A, Logeart D, Tartiere JM. "Diastolic" heart failure, overlooked systolic dysfunction, altered ventriculo-arterial coupling or limitation of cardiac reserve? *Int J Cardiol* 2008;**128**(3):299–303.

23. Coudray A, Romand JA, Treggiari M, Bendjelid K. Fluid responsiveness in spontaneously breathing patients: a review of indexes used in intensive care. *Crit Care Med* 2005; **33**(12):2757–62.

24. Bendjelid K, Romand JA. Fluid responsiveness in mechanically ventilated patients: a review of indices used in intensive care. *Intens Care Med* 2003; **29**(3):352–60.

25. Crystal GJ, Silver JM, Salem MR. Mechanisms of increased right and left ventricular oxygen uptake during inotropic stimulation. *Life Sci* 2013;**93**(2–3):59–63.

26. Tune JD, Gorman MW, Feigl EO. Matching coronary blood flow to myocardial oxygen consumption. *J Appl Physiol* 2004;**97**(1):404–15.

27. Nef HM, Möllmann H, Akashi YJ, Hamm CW. Mechanisms of stress (Takotsubo) cardiomyopathy. *Nat Rev Cardiol* 2010;**7**(4):187–93.

28. Lyon AR, Rees PS, Prasad S, Poole-Wilson PA, Harding SE. Stress (Takotsubo) cardiomyopathy – a novel pathophysiological hypothesis to explain catecholamine-induced acute myocardial stunning. *Nat Clin Pract Cardiovasc Med* 2008;**5**(1):22–9.

29. Buckberg GD; RESTORE Group. The ventricular septum: the lion of right ventricular function, and

its impact on right ventricular restoration. *Eur J Cardiothorac Surg* 2006;**29** Suppl 1:S272–8.

30. Dell'Italia LJ. Anatomy and physiology of the right ventricle. *Cardiol Clin* 2012;**30(2)**:167–87.

31. Haddad F, Hunt SA, Rosenthal DN, Murphy DJ. Right ventricular function in cardiovascular disease, part I: anatomy, physiology, aging, and functional assessment of the right ventricle. *Circulation* 2008;**117(11)**:1436–48.

32. Feihl F, Broccard AF. Interactions between respiration and systemic hemodynamics. Part I: basic concepts. *Intens Care Med* 2009;**35(1)**:45–54.

33. Feihl F, Broccard AF. Interactions between respiration and systemic hemodynamics. Part II: practical implications in critical care. *Intens Care Med* 2009;**35(2)**:198–205.

34. Fessler HE, Brower RG, Wise RA, Permutt S. Effects of positive end-expiratory pressure on the canine venous return curve. *Am Rev Respir Dis* 1992;**146(1)**:4–10.

35. Qvist J, Pontoppidan H, Wilson RS, Lowenstein E, Laver MB. Hemodynamic responses to mechanical ventilation with PEEP: the effect of hypervolemia. *Anesthesiology* 1975;**42(1)**:45–55.

36. Jellinek H, Krenn H, Oczenski W, et al. Influence of positive airway pressure on the pressure gradient for venous return in humans. *J Appl Physiol* 2000;**88(3)**:926–32.

37. Peters J, Hecker B, Neuser D, Schaden W. Regional blood volume distribution during positive and negative airway pressure breathing in supine humans. *J Appl Physiol* 1993;**75(4)**:1740–7.

38. Butler J. The heart is in good hands. *Circulation*. 1983;**67(6)**:1163–8.

39. Whittenberger JL, McGregor M, Berglund E, Borst HG. Influence of state of inflation of the lung on pulmonary vascular resistance. *J Appl Physiol* 1960;**15**:878–82.

40. Brower R, Wise RA, Hassapoyannes C, Bromberger-Barnea B, Permutt S. Effect of lung inflation on lung blood volume and pulmonary venous flow. *J Appl Physiol* 1985;**58(3)**:954–63.

41. Bendjelid K, Schütz N, Suter PM, et al. Does continuous positive airway pressure by face mask improve patients with acute cardiogenic pulmonary edema due to left ventricular diastolic dysfunction? *Chest* 2005;**127(3)**:1053–8.

42. Jubran A, Mathru M, Dries D, Tobin MJ. Continuous recordings of mixed venous oxygen saturation during weaning from mechanical ventilation and the ramifications thereof. *Am J Respir Crit Care Med* 1998;**158(6)**:1763–9.

43. Lemaire F, Teboul JL, Cinotti L, et al. Acute left ventricular dysfunction during unsuccessful weaning from mechanical ventilation. *Anesthesiology* 1988;**69(2)**:171–9.

44. Boerma EC, van der Voort PH, Ince C. Sublingual microcirculatory flow is impaired by the vasopressin-analogue terlipressin in a patient with catecholamine-resistant septic shock. *Acta Anaesthesiol Scand* 2005;**49(9)**:1387–90.

Chapter

13

Integrative approach for hemodynamic monitoring

Christoph K. Hofer, Steffen Rex, and Michael T. Ganter

Introduction

In the perioperative setting, hemodynamic monitoring in combination with cardiovascular and fluid management aims at preventing tissue hypoperfusion with consecutive cellular hypoxia and organ failure.[1] Therefore, typical targets in hemodynamic monitoring are *perfusion pressure* of the cardiovascular system, *cardiac function* as driving force of oxygen delivery, *preload* as major determinant of cardiac function, and *tissue oxygenation*.

Traditionally, hemodynamic monitoring can be classified *routine, expanded, and advanced*. Electrocardiography (ECG), non-invasive blood pressure measurement (NIBP) and pulse-oximetry are considered *routine monitoring*. Expanded monitoring includes invasive arterial blood pressure (IBP) and central venous pressure (CVP) measurements, whereas *advanced monitoring* implies primarily cardiac output (CO) assessment. Unfortunately, clinical examination is often neglected as one of the most important monitoring tools. Furthermore, recent developments of advanced non- or minimally invasive monitoring devices[2] blur the traditional graduation of hemodynamic monitoring. A standardized approach for hemodynamic monitoring integrates all available hemodynamic information and is tailored according to the need of specific patient groups and related procedures considering institutional logistics.

The aim of this chapter is to give an overview of hemodynamic monitoring in five sections ("steps") considering the traditional classification emphasizing the potential application of non- and minimally invasive advanced technology.

Integrative approach in five steps

Step 1: Indications for hemodynamic monitoring

While clinical examination and routine hemodynamic monitoring should be used as a standard in every patient undergoing surgery or any other invasive procedure, two major indications for expanded and advanced hemodynamic monitoring can be identified:

1. *The patient "at risk" for hemodynamic instability*

and

2. *The "hemodynamically unstable" patient*

The *patient at risk* is expected to require, whereas the *hemodynamically unstable patient* already requires on-going fluid resuscitation and/or pharmacologic support to maintain adequate tissue perfusion. Today, goal-directed hemodynamic management is standard of care in hemodynamically unstable patient.[3] In patients at risk, however, the value of pre-emptive goal directed "optimization" is still a matter of debate, although there is a growing body of evidence showing a beneficial postinterventional outcome especially in terms of reduced morbidity.[4]

Hemodynamic instability typically results from factors related to the *patient and/or factors related to the intervention* (Figure 13.1). *Patient factors* include advanced age with impaired physiological reserve, active disease states, associated co-morbidities such as cardiac disease (e.g., coronary artery, hypertensive and valvular disease with consecutive symptomatic arrhythmias, heart failure and/or myocardial ischemia), diabetes, impaired renal and liver function as well as respiratory dysfunction. Examples for active diseases are on-going gastrointestinal bleeding

Perioperative Hemodynamic Monitoring and Goal Directed Therapy, ed. Maxime Cannesson and Rupert Pearse. Published by Cambridge University Press. © Cambridge University Press 2014.

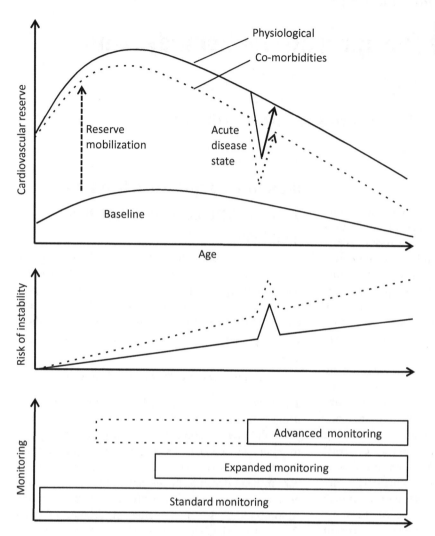

Figure 13.1. Risk of hemodynamic instability as a function of age and co-morbidities.

or inflammatory states (SIRS, sepsis) resulting in vasoplegia and/or intravascular fluid deficit. *Factors related to the intervention* include major blood loss, direct mechanical compression of the cardiovascular system (e.g., heart or caval compression, pneumoperitoneum), and stress reaction due to the major surgical "trauma."

In general, four groups of different etiologies for hemodynamic instability can be identified (Figure 13.2). In order to provide the right level of hemodynamic monitoring, each single patient has to be carefully assessed preoperatively. Together with the planned intervention, the risk for perioperative hemodynamic instability is then being estimated. Extended hemodynamic monitoring is being widely applied according to the patients' ASA physical status and the scheduled surgical intervention. However,

no specific, broadly applicable scoring system has yet been established for the advanced hemodynamic monitoring. The following tools are being used to assess patients' risk: the stratified clinical examination (see "step 2"), simple measures such as functional capacity[5] ("metabolic equivalents") determined by the ability to climb stairs (Table 13.1), the modified LEE risk-index[6] (Table 13.2) and "historical" definitions of "high-risk" patients[7] (Table 13.3).

Step 2: Use of clinical examination and observation

Physical examination and observation with frequent reassessment is an important part of monitoring that is often disregarded today. However, clinical assessment of hemodynamics is indispensable and helps to classify the risk for hemodynamic instability during the preanesthetic visit, may point at developing hemodynamic instability and is often required to diagnose hemodynamic failure. Clinical signs include:

- Impaired mental status (e.g., confusion, somnolence or coma) in an unsedated patient
- Mottled and cold skin, dry mucous membranes, decreased turgor of the skin
- Prolonged capillary refill time >3 seconds after pressure release
- Decreased pulse pressure
- Urine output lower than 0.5 mL/kg h^{-1}

They may all be interpreted as signs of early hypoperfusion[8] and may be used – in combination with lung auscultation for rales – to differentiate

Table 13.1. Clinical assessment of functional capacity

1 MET	Can eat, dress, use toilet Can walk indoors Can walk 1–2 blocks on ground level Can do light work around the house
4 METS	Can climb a flight of stairs Can walk up a hill Can do heavy work around the house
10 METS	Can do strenuous sports
1 MET	1 metabolic equivalent = O$_2$ consumption of 3.5 mL/kg min^{-1}
4 METS	At risk

between forward and backward cardiac failure (Figure 13.3).[9] Physical examination is most helpful in the pre- and postanesthetic period. During an intervention, clinical signs can be masked by a variety of factors such as anesthesia or drug administration altering fluid status (e.g., diuretics). Furthermore, large parts of the body are inaccessible, lighting

Table 13.2. Modified risk index

1. High-risk surgical procedures	*1 point*
• Intraperitoneal and intrathoracic • Suprainguinal vascular	
2. History of ischemic heart disease	*1 point*
• History of myocardial infarction • History of positive exercise test • Current complaint of chest pain • Use of nitrate therapy • ECG with pathological Q waves	
3. History of congestive heart failure	*1 point*
• Pulmonary edema • Paroxysmal nocturnal dyspnea • Bilateral rales or S3 gallop • Chest radiograph showing pulmonary vascular redistribution	
4. History of cerebrovascular disease	*1 point*
5. Preoperative treatment with insulin	*1 point*
6. Preoperative serum creatinine 2 mg/dL	*1 point*

Risk
- Increasing risk for perioperative complications with increasing number of points.
- Risk for cardiac event: 1 point: 1.5%; 2 points: 6%; 3 and > 3 points: 11.5%

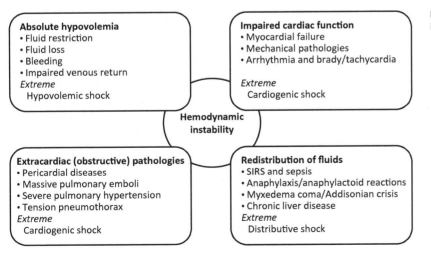

Figure 13.2. Basis of hemodynamic instability.

Table 13.3. Potential clinical patient-related criteria for high-risk of peri-interventional hemodynamic instability

1. Age > 70 years with limited physiological reserve in one and more vital organ functions
2. Cardiorespiratory disease: acute myocardial infarction, decompensated left heart failure, progressive chronic obstructive pulmonary disease with the risk of pulmonary artery hypertension or stroke
3. Late-stage vascular disease including aorta
4. Acute renal failure: Urea > 20 mmol L^{-1} or creatinine > 260 mmol L^{-1}. Respiratory failure: PaO_2 < 8 kPa on FiO_2 > 0.4 or mechanical ventilation > 48 hours
5. Bacteremia and sepsis
6. Acute abdominal "catastrophe" including severe peritonitis, perforated viscus, and pancreatitis

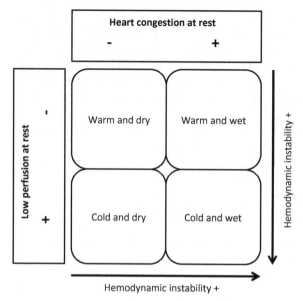

Figure 13.3. Simplified evaluation of cardiac function at the bedside.

conditions are poor, patients are covered, and warm blankets are applied.

Step 3: Use of routine hemodynamic monitoring

Routine hemodynamic monitoring consists of *ECG, NIBP, and pulse oximetry* as well as *capnography* in a patient under general anesthesia:

1. *ECG* is employed to continuously assess heart rate, rhythm and myocardial perfusion. Thereby, abnormal rate (i.e., tachy- and bradycardia), arrhythmias and myocardial ischemia, or infarction can be diagnosed. ST-segment alterations may indicate regional myocardial hypoperfusion that can result in systemic cardiovascular compromise. For reliable ST-segment and ST-trend analysis, at least a two-lead ECG (multi-lead technique) is required, i.e., lead II and V5. This allows detection of roughly 80% of all occurring ST-segment changes. An additional third lead (V4) further increases ECG sensitivity.[10]

2. *NIBP* is typically being assessed by oscillometry on an intermittent, automated basis, and mean arterial blood pressure (MAP) is considered the best representation of the perfusion pressure. Unfortunately, stable MAP within a narrow range does not necessarily indicate preserved and adequate organ blood flow. *First,* considering MAP as product of CO and systemic vascular resistance (SVR), it is evident that a decreased CO is initially being compensated by an increase in SVR due to a boosted sympathetic outflow thereby preserving MAP. This may result in an impaired end-organ perfusion. *Second,* local autoregulation of organ blood flow helps to support adequate organ blood flow over a wide blood pressure range. However, there is a large individual variability on a critical lower blood pressure, especially in the aged patient and in the patient with co-morbidities. Absolute blood pressure threshold values cannot be given ensuring adequate organ perfusion.[11] Nevertheless, blood pressure drops below 20%–30% of baseline have to be considered critical and MAP below 65 mmHg is widely accepted as critical threshold in goal directed protocols combined with other hemodynamic parameters.[12,13]

3. *Pulse oximetry* has been established as routine monitoring more than 30 years ago aiming at the prevention of hypoxemia. While pulse oximetry has been shown to reliably diagnose and reduce the incidence of hypoxemia, no impact on patient outcome has ever been established.[14,15] It has to be emphasized that the recognition of a developing hypoxemia can be delayed, due to the fact that oxygen saturation may be preserved for a long time: as a result of the sigmoid shape of the oxygen binding curve, pulse oximetry is

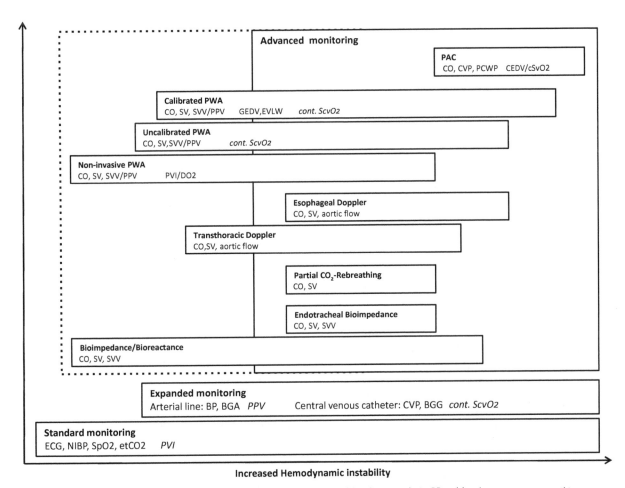

Increased Hemodynamic instability

Figure 13.4. Integrative approach for hemodynamic monitoring. BGA = blood gas analysis, BP = blood pressure, c = continuous, CEDV = continuous end-diastolic volume, CO = cardiac output, CVP = central venous pressure, ECG = electrocardiography, etCO$_2$ = end-expiratory carbon dioxide concentration, EVLW = extravascular lung water, GEDV = global end-diastolic volume, NIBP = non-invasive blood pressure, PAC = pulmonary artery catheter, PCWP = pulmonary capillary wedge pressure, PPV = pulse pressure variation, PVI = plethysmographic variability index, SpO$_2$ = peripheral oxygen saturation, SvO$_2$ = mixed venous oxygen saturation, ScvO$_2$ = central venous oxygen saturation, SV = stroke volume, SVV = stroke volume variation, TEE = trans-esophageal echocardiography, TTE = transthoracic echocardiography.

"only a sentry standing on the edge of the cliff of desaturation. It gives no warning as we approach the edge of the cliff; it only tells us when we have fallen off."[16] In addition to measuring oxygen saturation, some new pulse oximetry technologies provide additional, functional hemodynamic parameters.

4. *End-expiratory CO$_2$* levels assessed by *capnography* are usually applied to monitor adequate ventilation and may indirectly reflect CO. Low levels indicate large dead space or low CO with impaired tissue perfusion; increasing levels during cardiopulmonary

resuscitation may reflect the success of the treatment efforts and may serve as a prognostic parameter.[17,18]

Routine monitoring is applied to detect a beginning hemodynamic instability in "low-risk" patients. Based on the available information, initial measures to stabilize a patient can be started. To further the initiation of goal directed optimization, at least functional parameters derived from the pulse oximetry are required, or advanced technologies that allow the assessment of systemic flow (Figure 13.4) have to be used.

Combination with non-invasive advanced technologies

1. Bioimpedance (for example, *BioZ*, SonoSite, Bothel WA) and bioreactance (*NICOM*, Cheetha Medical Inc., Vancouver, WA) could be used conveniently in combination with standard monitoring for assessment of *CO and functional hemodynamics*, since the only prerequisite is the placement of cutaneous electrode patches.[19,20]

2. Non-invasive pulse wave analysis allows the continuous *non-invasive assessment of blood pressure (cNIBP) and CO*. The *Nexfin HD monitoring* (BMEYE B.V, Amsterdam, the Netherlands)[21] enables additional continuous *oxygen delivery* determination in combination with the Masimo Rainbow technology (Masimo Corp, Irvine, CA). This technique provides – apart from standard pulse oximetry – non-invasive hemoglobin measurement. Moreover, carboxy- and met-hemoglobin can be determined and *functional hemodynamics* (Pleth Variability Index; PVI) can be determined.[22] Quite comparable to the Nexfin monitor is the CNAP technique (CNSystems, Graz, Austria) for cNIBP monitoring and non-invasive assessment of functional hemodynamics by pulse pressure variation (PPV).[23] However, for CO assessment, the CNAP sensor must be connected to another monitor, the LiDCOrapid device (LiDCO Group Plc, London, UK).

Non-invasive advanced technologies are appealing, but limitations of the techniques have to be considered, clear indications are missing, and the devices are not widely used in clinical practice so far. However, these devices may be useful in the future, applying goal directed therapy in patients with a moderate risk for perioperative complications and hemodynamic instability.

Step 4: Use of expanded hemodynamic monitoring

The placement of arterial and central venous lines is the most commonly performed procedure in patients at risk for hemodynamic instability and hemodynamically unstable patients.

1. For *invasive arterial blood pressure (IBP) measurement*, the radial artery is generally preferred to the femoral one, as a result of better accessibility and lower rate of adverse events. However, even radial cannulation may rarely cause severe complications such as ischemia of the hand. IBP is referred to as the most accurate blood pressure measurement, but valid only when the technique is being used correctly, i.e., the electro-mechanical transducer is placed at the level of the right heart atrium and resonance problems of the required tubing system are minimized. Interestingly, IBP and NIBP measurements (especially MAP) are comparable in hemodynamic stable situations and as long as NIBP prerequisites are met, i.e., adequate relationship between cuff size and upper-arm circumference.[24] However, IBP is superior to NIBP in low blood pressure and low flow states.[25] The continuous monitoring detects blood pressure changes more rapidly than the conventional intermittent technique and functional hemodynamics (e.g., pulse pressure variation) may be measured in currently available IBP devices by integrating pulse wave analysis algorithms. However, continuous NIBP is available today, a fact that will change the indication of the IBP use. Limitations of pressure monitoring have to be considered, since blood pressure does not reflect organ blood flow. Therefore, in a developing hemodynamic instability, blood pressure is a late sign for impaired tissue hypoperfusion, since it is typically maintained normal for a certain period of time (increased sympathetic activity); meanwhile, organ blood flow may already be severely compromised.

2. Standard central venous lines are placed for reliable medication (i.e., vasoactives and inotropes; please recall that large bore cannulas are required for rapid fluid administration), to measure *central venous pressure (CVP)* and to withdraw central venous blood specimens (e.g., central venous blood gas analysis). Despite the scientific fact that CVP is considered a weak estimate of preload,[26,27] CVP is still widely used in clinical practice and recommended in different guidelines to manage fluid status.[28] The use of CVP should not be discouraged, since this parameter is easily accessible and a high CVP is an indicator of an underlying pathology, whereas a low to "normal" CVP cannot be exploited. Right ventricular filling pressures represent left ventricular filling only under ideal conditions; they may not necessarily

reflect end-diastolic myocardial wall tension in a compliant system such as the heart of an individual patient. Moreover, CVP is strongly influenced by surrounding pressure conditions. CVP changes in combination with other hemodynamic parameters are most useful in daily clinical practice. For example, a significant, rapid increase of CVP during fluid administration may serve as a warning sign for a congestion of the vascular system.

3. Arterial and central venous *blood gas analysis* (aBGA, cvBGA) play a central role in expanded hemodynamic monitoring, since BGA may provide some insights in tissue perfusion. Inadequate tissue perfusion, i.e., impairment of oxygen delivery and regional hypoxia induces a change of the energy supply from aerobic to anaerobic metabolism. Anaerobic metabolism results in the formation of large amounts of hydrogen ions, and a metabolic lactic acidosis develops with decreased pH and increased *lactate* level (>2 meq/L). Independent of global hypoperfusion and anaerobic metabolism, lactate levels may also be elevated during administration of large amounts of lactated Ringer's solution and reduced hepatic clearance of lactate. On the other hand, *pH* is a function of the available amount of plasma bicarbonate and arterial CO_2. The interaction between *pH, HCO_3- and PaCO_2* is explained by the Henderson–Hasselbalch equation. Typically, levels of bicarbonate and base excess decrease during the development of tissue hypoperfusion and progressive metabolic lactic acidosis, because plasma bicarbonate acts as hydrogen ion buffer. *Base excess* is defined as the amount of base required to raise 1 L of blood to a pH predicted from actual PCO_2 and is a derived parameter from bicarbonate and pH. Base excess has been shown to be a better indicator of global hypoperfusion and the development of metabolic acidosis than pH,[29,30] primarily because of the compensatory physiologic mechanisms to maintain the pH in a normal range. However, base excess can also be altered by etiologies other than global hypoperfusion. For example, hypercholemic metabolic acidosis induced by infusion of normal saline, diabetic ketoacidosis, and acidosis due to chronic renal failure may result in a decreased base excess (increased base deficit).

The oxygen saturation of venous blood is either measured in the pulmonary vein (mixed venous oxygen saturation = SvO_2) or in the superior vena cava (central venous oxygenation saturation = $ScvO_2$) using co-oximetry in order to determine the balance between systemic oxygen delivery and consumption (i.e., tissue oxygen extraction). Hypoperfusion due to hypovolemia for example results in a decreased oxygen delivery. SvO_2 reflects the oxygen extraction of the total body, $ScvO_2$ only that of the brain and the upper part of the body. Under physiologic conditions, $ScvO_2$ values are lower than SvO_2 values (higher oxygen extraction by the brain), whereas in a sedated patient after major abdominal surgery SvO_2 values may be significantly lower (higher oxygen extraction by the intestines). Thus, it has been argued that SvO_2 and $ScvO_2$ may not necessarily be used interchangeably.[31,32] However, since trends of these two parameters show a good correlation, SvO_2 and $ScvO_2$ are helpful tools for the fluid assessment and resuscitation in complex hemodynamic situations.[13]

Expanded monitoring is routinely used to detect hemodynamic instability in patients at risk and is essential to guide treatment in patients with obvious hemodynamic instability. No direct information on flow characteristics, but some functional hemodynamic parameters, can be obtained from traditional expanded monitoring tools. Thereby, goal directed optimization is possible in patients with moderate risk.

Combination with minimally invasive advanced technologies

To provide information on blood flow in patients on expanded hemodynamic monitoring, the following minimally invasive advanced technologies may be used.

1. Uncalibrated pulse wave analysis devices such as the FloTrac/Vigileo (Edwards LifeSciences, Irvine, USA)[33] or the Pulsioflex device (Pulsion Medical Systems, Munich, Germany) can be used for CO and functional hemodynamic monitoring after connection of the dedicated equipment to the arterial line already in place. The major indication for these devices that can be considered is clearly goal directed optimization in the perioperative period.

2. Dedicated central venous lines that allow the continuous $ScvO_2$ monitoring[13] could be used

instead of the traditional central venous lines. In contrast to intermittent cvBGA withdrawal, early "online" detection of a developing hypoperfusion is possible. However, they require specific monitoring devices. Clear indications for a routine use in the perioperative setting are missing so far.

Step 5: Use of advanced hemodynamic monitoring

All advanced hemodynamic monitoring devices offer – as already presented in the previous steps – CO assessment and functional hemodynamic parameters:

1. *CO* is the main parameter of advanced hemodynamic monitoring, represents global blood flow and determines oxygen delivery. Recall that "normal" and "threshold values" for CO were initially derived from circulatory studies in animals and volunteers, performed after the clinical introduction of the pulmonary artery catheter.[34] Furthermore, normal values cannot be defined, because CO varies as a result of individual metabolic demands. However, more important than absolute CO values is the assessment of CO trends that are being used for goal directed therapy and for detection of early hemodynamic instability.

2. The assessment of *functional hemodynamics* relies on cyclic changes of the intrathoracic pressure induced by positive pressure ventilation.[35,36] These changes induce variations in stroke volume (SV), mainly as a result of reduced venous return. According to the technique used, maximal and minimal SV, pulse pressure or plethysmographic changes are recorded and presented as an indexed parameter, i.e., SV variation (SVV), pulse pressure variation (PPV), or plethysmographic indices such as pleth variability index (PVI). Functional hemodynamics allow determination of the actual individual position on the Frank–Starling curve: on the ascending limb of the Frank–Starling curve, cyclic intrathoracic pressure changes induce large changes in preload and SV, whereas on the plateau of the Frank–Starling curve, only small SV changes occur. A growing number of studies have demonstrated that functional hemodynamic parameters allow reliable prediction of fluid responsiveness. By contrast, static preload parameters fail to do so. However, severe arrhythmias, right ventricular failure, spontaneous breathing activity, and low tidal volume (<8 mL kg^{-1}) may strongly

impact on the reliability of these parameters[37] and limit the broader application.

3. In addition to CO and functional hemodynamics, some of the devices allow the assessment of *volumetric parameters* as well as *oxygen consumption* that can support treatment decisions in complex clinical situations.

Advanced monitoring can be classified according to their underlying technology into four groups. According to their invasiveness, the pulmonary artery catheter represents the most invasive technique (Figure 13.5). In contrast to minimally invasive advanced hemodynamic monitoring, the following invasive techniques require the presence of a specific patient condition (e.g., the sedated and intubated patient) or the invasive placement of a tool (e.g., dedicated endotracheal tube, dedicated femoral arterial line). Principles and limitations of all groups are summarized below, as they present the most important factors for the clinical use in different clinical settings. However, detailed description of the techniques and aspects of validation, i.e., accuracy and precision of the different techniques are covered in the following chapters.

1. *Bioimpedance and Bioreactance* (*BioZ*, SonoSite, Bothel WA; and *NICOM*, Cheetha Medical Inc., Vancouver, WA, respectively) apply a high frequency, low-alternating electrical current to the thorax via skin electrodes. From changes in electrical conductivity (i.e., impedance) induced by cyclic variations of circulating blood volume, SV and CO are assessed using algorithms that consider geometrical models for left ventricular and aortic volumes.[19,20] Instead of externally applied electrodes, a recently released device uses a dedicated endotracheal tube (ECOM, ConMed, Utica, NY).[38] With this approach, the electrodes on the tube can be placed close to the aorta, but problems of signal processing may be of major concern. While all bioimpedance devices assess electrical amplitude changes, *bioreactance* targets an electrical frequency change that aims at providing more stable and reliable CO and SVV assessment by reducing the signal-to-noise ratio. Limitations of these techniques are not only related to the quality of signal detection and electrical interference with other devices used in the perioperative setting, but also the quality of algorithms utilized in the available devices when cardiovascular alterations or lung pathologies such as extravascular fluid collections are present.

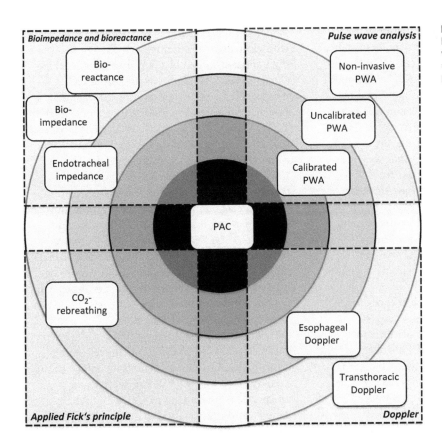

Figure 13.5. Classification of advanced hemodynamic monitoring according to working principles and invasiveness. PAC = pulmonary artery catheter, PWA = pulse wave analysis.

2. The *partial CO_2-rebreathing* technique (NICO system, Novametrix Medical Systems, Wallingford, USA) uses the Fick's principle modified to determine CO by CO_2 production and elimination,[39,40] flow, airway pressure, and CO_2 concentration sensors as well as a rebreathing loop reconnected to the endotracheal tube. In cycles of 3 minutes partial rebreathing is induced. CO is determined from CO_2 measurements before and during this cycle. Major limitations are the requirement of fixed ventilator settings and ventilation–perfusion mismatches that are present with relevant pulmonary pathologies.

3. *Esophageal Doppler* devices assess blood flow (and changes of flow) of the descending aorta and CO is calculated from the resulting velocity time integral of the Doppler signal and the aortic cross sectional area. This area is being estimated by the actually available devices such as the CardioQ™ (Deltex Medical Ltd, Sussex, UK) from nomograms. Typical limitations that have to be considered are the assumption of a fixed partition between cephalic and caudal blood flow for CO

determination[41] as a result of flow assessment at the descending aorta and the need to probe repositioning for optimal Doppler signal quality that renders esophageal Doppler measurements highly operator-dependent[42] and restricts the ability to continuously assess CO. The *transthoracic Doppler* (USCOM, Sydney, Australia) derives CO from aortic or pulmonary arterial flow measurements.[43] Again, continuous assessment is difficult to achieve and, for both techniques, a considerable level of experience is required for acceptable results.

4. *Pulse wave analysis devices* apply the same fundamental principle and derive SV, CO, and functional hemodynamics from the arterial pressure wave signals at short time intervals ranging from "online" beat-to-beat to several seconds. Typically, a "three-element-Windkessel" model based on Ohm's law (with the components vascular compliance, peripheral arterial resistance, and aortic impedance) and/or the "Wesseling approach" (that assumes a correlation between SV and the area under the systolic part of the pressure

115

curve) is being used in the devices' proprietary algorithms. As already mentioned, two *completely non-invasive systems* are available: the ccNexfin device (BMEYE B.V., Amsterdam, NL)[21,23] applies photoelectrical plethysmography in combination with the so-called "volume-clamp" technique using dedicated finger cuffs in order to determine CO and the continuous NIBP monitoring, the CNAP system (CNSystems, Graz, Austria) that was upgraded using the LiDCO algorithm for continuous CO assessment. *Uncalibrated devices*, on the other hand, assess arterial pressure signal by a conventional arterial catheter. Most prominent examples are the FloTrac/Vigileo monitoring system that uses a specific electro-mechanic transducer,[33] the Pulsioflex device with a proprietary transducer system, and the LiDCOrapid device that requires chip cards for unlocking the monitor.[44] All systems use nomogram-based mathematical algorithms to estimate CO, the LiDCOrapid and Pulsioflex system can be manually calibrated with an external CO reference technique. For all calibrated devices, however, external calibration with a reference CO (assessed via thermo- or lithium dilution) is mandatory. The PiCCOplus system (Pulsion Medical Systems, Munich, Germany) and the EV1000/VolumeView system (Edwards LifeSciences, Irvine, CA) require a thermistor-tipped catheter that is usually introduced into the femoral artery and a central venous access in order to perform calibration by transpulmonary thermodilution (TPTD).[45,46] For the LiDCOplus system (LiDCO Group Plc, London, UK), a lithium detector is attached to the arterial line and lithium dilution for calibration.[47] Major limitations of pulse wave analysis devices are damping and resonance phenomena of devices that require an arterial line for signal detection, whereas movement artifacts and sensor dislocation of completely non-invasive devices reduce optimal signal detection. Pronounced arrhythmia may limit the use of pulse wave analysis, although latest generations of pulse wave analysis devices allow filtering premature ventricular contractions.[48] However, sudden changes of vascular tone are of concern that may result in reduced accuracy of all devices; This issue is primarily a limitation for uncalibrated devices; calibrated devices can be recalibrated to reflect the actual vascular situation.

When lithium dilution is performed, interference with electrolyte and hematocrit changes as well as high concentrations of neuromuscular blocking agents have to be considered. Besides CO measurement, important additional parameters, so-called volumetric parameters, are provided by TPTD using PiCCO and EV1000, i.e., *global end-diastolic volume (GEDV)* and *extravascular lung water (EVLW)*. Both parameters are calculated from CO and different passage times of the thermal indicator traveling through the central intravascular compartments (i.e., right atrium and ventricle, pulmonary vessels, left atrium, and ventricle).[49] GEDV has shown to be a better estimate of cardiac preload than the traditional filling pressures.[26] However, GEDV cannot be used as a functional hemodynamic parameter for the assessment of fluid responsiveness. EVLW is a validated parameter of lung edema.[50] A good correlation with the development of lung edema has been observed in different clinical settings and it can be used to differentiate the etiology of lung edema. Moreover, EVLW can serve as an independent prognostic parameter in ARDS patients and may be used to guide therapy in these patients in order to improve outcome.[51] Of note, the accuracy of GEDV and especially EVLW measurements may be affected when a major part of the pulmonary vessels is excluded from flow (i.e., massive emboli, pneumonectomy) and large aortic aneurisms are present.[52]

As mentioned previously, dedicated CV lines that allow *continuous assessment of ScvO$_2$* can be attached to both monitoring systems, the PiCCOplus and the EV1000 device.

5. Despite the availability of all non- and minimally invasive advanced techniques, the *pulmonary artery catheter (PAC)* is still an important tool in complex hemodynamic situations (such as critically ill patients with right heart failure). CO can be determined by pulmonary artery thermodilution using the thermal bolus technique. Today, however, the automated continuous CO assessment is mostly being used (e.g., Vigilance catheters, Edwards LifeSciences, Irvine, CA or Opti-Q catheters, Abbott, Abbott Park, IL). Intermittent, minimal changes of pulmonary artery temperature, induced by small amounts of heat released at the thermal filaments of the PAC,

are assessed at a distal thermistor.[53] After cross-correlation of in- and output signals, a thermodilution curve is established and the averaged value of several intermittent measurements is displayed as the continuous CO (CCO). CCO assessment is delayed to some extent and rapid CO changes may not be detected. Another limitation for the PAC is its invasiveness and, with the availability of less or completely non-invasive alternatives, therefore, the worldwide PAC use has considerably decreased. However, a major advantage of the PAC is the assessment of *pulmonary artery pressure (PAP)* and the combined measurement of right and left heart filling pressures, i.e., *CVP and pulmonary capillary wedge pressure (PCWP)*. The fact that pressure measurements *are weak surrogate markers of preload* has been stressed already for CVP in the paragraph on expanded monitoring. Let us emphasize here again that an explanation for this finding is that both CVP and PCWP measurements are heavily influenced by changes of intrathoracic pressure (e.g., the combined effect *of underlying lung pathologies and* mechanical *ventilator settings in cr*itically ill patients) or intra-abdominal pressure (e.g., patient constitution, development of an acute abdominal compartment syndrome). Moreover, prevalent valve pathologies may limit the use of CVP and PCWP as preload estimates. Still, PCWP can be useful to assess a hydrostatic component of pulmonary edema, and it may help – in combination with CVP – to discriminate between right and left heart backward failure. However, CVP and PCWP cannot be used as functional hemodynamic parameters, since they are not able to predict fluid responsiveness.

Further important hemodynamic parameters that can be assessed using a specific PAC include continuous SVO_2 monitoring or continuous end-diastolic volume (CEDV). CEDV is determined using the pulmonary artery thermodilution curve and indicator detention times.[26] In contrast to GEDV, which includes all four heart chambers, CEDV reflects the right heart chambers and it is has also shown to be a preload estimate superior to CVP and PCWP.

Advanced hemodynamic monitoring devices can be used according to their indications, limitations, and invasiveness. As a rule of thumb, with increasing invasiveness, it can be assumed that accuracy and precision of CO assessment improves. However, in clinical practice, the increased robustness of continuous measurement is limited for non-invasive devices and limited to some extent for some minimally invasive devices. Therefore, different types of techniques have to be used for different patient groups in different settings, for example:

1. Non-invasive or mini-invasive and uncalibrated pulse wave analysis or Doppler: perioperative goal directed optimization.
2. Calibrated pulse wave analysis: treatment of critically ill patients such as cardiogenic shock or ARDS patients.
3. Pulmonary artery catheter: treatment of critically ill patients when limitations for the use of less invasive techniques exist or the continuous PAP or SVO_2 assessment are requested.

When an unclear hemodynamic situation occurs, it has to be emphasized that transesophageal echocardiography (TEE) is an indispensable tool for diagnosis and to guide treatment.

Summary

An integrative approach for perioperative, hemodynamic monitoring allows allocation of adequate monitoring tools efficiently, according to the risk of hemodynamic instability. Despite the fact that various monitoring technologies can – and have to – be used, clinical examination of the patient is fundamental, and standard monitoring has to be applied to every patient. *Non-invasive advanced monitoring* may be used before expanded monitoring tools are inserted; however, clear indications have yet to be defined. Indications for *minimally invasive advanced monitoring* are better defined and consist of perioperative, pre-emptive, goal directed guidance and therapy. *More invasive devices* providing additional hemodynamic information are restricted to the most critically ill patient. In severely hemodynamically unstable patients, when limitations for minimally invasive devices are present, the use of a PAC and TEE are still considered standard of care.

References

1. Takala J. The pulmonary artery catheter: the tool versus treatments based on the tool. *Crit Care* 2006;**10**:162.

2. Vincent J-L, Rhodes A, Perel A, *et al.* Clinical review: update on hemodynamic monitoring – a consensus of 16. *Crit Care* 2011;**15**:229.

3. Werdan K, Russ M, Buerke M, *et al.* Cardiogenic shock due to myocardial infarction: diagnosis, monitoring and treatment: a German–Austrian S3 Guideline. *Intens Med* 2011;**48**:291–344.

4. Grocott MP, Dushianthan A, Hamilton MA, et al. Perioperative increase in global blood flow to explicit defined goals and outcomes after surgery: a Cochrane Systematic Review. *Br J Anaesth* 2013;**111**:535–48.

5. Hlatky MA, Boineau RE, Higginbotham MB, *et al.* A brief self-administered questionnaire to determine functional capacity (the Duke Activity Status Index). *Am J Cardiol* 1989;**64**:651–4.

6. Ackland GL, Harris S, Ziabari Y, *et al.* Revised cardiac risk index and postoperative morbidity after elective orthopaedic surgery: a prospective cohort study. *Br J Anaesth* 2010;**105**:744–52.

7. Boyd O, Jackson N. How is risk defined in high-risk surgical patient management? *Crit Care* 2005;**9**:390–6.

8. Lima A, van Bommel J, Jansen TC, *et al.* Low tissue oxygen saturation at the end of early goal-directed therapy is associated with worse outcome in critically ill patients. *Crit Care* 2009;**13 Suppl 5**:S13.

9. Mehra MR. Optimizing outcomes in the patient with acute decompensated heart failure. *Am Heart J* 2006;**151**:571–9.

10. Landesberg G. Monitoring for myocardial ischemia. *Best Pract Res Clin Anaesthesiol* 2005;**19**:77–95.

11. Murphy GS, Hessel EA, 2nd, Groom RC. Optimal perfusion during cardiopulmonary bypass: an evidence-based approach. *Anesth Analg* 2009;**108**:1394–417.

12. Varpula M, Tallgren M, Saukkonen K, et al. Hemodynamic variables related to outcome in septic shock. *Intens Care Med* 2005;**31**:1066–71.

13. Rivers E, Nguyen B, Havstad S, et al. Early goal-directed therapy in the treatment of severe sepsis and septic shock. *N Engl J Med* 2001;**345**:1368–77.

14. Moller JT, Jensen PF, Johannessen NW, et al. Hypoxaemia is reduced by pulse oximetry monitoring in the operating theatre and in the recovery room. *Br J Anaesth* 1992;**68**:146–50.

15. Pedersen T, Dyrlund Pedersen B, Moller AM. Pulse oximetry for perioperative monitoring. *Cochrane Database Syst Rev* 2003: CD002013.

16. Tremper KK, Barker SJ. Pulse oximetry. *Anesthesiology* 1989;**70**:98–108.

17. Falk JL, Rackow EC, Weil MH. End-tidal carbon dioxide concentration during cardiopulmonary resuscitation. *N Engl J Med* 1988;**318**:607–11.

18. Sanders AB, Kern KB, Otto CW, *et al.* End-tidal carbon dioxide monitoring during cardiopulmonary resuscitation. A prognostic indicator for survival. *JAMA* 1989; **262**:1347–51.

19. de Waal EEC, Konings MK, Kalkman CJ, *et al.* Assessment of stroke volume index with three different bioimpedance algorithms: lack of agreement compared to thermodilution. *Intens Care Med* 2008;**34**:735–9.

20. Squara P, Denjean D, Estagnasie P, *et al.* Noninvasive cardiac output monitoring (NICOM): a clinical validation. *Intens Care Med* 2007;**33**:1191–4.

21. Bubenek-Turconi SI, Craciun M, Miclea I, Perel A. Noninvasive continuous cardiac output by the nexfin before and after preload-modifying maneuvers: a comparison with intermittent thermodilution cardiac output. *Anesth Analg* 2013;**117**:366–72.

22. Desebbe O, Boucau C, Farhat F, et al. The ability of pleth variability index to predict the hemodynamic effects of positive end-expiratory pressure in mechanically ventilated patients under general anesthesia. *Anesth Analg* 2010;**110**:792–8.

23. Monnet X, Dres M, Ferre A, *et al.* Prediction of fluid responsiveness by a continuous non-invasive assessment of arterial pressure in critically ill patients: comparison with four other dynamic indices. *Br J Anaesth* 2012;**109**:330–8.

24. Bur A, Hirschl MM, Herkner H, *et al.* Accuracy of oscillometric blood pressure measurement according to the relation between cuff size and upper-arm circumference in critically ill patients. *Crit Care Med* 2000;**28**:371–6.

25. Cohn JN. Blood pressure measurement in shock. Mechanism of inaccuracy in ausculatory and palpatory methods. *JAMA* 1967;**199**:118–22.

26. Hofer CK, Furrer L, Matter-Ensner S, *et al.* Volumetric preload measurement by thermodilution: a comparison with transoesophageal echocardiography. *Br J Anaesth* 2005;**94**:748–55.

27. Kumar A, Anel R, Bunnell E, *et al.* Pulmonary artery occlusion pressure and central venous pressure fail to predict ventricular filling volume, cardiac performance, or the response to volume infusion in normal subjects. *Crit Care Med* 2004;**32**:691–9.

28. Jones AE, Puskarich MA. The Surviving Sepsis Campaign Guidelines 2012: Update for Emergency Physicians. *Ann Emerg Med* 2014; **63**(1):35–47.

29. Davis JW, Shackford SR, Mackersie RC, Hoyt DB. Base deficit as a guide to volume resuscitation. *J Trauma* 1988;**28**:1464–7.

30. Englehart MS, Schreiber MA. Measurement of acid–base resuscitation endpoints: lactate, base deficit, bicarbonate or what? *Curr Opin Crit Care* 2006; **12**:569–74.

31. Marx G, Reinhart K. Venous oximetry. *Curr Opin Crit Care* 2006;**12**:263–8.

32. Dueck MH, Klimek M, Appenrodt S, Weigand C, Boerner U. Trends but not individual values of central venous oxygen saturation agree with mixed venous oxygen saturation during varying hemodynamic conditions. *Anesthesiology* 2005;**103**:249–57.

33. Senn A, Button D, Zollinger A, Hofer CK. Assessment of cardiac output changes using a modified FloTrac/Vigileo algorithm in cardiac surgery patients. *Crit Care* 2009;**13**:R32.

34. Shoemaker WC, Appel PL, Kram HB. Hemodynamic and oxygen transport responses in survivors and nonsurvivors of high-risk surgery. *Crit Care Med* 1993;**21**:977–90.

35. Cannesson M, Aboy M, Hofer CK, Rehman M. Pulse pressure variation: where are we today? *J Clin Monit Comput* 2011; **25**:45–56.

36. Michard F, Teboul JL. Using heart–lung interactions to assess fluid responsiveness during mechanical ventilation. *Crit Care* 2000;**4**:282–9.

37. De Backer D, Heenen S, Piagnerelli M, Koch M, Vincent JL. Pulse pressure variations to predict fluid responsiveness: influence of tidal volume. *Intens Care Med* 2005; **31**:517–23.

38. Fellahi JL, Fischer MO, Rebet O, *et al.* A comparison of endotracheal bioimpedance cardiography and transpulmonary thermodilution in cardiac surgery patients. *J Cardiothorac Vasc Anesth* 2012;**26**:217–22.

39. Jaffe MB. Partial CO_2 rebreathing cardiac output – operating principles of the NICO system. *J Clin Monit Comput* 1999;**15**:387–401.

40. Ng J-M, Chow MY, Ip-Yam PC, *et al.* Evaluation of partial carbon dioxide rebreathing cardiac output measurement during thoracic surgery. *J Cardiothorac Vasc Anesth* 2007;**21**:655–8.

41. Leather HA, Wouters PF. Oesophageal Doppler monitoring overestimates cardiac output during lumbar epidural anaesthesia. *Br J Anaesth* 2001;**86**:794–7.

42. Lefrant JY, Bruelle P, Aya AG, et al. Training is required to improve the reliability of esophageal Doppler to measure cardiac output in critically ill patients. *Intensive Care Med* 1998;**24**:347–52.

43. Thom O, Taylor DM, Wolfe RE, *et al.* Comparison of a suprasternal cardiac output monitor (USCOM) with the pulmonary artery catheter. *Br J Anaesth* 2009;**103**:800–4.

44. Feltracco P, Biancofiore G, Ori C, Saner FH, Della Rocca G. Limits and pitfalls of haemodynamic monitoring systems in liver transplantation surgery. *Minerva Anestesiol* 2012;**78**:1372–84.

45. Reuter DA, Huang C, Edrich T, Shernan SK, Eltzschig HK. Cardiac output monitoring using indicator-dilution techniques: basics, limits, and perspectives. *Anesth Analg* 2010;**110**:799–811.

46. Kiefer N, Hofer CK, Marx G, *et al.* Clinical validation of a new thermodilution system for the assessment of cardiac output and volumetric parameters. *Crit Care* 2012;**16**:R98.

47. Cecconi M, Dawson D, Grounds RM, Rhodes A. Lithium dilution cardiac output measurement in the critically ill patient: determination of precision of the technique. *Intens Care Med* 2009;**35**:498–504.

48. Cannesson M, Tran NP, Cho M, *et al.* Predicting fluid responsiveness with stroke volume variation despite multiple extrasystoles. *Crit Care Med* 2012;**40**:193–8.

49. Della Rocca G, Costa MG, Pietropaoli P. How to measure and interpret volumetric measures of preload. *Curr Opin Crit Care* 2007;**13**:297–302.

50. Kirov MY, Kuzkov VV, Kuklin VN, Waerhaug K, Bjertnaes LJ. Extravascular lung water assessed by transpulmonary single thermodilution and postmortem gravimetry in sheep. *Crit Care* 2004;**8**:R451–8.

51. Sakka SG. Extravascular lung water in ARDS patients. *Minerva Anestesiol* 2013;**79**:274–84.

52. Michard F. Bedside assessment of extravascular lung water by dilution methods: temptations and pitfalls. *Crit Care Med* 2007;**35**:1186–92.

53. Vincent JL. The pulmonary artery catheter. *J Clin Monit Comput* 2012;**26**:341–5.

Evaluation of a cardiac output monitor

Lester A. H. Critchley

Introduction

Reliable bedside cardiac output monitoring has been sought in clinical practice since the 1980s when the technology became available to support it. A number of monitoring modalities have been developed over the last few decades that include electrical bioimpedance and reactance, arterial pressure wave analysis, continuous wave Doppler ultrasound, and "heated wire" continuous thermodilution catheters.[1] However, the clinical evaluation of these technologies has resulted in much controversy, especially the issue of assessment of reliability.[2] In this chapter I will review the main aspects of their assessment with special attention paid to validation and statistical methods.

General considerations

There are several aspects to evaluating a clinical monitor. Commonly asked questions include: Is it safe? Is it easy to use? And how much does it cost? The clinician needs a guide so that a thorough evaluation is performed.

Intended use

Not all cardiac output monitors are equal in what they can do and provide. Neither are the requirements of different clinical settings. In the trauma room one may require a cardiac output monitor that can rapidly tell one whether the patient is responding appropriately to fluid replacement therapy, whereas in the postoperative high dependency unit one requires a cardiac output monitor that alarms if the patient's hemodynamic status changes suddenly. A Doppler monitor that provides reliable hemodynamic data, but is also highly operator dependent, may perform well in the trauma room setting, but when continuous surveillance of hemodynamic status on a high dependency unit is needed, continuous bioreactance or arterial pulse contour monitoring may perform better. Therefore, one needs to consider whether one's chosen cardiac output monitor has the right characteristics to fit the monitoring requirements of the intended clinical setting.

How easy is it to use?

The first continuous automated non-invasive cardiac output monitor to be marketed was a bioimpedance device called the BoMed.[3] It was very attractive to users because its operation involved attaching electrodes to the chest wall, switching the device on, and imputing data such as patient's height and weight. It produced a numerical readout every 16-heart beats. Unfortunately, its data proved to be unreliable. However, for many patient monitoring situations a device that can be easily attached to the patient and provides continuous data with very little user effort or skill is highly desirable. Compared with thermodilution cardiac output that requires placement of a pulmonary artery catheter and intermittent injections of saline, the BoMed was much easier to use and it provided continuous readings. Many cardiac output monitoring systems available today require constant attention, and thus are inappropriate as surveillance monitors. For example, pulse contour systems require arterial access and are prone to dampening.

Furthermore, some cardiac output techniques require skills that need to be learnt. External Doppler devices such as the USCOM (USCOM Ltd., Sydney, Australia) can provide reliable data, but also require a level of operator skill to be used properly, and this may limit use. However, the USCOM does provide a level of sophistication not found in most other cardiac

Perioperative Hemodynamic Monitoring and Goal Directed Therapy, ed. Maxime Cannesson and Rupert Pearse. Published by Cambridge University Press. © Cambridge University Press 2014.

output monitoring systems. Its interactive screen facilitates probe focusing and data trending.[4]

Clinical safety

For many years the pulmonary artery catheter was the clinical standard in cardiac output monitoring. However, its invasive nature and the potential complications associated with its use has resulted in a significant decline in its use[5] and new less invasive technologies have been developed that have replaced it.[1] Today, clinical safety is less of an issue, as most cardiac output devices are minimally invasive. Arterial line and esophageal probe insertion both have an excellent safety record. Even thermodilution can be performed using a transpulmonary method which greatly reduces associated risk (i.e., PiCCO, Pulsion, Munich, Germany). Hence, routine cardiac output monitoring has become much safer and more acceptable.

Costs and availability

When buying a new cardiac output monitoring system, running costs should be considered. In addition to the price of the monitor, most systems require disposable items to operate. Esophageal Doppler requires disposable probes, which are designed for one patient use. The FloTrac-Vigileo (Edwards LifeSciences, Irvine, CA, USA) uses a disposable pressure transducer. The PiCCO uses a femoral artery catheter that also acts as a thermodilution catheter. The LiDCO (LiDCO Ltd., London, England) and PRAM system (Vytech, Padova, Italy) work on a credit card system to buy user time. The NICOM uses purpose-made skin electrodes. Most of these disposables are priced around the same cost as the thermodilution catheter. The only system that does not require disposable items is the USCOM. Financing one's supply of these consumables can become a problem and may limit use of the monitor. Manufacturers will claim that it is a necessary evil to sustain the company financially and repay their investment in the research and development of the monitor.

Combining data sources

Finally, one needs to consider how the cardiac output monitor will interface with other hemodynamic devices and systems. Hybrid hemodynamic parameters such as systemic vascular resistance, cardiac work and oxygen delivery are becoming more widely used in clinical practice. Their generation requires the combination of cardiac output with other hemodynamic variables such as blood pressure, hemoglobin level, and oxygen saturation and this may require integration with data sources from other devices. Therefore, when evaluating a new cardiac output monitor, accessibility to these hybrid parameters also need to be considered.

Summary

Thus, when evaluating a new cardiac output monitor, one needs to consider (i) where it is going to be used and what are your monitoring requirements, (ii) how easy is it use, (iii) your budget and most importantly (iv) who will be using it.

Reliability and clinical validation

The aim of clinical validation is to determine whether a new monitor measures cardiac output reliably, which is done by comparing its performance with that of an accepted clinical standard such as thermodilution cardiac output. If the new monitor performs as well or better than the reference method, it can be accepted into clinical practice.

However, there are two important parts to clinical validation:

(i) The accuracy of individual readings, and
(ii) The ability to detect changes, or trends between readings.

The type of clinical data and statistical analysis needed to evaluate these two parts are different.

If one's objective is to diagnose a low or high cardiac output, then the accuracy of individual readings in relation to the true value is of greatest importance. However, if one's objective is to show a change in hemodynamic response to a therapeutic intervention, then serial cardiac output readings are needed and their absolute accuracy becomes less important, providing the readings reliably show changes. This division may at first seem unnecessary, but a monitor that does not measure cardiac output accurately may still be useful clinically if it detects changes reliably. As most bedside cardiac output monitors used today are now able to measure cardiac output continuously, the ability to detect trends reliably has become very relevant. Unfortunately, in the past validation studies only addressed accuracy and not trending ability.[6]

Understanding errors

The error that arises when measuring cardiac output has two fundamental components:

(i) Random error that arises from act of measuring and

(ii) Systematic error that arises from the measurement system.

If I use a measuring tape to measure the heights of patients attending a clinic, my readings may vary by a few millimeters from the true height of each patient. This is random error. But if the measuring tape becomes elongated by 2 to 3 centimeters, then every reading I take will consistently under-read the height of each patient by a few centimeters. This is a systematic error. The division of measurement error into random and systematic components plays an important role in validation statistics, because random errors affect all readings equally, whereas systematic errors remain constant within each group of readings.

One of the main causes of systematic error is imprecise calibration. Calibration is performed by (a) measuring cardiac output using a second method such as thermodilution, or (b) using population data to estimate cardiac output from the patient's demographics (i.e., age, height, weight and gender). Unfortunately, cardiac output and related parameters vary between individuals. In the Nidorf normogram used to predict aortic valve size when using Doppler cardiac output (i.e., USCOM) the range of possible values about the mean for valve size at each height is ±16%.[7] This gives rise to a significant systematic error between patients, which impacts upon accuracy when Bland–Altman comparisons are made against a reference method.[8] However, reliability during trending may still be preserved because trending involves a series of readings from a single patient. Providing the systematic error remains constant, and the random measurement errors between the series of readings are acceptably low, the monitor will detect any changes in cardiac output reliably.

How to present errors

The accepted measurement of variation in normally distributed data is the standard deviation. In validation statistics, errors are presented as (i) percentages of mean cardiac output and (ii) 95% confidence intervals, which approximates to two standard deviations. The term precision error is used, and should not be confused with the percentage error, which is one of the outcomes of Bland–Altman analysis.

Statistical approaches

Simple comparisons against a reference method

Validation in the clinical setting is usually performed by comparing readings from the method being tested against a reference method. Traditionally, thermodilution cardiac output performed using a pulmonary artery catheter has been used. The average of three thermodilution readings is used, and aberrant readings that differ by more than 10% are rejected, in order to improve the precision. However, thermodilution is not a gold standard method and significant measurement errors, both random and systematic, arise when it is used. It is generally accepted that thermodilution has a precision error of ±20%. True gold standard methods, such as aortic flow probes, have precision errors of less than ±5%. Thus, thermodilution is an imprecise reference method and this has greatly influenced the statistics used in validation. Most of the benchmarks against which the outcomes of validation studies are judged are based on this precision of ±20%.

Other more precise and gold standard reference methods could be used, such as the Fick method or a flow probe surgically placed on the aorta. However, in the clinical setting their use is inappropriate and thus the current clinical standard for cardiac output measurement remains thermodilution using a pulmonary artery catheter. The current decline in its clinical use has left a void. Thus, some recently published validation studies have either used transpulmonary thermodilution with the PiCCO system or esophageal Doppler monitoring using the CardioQ as reference methods.

Precision error of thermodilution

Recently, the precision of ±20% for thermodilution has come under scrutiny. The reason that thermodilution is said to have a precision error of ±20% can be attributed to our 1999 publication on bias and precision statistics, which first proposed percentage error.[9] In the 1990s consensus of opinion was that, for a monitor to be accepted into clinical use, it should be able to detect at least a change in cardiac output of 1 L/min when the mean cardiac output was 5 L/min, which was a 20% change.[10,11] Furthermore, Stetz and colleagues' meta-analysis of studies from the 1970s validating the thermodilution method suggested that it had a precision of 13%–22%.[12] Thus 20% was proposed. The 30% benchmark percentage error that everyone today quotes was based on this precision error of ±20% for thermodilution. However, it now seems that the precision of thermodilution can be very variable and depends on the type of patient and measurement system used.[13] Recently, Peyton and Chong have suggested that the precision of thermodilution may be as large as ±30%.[14]

Study design

Study design becomes relevant when ability to detect trends, in addition to accuracy, is investigated. To determine accuracy, one needs only a single pair of cardiac output readings, test and reference, from each patient. Test refers to the new method being validated and reference to the clinical standard thermodilution, though ideally a gold standard method should be used. Readings, test and reference, should ideally be performed simultaneously, because cardiac output is not a static parameter and fluctuates between cardiac cycles. The size of the study usually includes 20 or more pairs of readings.

Study design becomes more complicated if the ability to detect trends is also being investigated. A series of paired readings from the same patient are now needed that show changes in cardiac output. A wide range of values of cardiac output readings is also needed. A new parameter called delta cardiac output (ΔCO) is calculated for both test and reference data, which is calculated from the difference between consecutive readings. Trend analysis is performed on the ΔCOs. The data can be collected (a) at random or (b) at predetermined time points. Readings collected at random can lead to uneven data distribution. Thus, a more rigid protocol with data being collected at predetermined time points tends to be used. Commonly, six to ten time points are used. A typical protocol for a patient having cardiac surgery might be: (T1) – before anesthesia, (T2) – after induction, (T3) – after sternotomy, (T4) – after bypass, (T5) – after closure of the chest and (T6–8) – at set times on the intensive care.

Graphical presentation and analysis

Data format

The simplest format to use is the unchanged cardiac output data (CO). However, sometimes authors choose to normalize data by either presenting the cardiac output as a percentage of a baseline, and this is popular for trend data (ΔCO), or indexing against usually body surface area (CI). These data transformations can help if data from subjects of varying body sizes are grouped together, such as from children. Our preference is to use CO.

Scatter plot

Validation data first should be plotted on a graph that shows the relationship between the test and reference cardiac output readings. The simplest approach is to plot the data on a scatter plot where the x-axis represents the reference readings and the y-axis represents the test readings (Figure 14.1). The data points should lie within close proximity to the line of identity $x = y$ for there to be good agreement. A regression line can be added. However, correlation is not performed if the aim of the analysis is to assess the agreement between two methods rather than assessing trending ability. This point was highlighted by Bland and Altman when they published their well-known method of showing agreement.[15]

Bland–Altman plot

The agreement between two measurement techniques, test and reference, is evaluated by calculating the bias, which is the difference between each pair of readings, test minus reference. In the Bland–Altman plot the bias of each pair of readings (y-axis) is plotted against the average of the two readings (x-axis) (Figure 14.2). Then, three horizontal lines are added to the plot: (a) The mean bias for all the data points and (b) the two 95% confidence interval lines for the bias (1.96 × standard deviation of the bias) known as the "Limits of Agreement." Sufficient information should also be provided to allow the calculation of percentage error.

Modifications to the plot

(i) Some investigators argue that the best estimate of cardiac output (x-axis), or the reference value, should be used instead of the average.

(ii) When the study protocol collects more than one set of data from each patient, the limits of agreement should be adjusted for repeated

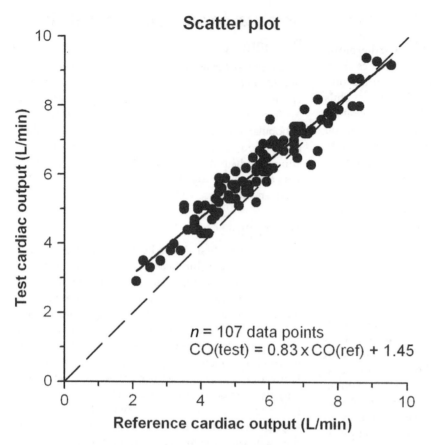

Figure 14.1. Scatter plot showing test and reference cardiac output (CO) data points. The regression line (solid) crosses *y*-axis at 1.45 L/min, indicating an offset in calibration between the two methods. A line of identity (dashed) $y = x$ is added. There is good agreement between the test and reference methods because data points lie close to the regression line. The correlation coefficient (*r*) is not provided.

measures. The effect of having multiple readings from the same subject is to reduce the influence of systematic errors, thus decreasing the standard deviation of the bias and narrowing the limits of agreement. As a consequence, the limits become falsely reduced. Two recent articles describe how to perform a correction for repeated measures.[16,17] The models used in the two corrective methods are slightly different.

(iii) The Bland–Altman plot assumes that both the test and reference methods have the same calibrated scales for measuring cardiac output. Otherwise, the distribution of data will be sloping and the limits of agreement falsely wide. Bland and Altman described a logarithmic transformation to deal with this scenario.[15]

Which parameters should be presented?

In the past many authors have not known how to present their cardiac output data from validation studies in a meaningful and useful manner. When presenting data on a scatter plot, one should include the number of data points in the plot. Attention also needs to be given to the scale used on the axis so that false impressions of the spread of the data are avoided. Ideally, the axes should be of equal scale and range from zero to the maximum value of cardiac output. If a regression line is added, the equation of the line should be shown. Correlation analysis is not required unless serial data that shows trending is being used.

Similar issues apply to the Bland–Altman plot. In particular, the range of cardiac output on the *x*-axis and the range of values for bias need to be appropriate. If several plots comparing data from several devices or patient groups are shown, the scales on each plot should be equivalent.

The important data measured using the Bland–Altman analysis are:

(i) The mean bias

(ii) The standard deviation of the bias which is presented as the 95% confidence intervals or Limits of Agreement

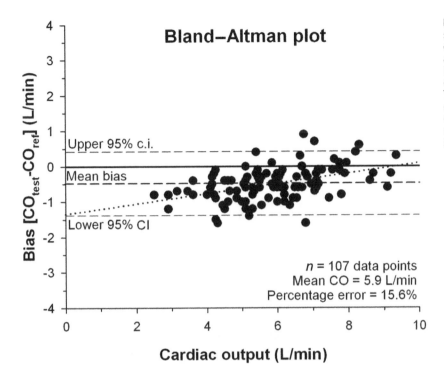

Figure 14.2. Bland and Altman plot showing test and reference cardiac output (CO) data points. The mean bias and limits of agreement lines (dashed) have been added to plot. 95% of the data points fall between these limits. The percentage error has been calculated from the mean CO and limits of agreement. Note the slightly skewed distribution of the data shown by the sloping regression line (dotted).

(iii) The mean cardiac output, and

(iv) A calculated parameter called the percentage error.

The study size (n) and percentage error at least should be presented with the Bland–Altman plot.

Percentage error and the 30% benchmark

The percentage error is calculated using the formula "1.96 × standard deviation of the bias / mean cardiac output" and is expressed as a percentage. It represents a normalized version of the limits of agreement. The percentage error enables one to compare data from different studies when the ranges of cardiac outputs are different. Even today, many authors still fail to present the percentage error.

Following a meta-analysis of data from cardiac output studies published pre-1997 that used Bland–Altman analysis, we proposed that, when the percentage error was less than 28.4%, it was reasonable to accept the new test method. However, the reference method had to be thermodilution with an estimated precision was ±20%.[9] Our work led to the 30% benchmark for percentage error quoted in many publications over the last decade. An error-gram was published in our 1999 paper to allow for adjustment

to this threshold when reference methods of different precision errors were used.

Showing reliable trending

To assess the trending ability of a new monitor against a reference method, one uses serial cardiac output readings. The simplest way to show trending is to plot the test and reference methods together against time (Figure 14.3). However, time plots only show data from a single subject, so to confirm reliable trending, data from several subjects needs to be shown. Time plots provide only graphical evidence of trending and therefore an objective measure of trending is also needed.

The four-quadrant plot

The variable commonly used to assess trending in statistical analysis is the delta cardiac output (ΔCO), the difference between successive readings, or the change in cardiac output ($CO_b - CO_a$). Bland–Altman analysis does not show trending, so other analytical methods are used. There is limited consensus on which analytical method should be used.[6] In clinical trials concordance, using a four-quadrant plot has become the popular method.

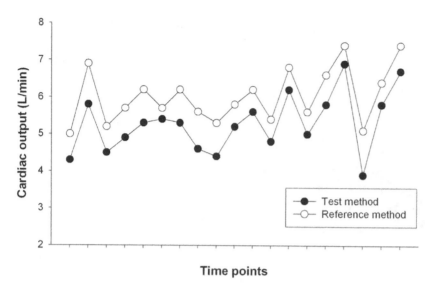

Figure 14.3. Time plot showing the relationship between test and reference cardiac output readings over time. Data pairs come from a single patient collected at intervals during surgery. The test method follows changes in reference cardiac output, despite the test method under-reading by approximately 0.75 L/min. Thus, reliable trending ability is demonstrated in the patient.

The four quadrant plot is simply a scatter plot showing delta cardiac output (ΔCO) for the test method against the reference method. Because the changes in cardiac output are used, the *x*- and *y*-axes pass through zero (0,0) at the center of the plot. The delta data points should lie along the line of identity ($y = x$) if good trending is present (Figure 14.4). The earliest references to this method appeared in the mid 1990s.[18,19]

Concordance analysis

The concordance is measured as the proportion of data points in which either both methods change in a positive direction (i.e., increase and lie within the right upper quadrant) or change in a negative direction (i.e., decrease and lie within the left lower quadrant). Data points that do not concord (i.e., change in different directions) lie within the upper left or lower right quadrants. The concordance rate is the percentage of data points that are in concordance or agree, regarding the direction of change of cardiac output.

The central exclusion zone

One of the main problems encountered when using the four quadrant plot is that data points close to its center, which represent relatively small cardiac output changes, often do not concord because random error effects are of similar magnitude to the cardiac output changes. This phenomenon results in statistical noise that adversely affects the concordance rate. Perrino and colleagues introduced a central exclusion zone to filter out these random error effects.

Receiver operator characteristic (ROC) curve analysis of Perrino and colleagues data was performed to predict the most desirable exclusion zone.[18] For a mean cardiac output of 5.0 L/min, these authors recommended an exclusion zone of 0.75 L/min or 15%. In the above example it can be seen that, after central zone exclusion of data, most of the remaining data lie within the upper right (i.e., positive changes) and lower left (i.e., negative changes) quadrants of concordance. The concordance rate is 98%, as one data point lies outside these quadrants. Without the zone, the rate would be lower.

When performing concordance analysis, one needs to know what is an acceptable rate? In a recent publication on trend analysis, we analyzed data from nine studies that used concordance analysis. From this data we concluded that, for good trending ability to be shown against thermodilution as a reference method, the concordance rate should be 92% or above.[6]

Polar plots

Concordance analysis and the four quadrant plot have limitations. The changes in cardiac output between the test and reference methods can be very different, yet concord if both have the same direction of change and if the magnitude of the change in cardiac output plays no part in the analysis other than determining what data are excluded. To address these issues, we developed a method of concordance analysis based on converting the data to polar coordinates. The polar angle represented agreement, whilst the radius

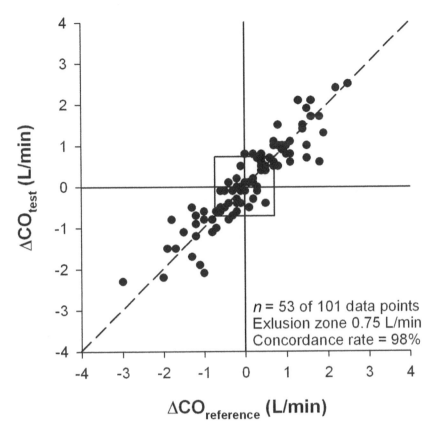

Figure 14.4. Four quadrant scatter plot comparing changes in test and reference cardiac output (ΔCO) readings. The plot is divided into four quadrants about the x- and y-axes that cross at the center (0,0). Data points lie along the line (dashed) of identity $y = x$. A square exclusion zone is drawn at the center to remove statistical noise. Concordance analysis is performed by counting the number of data points remaining after central zone exclusion that lie within the two quadrants of agreement (upper right and lower left). In the plot 98% of the data concords, thus trending ability is very good. Suprasternal and esophageal Doppler were being compared.

n = 53 of 101 data points
Exlusion zone 0.75 L/min
Concordance rate = 98%

represented the magnitude of change in cardiac output.[20] The polar data is generated from the ΔCO (test) and ΔCO(reference). Descriptions on how to draw polar plots are found in our paper.

Our earliest description of polar plots used a full 360-degree circle to show both positive and negative directional changes (Figure 14.5). The data points are seen to lie within the narrow ±30-degree sectors about the polar axes, signifying good trending ability. When 30-degree limits are used, the allowable differences in size of ΔCO are limited to a ratio of 1 to 2, rather than just direction of change.

The half-moon plot was later developed to show positive and negative ΔCO changes together (Figure 14.6).

The plot provides several parameters that describe trending:

(i) The mean polar angle which shows the deviation in agreement from the polar axis zero-degrees. It is a measure of offset in scales between the test and reference methods.

(ii) The radial limits of agreement which are 95% confidence intervals of the polar angles. If the angles lie within the 30-degree boundaries,

the ΔCO radial values differ by less than 1 to 2 (i.e., half to double) in 95% of paired readings.

(iii) The polar concordance rate, which for comparisons against thermodilution are set at 30-degrees, but there are currently limited data to support these limits.

The exclusion zone is used for similar reasons as in the four quadrant plot. However, as the radial distance is mean cardiac output rather than the hypotenuse of a triangle bounded by two cardiac output readings, reference and test, its radius needs to be a ratio of 1 to 1.4 smaller. Thus, rather than using 0.75 L/min or 15% as in the four quadrant plot, we used 0.5 L/min.

Making sense of study outcomes

If evidence-based approaches are to be adopted when using cardiac output monitoring in one's clinical practice, then data from clinical validation studies will need to be critically reviewed. Marketing information from most manufacturers of such devices provide lists of publications that they claim support

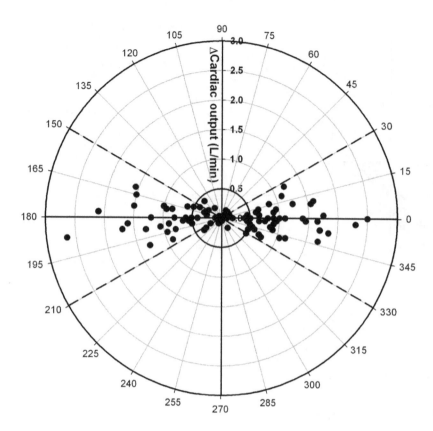

Figure 14.5. The polar plot displays ΔCO data. The axis of the plot lies at 0 degrees (and 180 degrees). It is equivalent to the line of identity $y = x$ on the scatter plot (Figure 13.5), except that the plot has been rotated clockwise by 45 degrees. Concordance limits are drawn at ±30 degrees. A circular exclusion zone of 0.5 L/min is drawn at the center. Data points that lie within these limits concord. Positive changes in cardiac output (ΔCO) (right half) and negative ΔCO (left half) are presented on opposite halves of the plot. The mean polar angle and radial limits of agreement for data have been omitted.

Polar plot set up:
Exclusion zone 0.5 L/min
n = 69 of 114 data pairs

Polar analysis:
Angular bias = –0.4 degrees
Radial limits (95% c.i.)
= –22 to 21 degrees
Polar concordance
(at <30 degrees) = 100%

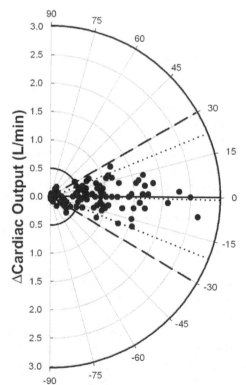

Figure 14.6. Half-moon polar plot showing the same data as the full-circle plot, but all within the same semicircle. The mean polar angle and radial limits of agreement are now shown. A central exclusion zone circle removes data points where the changes in cardiac output are small. Trending of cardiac output is good because most of the data points lie within the 30 degrees of the polar axis (0 degrees). Concordance is performed by counting the percentage of data points that lie within this zone. Outcomes of the polar analysis are provided with the plots. (Graphs drawn using Sigma Plot version 7.0.)

their product. In reviewing such data one needs to ask the following questions:

(i) Is the study design and data appropriate?
(ii) Have the correct statistics been used?
(iii) Have the correct criteria been applied to results?
(iv) And are the conclusions correct?

Patients and clinical settings

Study design is critical. (a) A sufficient number of patients should have been studied, though calculating the power of validation studies is not a simple matter. Comparison of study size with other similar validation studies may help. (b) Type of patients and clinical setting affect results. Situations where a wide range of cardiac outputs and conditions (i.e., peripheral resistance) are encountered provide a rigorous test of performance. (c) Some of the early and more favorable validation studies using pulse contour devices were performed in cardiac surgery patients in whom hemodynamics were kept relatively stable. It was only when the same devices were tested in more labile liver transplant patients with cirrhosis that the problem with these devices and peripheral resistance became apparent.[21]

Study design and appropriate analysis

The different statistical methods used in validation have been systematically covered previously. (a) If a simple test versus reference method comparison has been performed, then only Bland–Altman analysis is needed, but make sure the outcomes of the analysis are properly presented, including the percentage error. (b) If a sophisticated study design that allows trending to be assessed has been used, then concordance analysis using the four quadrant plot, and possibly a polar analysis, should have been used to show trending. Check that central exclusions zones have been applied to the ΔCO data. (c) Animal studies are slightly different because of extent and quality of data that can be collected, and here it is reasonable to use regression analysis to show trending ability.

Bland–Altman analysis

When interpreting the results of Bland–Altman analysis: (a) Make sure the precision error of the reference method is correct. Normally for thermodilution it is ±20%, but other modalities may have different precisions and criteria may need correcting, such as the 30% for percentage error. (b) Make sure

all the outcomes of the Bland–Altman analysis have been presented. The key to interpreting Bland–Altman is the percentage error which needs the mean cardiac output and limits of agreement to be calculated. (c) Make sure that the limits of agreement have been corrected for repeated measures if indicated.[16,17]

Concordance analysis

When interpreting the results of concordance analysis: (a) Make sure central exclusion zones have been used. These should be shown on the four quadrant plot. (b) Make sure the exclusion criteria used in the plot are appropriate, usually set at 15% or 0.75 L/min when mean cardiac output is 5 L/min. (c) Make sure the precision error of the reference method is known as this will affect the threshold criteria for good trending. (d) When thermodilution is the reference method, a concordance rate of above 90%–95% signifies good trending ability of the test method.

Sample size

To overcome issues with study and power sample size, one can estimate 95% confidence intervals for the concordance rate. The standard deviation of the number of data sets that agree can be calculated using $SD(np) = \sqrt{np(1-p)}$, where n is the number of data sets and p is the proportion that concord, and this is used to determine the confidence intervals. If these confidence intervals do not cross the 90%–95% threshold for good trending, then the original sample size can be considered as sufficient.

Polar methods

Polar plots are relatively new to trend analysis so their usefulness and threshold criteria for good trending still need to be set. However, they are an excellent method of showing trend data from multiple patients and, for good trending, data should lie within the 30-degree radial limits.[20] They also show offsets in calibration between test and reference methods by the deviation of the mean polar angle from the polar axis.

Concluding statements

When reading authors' conclusions regarding their validation study data, be skeptical about what is written, as the statistical analyses are often incomplete and authors tend to exaggerate their findings. In general, the percentage error should be less than 30% for good agreement and the concordance rate should be above 90%–95% for good trending ability.

Animal data

Advantages

Testing in animal models has two big advantages:

(i) More invasive and precise gold standard reference methods of monitoring cardiac output can be used, such as a flow probe surgically placed on the ascending aorta. Thus, the limitations of comparing against thermodilution can be avoided. The original flow probes were electromagnetic, but today ultrasonic transit time flow probes are used.

(ii) The ranges of circulatory conditions and cardiac outputs that can be studied are much greater than in humans for ethical reasons. This enables the cardiac output monitor to be tested over a wide range of cardiac outputs and conditions.

Differences in statistical analysis

Bland–Altman and concordance analysis can still be used to assess accuracy and trending. However, the ability to perform multiple readings over a range of cardiac output and conditions against a gold standard method allows the test method to be fully assessed. Regression analysis and correlation now are the appropriate methods for analyzing the data. Regression plots from each animal experiment are used to show how the test method behaves over a range of cardiac outputs. The regression line defines the relationship between test and flow probe methods. Correlation reflects the repeatability and trending ability of the test method, rather than the agreement between methods. Either r or R^2 are quoted. R^2 is used when a relationship exists between the two methods. The correlation coefficient (R^2) ranges from 0 to 1, where a value > 0.9 signifies good correlation. Ideally, if the test and reference (i.e., flow probe) methods are correctly calibrated, their data should lie along the line of identity $y = x$, and correlation can also be performed along this line, which is known as Lin's concordance. Alternatively, the interclass correlation coefficient (ICC) is used. These methods were used in our 2005 paper to validate the suprasternal Doppler method in anesthetized dogs.[22] Occasionally, one may come across the standard error of the estimate, or SEE, being used in older pre-1980s publications. This is a variant of the correlation coefficient that was simpler to calculate and not normalized.

Permissions and acknowledgments

Adapted from a chapter written by the author under the Creative Commons Attribution 3.0 license: Critchley LA, Chapter 4. Minimally invasive cardiac output monitoring in the year 2012. In Aronow WS (ed.), *Arterial Bypass*, published by InTech, Rijeka, Croatia.

References

1. Marik PE. Noninvasive cardiac output monitors: a state-of the-art review. *J Cardiothorac Vasc Anesth* 2013;**27**:121–34.

2. Bein B, Renner J, Scholz J, Tonner PH. Comparing different methods of cardiac output determination: a call for consensus. *Eur J Anaesthesiol* 2006;**23**:710.

3. Bernstein DP. Continuous noninvasive real-time monitoring of stroke volume and cardiac output by thoracic electrical bioimpedance. *Crit Care Med* 1986;**14**(10):898–901.

4. Critchley LA, Huang L. USCOM – Window to the circulation: utility of supra-sternal Doppler in an elderly anaesthetized patient for a robotic cystectomy. *J Clin Monit Comput* 2014; **28**(1):83–93.

5. Koo KK, Sun JC, Zhou Q, et al. Pulmonary artery catheters: evolving rates and reasons for use. *Crit Care Med* 2011;**39**:1613–18.

6. Critchley LA, Lee A, Ho AM. A critical review of the ability of continuous cardiac output monitors to measure trends in cardiac output. *Anesth. Analg* 2010;**111**:1180–92.

7. Nidorf SM, Picard MH, Triulzi MO, et al. New perspectives in the assessment of cardiac chamber dimensions during development and adulthood. *J Am Coll Cardiol* 1992;**19**:983–8.

8. Chong SW, Peyton PJ. A meta-analysis of the accuracy and precision of the ultrasonic cardiac output monitor (USCOM). *Anaesthesia* 2012;**67**:1266–71.

9. Critchley LA, Critchley JA. A meta-analysis of studies using bias and precision statistics to compare cardiac output measurement techniques. *J Clin Monit Comput* 1999;**15**:85–91.

10. LaMantia KR, O'Connor T, Barash PG: Comparing methods of measurement: an alternative approach. *Anesthesiology* 1990;**72**:781–3.

11. Wong DH, Tremper KK, Stemmer EA, et al. Noninvasive cardiac output: Simultaneous comparison of two different methods with thermodilution. *Anesthesiology* 1990;**72**:784–92.

12. Stetz CW, Miller RG, Kelly GE, Raffin TA. Reliability of the thermodilution method in the determination of cardiac output in clinical practice. *Am Rev Resp Dis* 1982;**126**:1001–4.

13. Yang XX, Critchley LA, Joynt GM. Determination of the measurement error of the pulmonary artery thermodilution catheter using in-vitro continuous flow test rig. *Anesth Analg* 2011;**112**:70–7.

14. Peyton PJ, Chong SW. Minimally invasive measurement of cardiac output during surgery and critical care: a meta-analysis of accuracy and precision. *Anesthesiology* 2010;**113**:1220–35.

15. Bland JM, Altman DG. Statistical methods for assessing agreement between two methods of clinical measurement. *Lancet* 1986;**1** (**8476**):307–10.

16. Bland JM, Altman DG. Agreement between methods of measurement with multiple observations per individual. *J Biopharm Stat* 2007;**17**:571–82.

17. Myles PS, Cui J. Using the Bland–Altman method to measure agreement with repeated measures. *Brit J Anaesth* 2007;**99**:309–11.

18. Perrino AC, O'Connor T, Luther M. Transtracheal Doppler cardiac output monitoring: comparison to thermodilution during noncardiac surgery. *Anesth Analg* 1994;**78**:1060–6.

19. Perrino AC, Harris SN, Luther MA. Intraoperative determination of cardiac output using multiplane transesophageal echocardiography: a comparison to thermodilution. *Anesthesiology* 1998;**89**:350–7.

20. Critchley LA, Yang XX, Lee A. Assessment of trending ability of cardiac output monitors by polar plot methodology. *J Cardiothorac Vasc Anesth* 2011;**25**:536–46.

21. Biancofiore G, Critchley LA, Lee A, et al. Evaluation of an uncalibrated arterial pulse contour cardiac output monitoring system in cirrhotic patients undergoing liver surgery. *Brit J Anaesth* 2009;**102**:47–54.

22. Critchley LAH, Peng ZY, Fok BS, et al. Testing the reliability of a new ultrasonic cardiac output monitor, the USCOM using aortic flow probes in anaesthetized dogs. *Anesth Analg* 2005;**100**:748–53.

Chapter

15

Invasive hemodynamic monitoring systems

Paul E. Marik

The management of hemodynamically unstable patients requires an assessment of the cardiac output (CO) and the patients' intravascular volume status (cardiac preload). An assessment of the patient's intravascular volume status includes the ability to predict the hemodynamic response following a fluid challenge (volume responsiveness).[1] Fundamentally, the only reason to give a patient a fluid challenge is to increase stroke volume (volume responsiveness). If the fluid challenge does not increase stroke volume (SV), volume loading serves the patient no useful benefit and is likely to be harmful. The (accurate) measurement of SV and CO is therefore fundamental to the hemodynamic management of critically ill patients in the ICU and unstable patients in the operating room. Both fluid challenges and the use of inotropic agents/vasopressors should be based on the response of the SV to either of these challenges. Previously, static pressure measurements, namely the pulmonary capillary wedge pressure (PCWP) and the central venous pressure (CVP) have been used to guide fluid therapy. However, studies performed over the last two decades demonstrate that these techniques are unable to accurately assess volume status or fluid responsiveness.[2] The pulmonary artery catheter (PAC) has, until recently, been the most common clinical tool for assessment of a patient's hemodynamic status. However, recently less invasive technologies have been developed for this purpose. This chapter will review the PAC as well as other invasive technologies available for hemodynamic monitoring.

The pulmonary artery catheter

Pulmonary artery (PA) catheterization was first performed by Lewis Dexter in 1945.[3] He recognized that this procedure could be used to measure pressures and oxygen content in the right heart chambers, thus making it possible to diagnose a wide variety of congenital heart lesions. In 1947, Dexter and his colleagues found that it was possible to measure the pulmonary artery "wedge" pressure by positioning a PA catheter in a distal branch of a PA.[4] They demonstrated that, in the absence of mitral valve disease, the pressure recorded in the wedge position was the same as the filling pressure in the left ventricle. After observing a spinnaker on a sailboat off Santa Monica beach, the idea of a flow-directed PA catheter was developed by Swan and Ganz in 1970, allowing bedside placement.[5] As well as measuring right heart pressures and mixed venous oxygenation, the PAC was modified with a thermistor to allow measurement of cardiac output.[6] Further modifications enabled right atrial and ventricular pacing, with infusion ports, to allow administration of drugs. Later modifications allowed continuous cardiac output measurement, right ventricular ejection fraction and right ventricular end-diastolic volume estimations. Shortly after the publication by Swan et al. in 1970, the balloon tipped PA catheter became commercially available and it began to be used in a variety of clinical settings. The use of the PAC moved from the cardiac catheterization laboratory to the ICU and its use changed from being used as a diagnostic to a therapeutic tool. Clinicians began to use the hemodynamic data derived from the PAC to select, modify, and monitor medical treatments. After the introduction of the PAC, enthusiasm for the device increased and its use increased exponentially. Indeed, the PAC came to be considered the cornerstone of critical care and a hallmark of the ICU. In the 1980s 20% to 40% of seriously ill patients who were hospitalized were reported to undergo pulmonary artery catheterization.[7]

Perioperative Hemodynamic Monitoring and Goal Directed Therapy, ed. Maxime Cannesson and Rupert Pearse.
Published by Cambridge University Press. © Cambridge University Press 2014.

This phenomenon occurred, despite that fact that the safety, accuracy, and benefit of the device had never been established. Benefit was simply assumed.

While the use of the PAC increased worldwide, the use of the device was shrouded in controversy ever since its adoption in clinical medicine. In an editorial written by David Spodick in the *American Journal of Cardiology* in 1980 in response to an apparent increased mortality in patients with myocardial infarction managed with the PAC, he raised the question of whether "*invasive instrumentation will be deleterious or helpful to the patient*" and made the plea for a randomized controlled trial (RCT).[8] This was followed by the editorials written by Eugene Robin in which he called for a moratorium on the use of the PAC until RCTs were performed that demonstrated the safety and improved outcomes associated with the use of the PAC.[9,10] This was followed by a number of cohort studies, which suggested that the PAC may be harmful. Gore and coworkers reported a higher mortality in patients with an acute myocardial infarction with hypotension or congestive heart failure managed with a PAC than those who did not have a PAC.[11] In 1996 Connors et al. analyzed the use of the PAC from the SUPPORT database.[12] In this study, these investigators compared the use of the PAC versus no PAC during the first 24 hours in the ICU. Using propensity matching, this study demonstrated a 24% increased risk of death with the use of the PAC. Furthermore, the PAC was associated with an increased hospital length of stay and hospital cost.

The first large randomized, controlled, prospective, blinded (single) evaluation of the PAC was published by Sandham and colleagues in 2003.[13] These authors randomized 1994 high-risk patients 60 years of age or older, who were scheduled for major surgery to goal directed therapy guided by a PAC compared to standard care without a PAC. Hospital and 6-month mortality and length of stay were similar between the two groups. Except for pulmonary embolism, which was higher in the PAC group, morbidity was similar between groups. This was followed by the French multicenter study in which 676 patients with shock, ARDS or both were randomized to receive a PAC or not.[14] In this study use of the PAC did not significantly affect any outcome variable. In 2005 the PAC-Man and ESCAPE trials, evaluating the effectiveness of the PAC in general ICU patients and patients in congestive heart failure respectively, were published.[15,16] These trials were unable to demonstrate a benefit from the use of the PAC. In the

ESCAPE trial, in-hospital adverse events were more common in the PAC group, although no deaths were directly attributed to the use of the PAC. Shah et al. performed a meta-analysis of RCTs that had evaluated the clinical effectiveness of the PAC.[17] This meta-analysis, which included both large and small RCTs, could discern no benefit from the use of the PAC. Similarly, a meta-analysis conducted by the Cochrane group demonstrated no benefit from the use of the PAC in high-risk surgery patients (eight studies) and in general ICU patients (four studies).[18] In the USA, the use of the PAC peaked between 1993 and 1996 with a rate of 5.6 per 1000 hospital admissions declining to a rate of 1.99 per 1000 hospital admissions in 2004.[7] The decline in the use of the PAC appears to have followed the publication of the Conners study in 1996.[12] Koo et al. evaluated the use of the PAC in ICUs in Hamilton, Canada between 2002 and 2006.[19] In this study the rate of PAC use decreased from 16.4% to 6.5% over the 5-year time period. In a retrospective study (published in 2000) conducted in more than 10 000 patients included in a critical care database maintained by the Society of Critical Care Medicine, independent factors linked to PAC use were the setting of a surgical ICU and (for patients of white race) having a private medical insurance contract.[20] Importantly, the presence in the ICU of a full-time critical care physician was associated with reduced PAC use. Current utilization of the PAC in ICUs in the USA and Canada is unknown, but is likely to be less than 5%, with most PACs being placed in patients undergoing cardiothoracic surgery.

In summary, multiple randomized trials in diverse settings have demonstrated that the PAC does not improve patient outcome. While no monitoring tool, in and of itself, can improve patient outcome, the therapeutic interventions that result from the correct interpretation of data could theoretically achieve the desired patient outcomes. The failure of the PAC to improve patient outcomes implies that the PAC provides inaccurate or misleading data; that the information provided by the PAC is incorrectly interpreted; that the use of the PAC triggers harmful therapy or that the PAC is intrinsically harmful. Furthermore, it is possible that, even if the data is accurate and correctly interpreted, the PAC may be unhelpful in directing the management of critically ill patients due to the absence of effective evidence-based treatments, which are based on the information provided by the PAC. These concepts are reviewed below.

Risks from the PAC

The complications that may arise directly from the use of the PAC include pulmonary artery rupture, pulmonary artery thrombosis, intracardiac knotting of the catheter, pulmonary hemorrhage, right atrial thrombosis, catheter-related bloodstream infection, internal jugular/subclavian vein stenosis or thrombosis, atrial and ventricular arrhythmia, electromechanical dissociation, and right-sided endocarditis. These risks may not be trivial. A study of 70 critically ill patients demonstrated that 4% died from complications related to the PAC and that between 20% and 30% had major complications related to the PAC.[21] Fatal air embolism related to the PAC introducer has been reported.[22–24]

Technical and interpretive issues likely trigger inappropriate therapies. Errors in zeroing and obtaining baseline measurements are exceedingly common and may result in changes in PA pressure of up to 6 mmHg.[25,26] Damped tracings and catheter "fling" may not be recognized.[27] The patient's position is frequently not standardized, leading to further errors in measurement.[27] These errors are compounded in patients on mechanical ventilators where the use of positive pressure ventilation, spontaneous breaths, and the use of PEPP make analysis of the PAP and PCWP challenging and unreliable.[25,28,29] Incorrect decisions regarding fluid management are often made, based on the results of erroneous measurements.

Does the PAC measure cardiac output accurately?

Adolph Fick described the first method of CO estimation in 1870.[30] Fick described how to compute an animal's CO from arterial and venous blood oxygen measurements. Fick's original principle was later adapted in the development of Stewart's indicator-dilution method in 1897,[31] and Fegler's thermodilution method in 1954.[32] The introduction of the PAC in 1970 and its subsequent use in performing thermodilution measurements in humans translated the ability to measure CO from the experimental physiology laboratory to multiple clinical settings.[6] The direct Fick method was the reference standard by which all other methods of determining CO were evaluated until the introduction of the PAC. Currently, the PAC is considered the "gold standard" against which other devices are compared. Remarkably, the accuracy of the CO measurements as determined by the PAC has never been established. Furthermore, electromagnetometry and ultrasound using aortic flowprobes most closely represent a true gold standard for determination of CO, but can only be performed in instrumented animals.[33–35] As no true gold standard exists, the bias and limits of agreement as determined by the Bland–Altman method should be reported when comparing two CO devices.[36] The correlation coefficient should not be used for assessing agreement between two methods of CO measurement, as there may be a good correlation between the two devices, but very poor accuracy.[36] Critchley and Critchley have suggested that, when comparing the CO measurement between two devices, the mean cardiac output (μ), the bias, the limits of agreement (95% CI), and the percentage error ($2SD/\mu$) should be reported.[37] These authors demonstrated that a percentage error of up to 30% was acceptable.[37]

Despite the ubiquitous use of the PAC, remarkably few studies have investigated the accuracy of the CO measurements as determined by thermodilution. Dhingra and coauthors compared the thermodilution CO with that measured by the Fick technique over a wide range of cardiac outputs.[38] The bias was -0.17 L/min with the upper and lower limits of agreement being 2.96 L/min and -3.30 L/min, respectively. The percentage error was 62%. Espersen et al. compared CO measurements in ten healthy individuals in the supine and sitting position and after exercise using thermodilution, Doppler, CO_2 rebreathing and the direct Fick method.[39] Thermodilution overestimated CO compared to the other techniques, which showed close agreement with each other.[39] When the thermodilution method was compared with the direct Fick method the bias was 2.3 L/min, with a percentage error of 56%. Rich and colleagues compared the CO measured by thermodilution with that measured by the Fick method and Bioreactance (NICOM, Cheetah Medical, Vancouver, WA) in patients with pulmonary hypertension.[40] CO measured by NICOM was significantly more precise than that measured by thermodilution (3.6 ± 1.7 vs. $9.9 \pm 5.7\%$, $P<0.001$). The bias and limits of agreement for the thermodilution and Fick CO measurements were -0.91 and 2.1 L/min respectively; the percentage error was 83%. Philips at al. compared thermodilution CO with surgically implanted ultrasonic flow probes in an ovine model.[33] The percentage bias and precision was -17% and 47%, respectively; the PAC under-measured dobutamine-induced CO changes by 20% (relative 66%) compared with the flow probe. This study found that the PAC was an inaccurate measure of CO and was unreliable for detection of CO changes less than 30%–40%.

Why are thermodilution cardiac output measurements inaccurate?

Intermittent bolus PA thermodilution requires the injection of a known quantity of cold indicator through the proximal lumen of the PAC into the right atrium. The indicator mixes with the surrounding circulation in the right ventricle and enters the pulmonary artery, where it produces a thermodilution curve detected by a thermistor located near the catheter tip. The modified Stewart Equation is then used to compute the CO. It is likely that multiple factors interact to affect the accuracy of the thermodilution CO calculation.[41] Occult warming of cold indicator before injection can produce indicator losses leading to overestimates of CO. Incompletely chilled "iced" injectate results in inaccurate measurements; each 1 °C increase in temperature contributes an approximate 3% error to the computed CO.[42] Furthermore, the catheter contains saline at an undetermined temperature in its dead space. Significant losses of thermal indicator arise from the dissipation of cold indicator through the intravascular portions of the catheter, which have been pre-warmed by the surrounding blood. For a 10-mL bolus of iced injectate, this indicator loss leads to an approximate 20% overestimate of the CO.[43] Several physical variables additionally influence the extent of indicator loss through the catheter.[44] In addition, cold indicator losses to surrounding tissue occur during intravascular transit, particularly during low flow states.[45]

Spontaneous or mechanical ventilation affects the actual CO; the SV can vary by as much as 50% at various phases of the respiratory cycle.[46,47] The averaging of multiple measurements at different phases of the respiratory cycle has therefore been proposed. It is unclear how many measurements are needed for sufficient accuracy and reproducibility, but it seems that three, although clinically mostly performed, is insufficient. PA thermodilution CO measurements are unreliable in the presence of tricuspid regurgitation. For thermodilution CO measurements to be "accurate," complete mixing of the thermal indicator must occur in the setting of unidirectional flow within the right ventricle. Incomplete mixing of cold injectate due to tricuspid regurgitation will lead to recirculation of indicator, increased total area under the thermodilution curve, and underestimation of CO.[35] In general, CO is underestimated in patients with tricuspid regurgitation.[35,48,49] This finding is important, as the incidence of tricuspid regurgitation is about 15% in the general population increasing to greater than 70% in elderly patients.[50–52] Furthermore, it should be noted that pulmonary artery catheterization itself increases the velocity of the tricuspid jet.[53]

Does the PCWP reflect volume status?

A commonly cited benefit of PAC is that it provides filling pressures, which can be used to identify fluid responsiveness and guide fluid administration. However, these filing pressures have been found to be neither uniformly accurate nor effective for fluid guidance. The PCWP suffers from the same limitation as the CVP.[2,54] Multiple studies have shown a poor relationship between the PCWP and circulating blood volume, SV and left ventricular end-diastolic volume.[55–60] Furthermore, the PCWP is unable to predict fluid responsiveness.[1,61,62] These data indicate that the PCWP should not be used to make decisions regarding fluid management. Furthermore, due to its inherent accuracy, the change in the SV following a fluid bolus cannot be used to construct a Frank–Starling Curve and guide further fluid challenges.

It is generally not recognized that changes in the PCWP following fluid administration cannot be clearly interpreted.[9] The variables that govern change in pressure can be derived from the Starling relationship and require an accurate estimate of end-diastolic volume and myocardial compliance. This means that finding a relatively low PCWP and only a small increase in pressure after a trial infusion of fluids does not mean that the patient requires additional fluid. In patients with large end-diastolic volumes and/or decreased myocardial compliance, giving additional fluid can lead to pulmonary edema. Conversely, with a stiff left ventricle, following fluid administration, the conclusion might be that the patient did not need additional fluid, whereas in reality fluids are required for optimal management.

Harm due to knowledge deficit

A 1990 study by Iberti et al., in which a 31-item examination on the PAC was completed by 496 North American "intensivists", found that only 67% of the answers were correct.[63] The instrument yielded similar results in Europe.[64] A 1996 survey of more than

1000 critical care physicians found that, although 83% of questions were answered correctly, a third of the respondents could not correctly identify the PCWP on a clear tracing and could not identify the major components of oxygen transport.[65] Large interobserver variability has been reported in the interpretation of PAC pressure tracings with little agreement between experts.[66-68] A survey of practicing cardiac anesthesiologists concluded that "*a large proportion of anesthesiologists who use the PAC disagree about PCWP estimation, and even those who agree may lack the confidence necessary to use it effectively.*"[69] What is most disturbing is that, when board certified intensivists are provided with the same PAC data, there is enormous variability in the intervention consequent to interpretation of the data.[66] Remarkably, while clinicians acknowledge that other practitioners have a poor understanding on the PAC and the interpretation of the hemodynamic profile derived from the PAC, they believe that they have a good understanding of the PAC and that in their hands the PAC is a useful and beneficial device. Similar problems concerning a knowledge deficit have been identified among critical care nurses.[70] Johnson and colleagues, using the same questionnaire as Iberti et al. in a cohort of ICU nurses, demonstrated only 42% of questions were answered correctly.[71] In this study 51% of respondents were unable to correctly identify the pressure change as the catheter was advanced from the right ventricle to the PA. It is clear that the "knowledge deficit" is a major factor explaining the lack of benefit (? harm) of the PAC, and is more important than any harm caused by the PAC itself.

The data obtained from the PAC is not useful in managing critically ill patients

A major factor explaining the lack of benefit of the PAC is that the data obtained is not useful in managing critically ill patients. Apart from being inaccurate, the CO itself has very little utility in guiding patient management. Attempts at increasing CO and achieving supra-normal levels of oxygen delivery have universally failed to positively impact patient outcome.[13,14,18,72] Indeed, the study by Hayes and colleagues demonstrated that such an approach is harmful.[73] The value of a CO/SV determination lies in its response to a therapeutic intervention (passive leg raising, fluid challenge, and inotropic agent). Due to the inherent inaccuracies of the device, the PAC cannot be used for

this purpose. Similarly, the PCWP is misleading and provides little useful information in guiding fluid management.

The PAC results in overtreatment

Survey studies in postoperative and intensive care units have demonstrated that the PAC provided new information or seemed to change therapy in 30%–62% of cases.[74-76] However, the clinical significance of these changes is uncertain and, in the absence of demonstrated benefit, it is likely that many of these interventions were not beneficial. Fellahi et al. demonstrated a significant independent increase in cardiac morbidity and in-hospital mortality in cardiac surgical patients who received dobutamine to improve CO based on PAC values.[77] Sandison et al. compared the outcome of patients undergoing non-elective abdominal aortic aneurysm in two different centers.[78] In the one center PACs were inserted in 96% of cases versus 18% in the other. The patients in the center with higher PAC usage received more crystalloid, colloid, and inotropes. Their incidence of renal failure was noted to be higher, as were their lengths of stay in both ICU and hospital. These data suggest that placement of a PAC may result in excessive and inappropriate therapeutic interventions that have the potential to harm patients.

Benefits of the PAC

The benefits of the PAC are somewhat difficult to define. In some patients the diagnosis between noncardiogenic and cardiogenic pulmonary edema is difficult to make. In such circumstances the PCWP has been used to make this distinction. However, with advancements in echocardiography, catheterization of the pulmonary artery for this purpose is seldom required. The PAC therefore appears to be a diagnostic/monitoring tool without any proven indication. It would appear that the role of the PAC is limited to diagnosing pulmonary hypertension (see below), intracardiac shunts (echocardiography may be better), and amniotic fluid embolism.[79]

Indications for the use of the PAC

Doppler echocardiography is frequently used to calculate the pulmonary artery systolic pressure (sPAP). However, the sPAP as determined by Doppler echocardiography is an inaccurate estimate of sPAP,[80,81] and this technology is not considered a reliable method for the diagnosis and management of pulmonary arterial hypertension.[82] Pulmonary artery catheterization is therefore required to confirm the diagnosis of pulmonary arterial hypertension (PAH), classify PAH, assess its severity and to test the vasoreactivity of the pulmonary circulation.[83,84] The hemodynamic parameters that define category 1 PAH are a mean PAP > 25 mmHg at rest, with a PCWP $\leq$ 15 mmHg and a pulmonary vascular resistance > 3 Woods units. It would therefore appear that the only clinical use of the PAC is for the accurate diagnosis of PAH and the distinction between category 1 PAH and category 2 PAH is secondary to left heart disease. Pulmonary artery catheterization has been recommended in patients with significant PAH (sPAP > 50 mmHg and/or RV enlargement) undergoing a major surgical intervention.[85] While this recommendation is not supported by high-quality evidence, it would appear to be logical, as the PA pressure is the only reliable hemodynamic parameter derived from the PAC and its use may allow for the rational titration of vasoactive agents.

A review of the practice guidelines regarding pulmonary artery catheterization published by the major American and European Societies provide conflicting recommendations. The International Consensus Conference on *Hemodynamic Monitoring in Shock* (2006) recommend against the routine use of the PAC for patients in shock [Level 1; quality of evidence high (A)].[86] An updated report by the American Society of Anesthesiologists Task Force on Pulmonary Artery Catheterization (2003) stated that *"routine catheterization is generally inappropriate for low- or moderate-risk patients,"* but recommend pulmonary artery catheterization in those *"high risk category ASA 4 or 5 and those with hemodynamic disturbances with a great chance of causing organ dysfunction or death."*[87] Furthermore, the report states *"the risk of PAC is both appropriate and necessary in selected surgical patients undergoing procedures associated with complications from hemodynamic changes or entering surgery with preexisting risk factors for hemodynamic disturbances (e.g., advanced cardiopulmonary disease)."* The 2009 American Heart Association practice guidelines state: *"hemodynamic monitoring should be strongly considered in patients whose volume and filling pressures are uncertain or who are refractory to initial therapy, particularly in those whose filling pressures and cardiac output are unclear. Patients with clinically significant hypotension (systolic blood pressure typically less than 90 mmHg or symptomatic low systolic blood pressure) and/or worsening renal function during initial therapy might also benefit."*[88] However, the updated 2012 European Society of Cardiology guidelines state: *"Right heart catheterization does not have a general role in the management of acute heart failure, but may help in the treatment of a minority of selected patients with acute (and chronic) heart failure. PAC artery catheterization should only be considered in patients: (i) who are refractory to pharmacological treatment; (ii) who are persistently hypotensive; (iii) in whom LV filling pressure is uncertain; or (iv) who are being considered for cardiac surgery. A primary concern is to ensure that hypotension (and worsening renal function) is not due to inadequate LV filling pressure, in which case diuretic and vasodilator therapy should be reduced (and volume replacement may be required). Conversely, a high LV filling pressure and/or systemic vascular resistance may suggest an alternative pharmacological strategy (e.g., inotropic or vasodilator therapy), depending on blood pressure. Measurement of pulmonary vascular resistance (and its reversibility) is a routine part of the surgical work-up before cardiac transplantation."*[89]

Are there any perioperative indications for a PAC?

Cardiac surgery

The quality of data relating to the PAC in cardiac surgery is particularly poor. Despite dramatic reductions in the routine use of the PAC in cardiac surgery to less than 20% of cases in Europe and less than 10% in Japan, some centers in North America still routinely use the device.[90,91] Almost two decades ago in a non-randomized study of 1094 consecutive patients having non-emergent cardiac surgery with either a PAC or a central venous catheter (CVC), Tuman et al. found no significant differences in any outcome variables.[92] Polonen et al. randomized 403 elective coronary artery bypass graft patients, all of whom received a PAC, to either goal directed therapy, aiming for a mixed venous saturation of >70% and lactate concentrations less than 2.0 mmol/L, or standard therapy where the PAC was used to measure and optimize filling pressures and cardiac index. Goal directed patients received more fluids and vasoactive drugs with a reduction in hospital stay, but no difference in major morbidity or mortality.[93] Resano et al. performed a retrospective analysis of low-risk patients having off-pump coronary artery surgery in

2414 patients, where 70% had a PAC and 30% had a central venous catheter.[94] Patients had similar baseline characteristics and there were no significant differences in any outcome, suggesting that central venous catheter placement is sufficient in most off-pump cases. Unfortunately, there are no large-scale randomized controlled trials in cardiac surgical patients. Common sense, a critical appraisal on the risks and unproven benefits of the use of the PAC, "clinical experience" and retrospective data would seem to suggest that low-risk cardiac surgery and most high-risk cases can be safely performed without routine insertion of the PAC.[95] Transesophageal echocardiography (TEE) is currently widely applied during and after cardiac surgery. Two-dimensional TEE provides valuable images of the heart and great vessels, and its roles in assessing valve function, right and left ventricular contractility, and left ventricular diastolic function are well established.

Vascular surgery

Valentine et al., in a small trial of 120 patients having aortic surgery, randomized patients to perioperative monitoring with a PAC and preoperative admission to the ICU for "hemodynamic optimization," compared with intravenous hydration on the ward and no PAC.[96] PAC patients received more fluid and more vasoactive drugs; however, there were no differences in ICU or hospital stay, postoperative complications or mortality. Despite this study being underpowered and using controversial goal directed therapy, the authors concluded that routine PAC in major vascular surgery is not beneficial. In the study by Sandison et al. (discussed above) use of the PAC in patients undergoing non-elective abdominal aortic aneurysm surgery was associate with worse outcomes.[78] In the absence of definitive data demonstrating its benefit, the PAC would appear to have a limited role in vascular surgery patients.

Transplant surgery

PAC monitoring during cardiac, lung, and liver transplantation is still widespread, despite almost no data to support or refute its use, and despite increasing use of intraoperative echocardiography.[97]

Transpulmonary thermodilution and pulse contour analysis

Transpulmonary thermodilution (TPTD) monitors measure and integrate a wide array of hemodynamic variables through intra-arterial and central venous catheterization alone. As such, they are considered less invasive than the PAC and provide additional data not available from the PAC. A significant advantage of TPTD is that the technology can be used in pediatric and neonatal patients, which is a major limitation of the PAC.[98–104] Currently, two TPTD systems are commercially available, the PiCCO (Pulse index Continuous Cardiac Output) monitor (Pulsion, Munich, Germany) and the EV1000 VolumeView clinical platform (Edwards Lifesciences (Irvine, CA). Both systems combine pulse contour analysis with TPTD CO to determine a number of hemodynamic parameters. Pulse contour analysis is based on the relation between the area under the arterial waveform, SV and arterial compliance.[105] Pulse contour stroke volume estimation involves analysis of the area under the systolic portion of the arterial waveform and analysis of the shape of the arterial waveform (dP/dt). Pulse contour analysis-derived CO estimation is then calibrated against a simultaneous TPTD measurement providing a calibration factor (K) for continuous CO determination by pulse contour analysis. The advantage of pulse contour analysis over intermittent thermodilution is that it provides beat-to-beat measures of SV, which are exceedingly useful in determining the dynamic response to a therapeutic intervention (PLR, fluid bolus, vasoactive agent, etc.) and for detecting sudden changes in hemodynamic status. In these situations, the precision and absolute accuracy of the values are less important that the trending ability. Pulse contour analysis is, however, inaccurate in patients with arrhythmias and in those with intra-aortic balloon counterpulsation or other forms of mechanical circulatory assist devices.

The hemodynamic data displayed by the PiCCO and EV1000 are similar; however, the formula used to calculate the derived values differs somewhat. Nevertheless, there appears to be good agreement between the variables derived from each device.[106] The PiCCO-2 system allows continuous monitoring of central venous oxygen saturation with the addition of a fiberoptic probe inserted through the distal lumen of the central venous catheter. TPTD requires both central venous (internal jugular or subclavian) and central arterial (femoral artery) catheterization. While many consider femoral artery catheterization invasive, the risks associated with the arterial catheter are extremely low, resulting in a very favorable risk–benefit ratio.[107–110] Furthermore, femoral arterial catheterization allows for the measurement of central arterial pressures.

Table 15.1. Summary of the hemodynamic parameters measured by transpulmonary thermodilution systems

Parameter	Description
CO	Cardiac output (intermittent)
CCO	Continuous cardiac output derived from pulse contour analysis
PPV	Pulse pressure variation. Normal less than 13%
SVV	Stroke volume variation. Normal less than 13%
EVLWI	Indexed extravascular lung water, a quantitative index of the amount of fluid in the lung (parenchyma) and an accurate diagnostic test for pulmonary edema. Normal < 10 mls/kg IBW
PVPI	Derived from the ratio of EVLW to pulmonary blood volume. Allows differentiation between hydrostatic from inflammatory pulmonary edema. Normal 1–3
GEDVI	Indexed global end-diastolic volume. This is a "virtual" measurement of the total volume of fluid in all four heart chambers at end-diastole. Normal 680–800 ml/m^2
ITBV	Intrathoracic blood volume index. GEDVI plus pulmonary blood volume. Normal 850–1000 ml/m^2
CFI	Cardiac function index is the ratio of CO to GEDVI. It provides an estimate of cardiac contractility and correlates closely with the ejection fraction. Normal 4.5–6.5 min^{-1}

Important differences in pressure readings may exist between the radial and femoral artery. In addition, due to redistribution of blood flow in shock, the radial artery is a poor site for monitoring heart–lung interactions during mechanical ventilation.[111,112]

The TPTD systems measure and display a wide array of hemodynamic data (see Table 15.1). All the parameters except the continuous CO, pulse pressure and stroke volume variation are "static" and are derived from the intermittent TPTD. The PAC is based on indicator transit through the right side of the heart with a sensor placed in the pulmonary artery. In contrast, in TPTD a known quantity of cold injectate is delivered via a central venous catheter, and mixing of the thermal indicator occurs as it passes through the right atrium and ventricle, pulmonary circulation, left atrium, ventricle, and aorta. A thermistor-tipped arterial line quantifies the change in temperature over time in a large proximal artery (femoral artery). A mono-exponential transformation of the curve with extrapolation of a truncated descending limb back to baseline allows calculation of area under the curve for CO measurement. TPTD suffers from many of the errors and limitations associated with CO determined by the PAC. Compared with PAC thermodilution, the greater transit time and distance between injectate delivery and measurement with TPTD will tend to increase the error associated with conductive loss and recirculation, while reducing the potential for the measured CO to be unrepresentative of its true value over the entire respiratory cycle.

Nevertheless, several studies have validated the CO measurements obtained by TPTD with the Fick method.[103,104]

Analysis of the slope and duration of the thermal indicator dilution curve after passage through both sides of the heart and pulmonary circulation enables estimation of additional hemodynamic parameters (see Figure 15.1). The extrapolated and log transformed slope of the indicator time concentration curve as it returns to baseline is represented by the exponential decay time. Assuming a model of the circulation in which the indicator solution has undergone mixing in a series of chambers, the exponential decay time is proportional to the volume of the pulmonary circulation. The mean transit time of the indicator solution is the time taken for half the indicator to pass the arterial detection point and is proportional to the total intrathoracic volume. These measurements are used to calculate the intrathoracic blood volume (ITBV), extravascular lung water (EVLW), and global end-diastolic volume (GEDV). The EVLW is indexed to ideal body weight, which is a better index of lung volume than body surface area.[113,114] EVLW has been well validated using the gravimetric and double indicator dilution techniques in both experimental models and in patients.[115–117] The EVLWI and pulmonary vascular permeability index (PVPI) have been shown to have very good discriminatory value in the diagnosis of pulmonary edema and in differentiating cardiogenic from non-cardiogenic pulmonary edema.[118,119] EVLWI appears to be the most

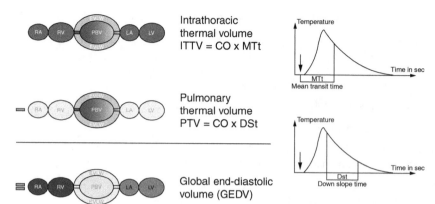

Intrathoracic thermal volume
ITTV = CO x MTt

Pulmonary thermal volume
PTV = CO x DSt

Global end-diastolic volume (GEDV)

Figure 15.1. Determination of transpulmonary thermodilution volumetric measurements
PTV = pulmonary thermal volume; volume in the biggest mixing chamber, i.e., the lungs (includes blood and water); ITTV = intrathoracic thermal volume; the total volume in which the indicator can be distributed (chambers between point of injection and detection); EVLW = extravascular lung water; volume of fluid in lung interstitium and alveoli; GEDV= global end-diastolic volume; total amount of fluid in all four chambers of the heart at end-diastole; CO = cardiac output.

accurate method of diagnosing ALI/ARDS.[120] Furthermore, EVLWI can be used to predict the development of ARDS/ALI and can accurately predict outcome in this syndrome.[102,114,119,121] While the GEDV as a single parameter has limitations in determining fluid responsiveness,[122] it is a good measure of preload and intrathoracic blood volume,[123–126] and is useful in assessing volume status and fluid responsiveness when interpreted in the context of other indices of fluid responsiveness.[1] The cardiac function index (CFI) is derived from the SV and GEDV and has been shown to correlate closely with ejection fraction.[127]

Mitchell et al. demonstrated an improved outcome of critically ill patients when fluid therapy was guided by EVLW (determined by double indicator technique) rather than by the PCWP.[128] The patients in the EVLW-guided treatment group were observed to have a less positive cumulative fluid balance, and a shorter duration of mechanical ventilation and ICU stay. The clinical utility of TPTD has been evaluated in patients undergoing cardiac surgery and in patients with subarachnoid hemorrhage (SAH). Goepfert et al. demonstrated that an algorithm based on the GEDVI reduced the need for vasopressors, catecholamines and

mechanical ventilation in patients undergoing cardiac surgery.[129] Optimization of CO and intravascular volume is of paramount importance in the management of patients with SAH. Mutoh and colleagues have developed a goal directed hemodynamic algorithm using TPTD in patients with SAH; the specific targets included a CI $\geq$ 3.0 L/m^2, a GEDVI of 700–900 mL/m^2 and an EVLW < 14 mL/kg.[130] Using this protocol, these authors have demonstrated a reduction in the incidence of vasospasm and cardiopulmonary complications compared with a protocol guided by the PAC.[131] These studies demonstrate that TPTD, when coupled with an evidenced-based therapeutic protocol has the potential to improve the outcome of critically ill and injured patients. The greater potential for TPTD to demonstrate benefit where the PAC failed is the integration of CO measurements with other potentially useful hemodynamic parameters. In addition, TPTD provides validated data that has important therapeutic implications (EVLW, GEDVI) and allows for the dynamic assessment of interventions that alter cardiac performance (pulse contour CO and PPV).

The author has no financial interest in any of the products mentioned in this chapter.

References

1. Marik PE, Monnet X, Teboul JL. Hemodynamic parameters to guide fluid therapy. *Ann Crit Care* 2011;**1**:1.

2. Marik PE, Cavallazzi R. Does the Central Venous Pressure (CVP) predict fluid responsiveness: an update meta-analysis and a plea for some common sense. *Crit Care Med* 2013;**41**:1774–81.

3. Dexter L, Haynes FW, Burwell CS, et al. Studies of congenital heart disease, I: technique of venous catheterization as a diagnostic procedure. *J Clin Invest* 1947;**26**:547–53.

4. Dexter L, Haynes FW, Burwell CS, et al. Studies of congenital heart disease, II: the pressure and oxygen content of blood in the right auricle, right ventricle, and pulmonary artery in control

patients with observations on the oxygen saturation and source of pulmonary "capillary" blood. *J Clin Invest* 1947;**26**:554–60.

5. Swan HJ, Ganz W, Forrester J, et al. Catheterization of the heart in man with use of a flow-directed balloon-tipped catheter. *N Engl J Med* 1970;**283**:447–51.

6. Ganz W, Donosco R, Marcus HS, et al. A new technique for measurment of cardiac output by thermodilution in man. *Am J Cardiol* 1971;**27**:392–6.

7. Wiener RS, Welch HG. Trends in the use of the pulmonary artery catheter in the United States, 1993–2004. *JAMA* 2007;**298**:423–9.

8. Spodick DH. Physiologic and prognostic implications of invasive monitoring: undetermined risk/benefit ratios in patients with heart disease. *Am J Cardiol* 1980;**46**:173–75.

9. Robin ED. Death by pulmonary artery flow directed catheter, time for a moratorium? *Chest* 1987;**92**:727–31.

10. Robin ED. The cult of the Swan–Ganz catheter. Overuse and abuse of the pulmonary flow catheters. *Ann Intern Med* 1985;**103**:445–49.

11. Gore JM, Goldberg RJ, Spodick DH, et al. A community-wide assessment of the use of pulmonary artery catheters in patients with acute myocardial infarction. *Chest* 1987;**92**:721–7.

12. Connors AF, Speroff T, Dawson NV, et al. The effectiveness of right heart catheterization in the initial care of critically ill patients. *JAMA* 1996;**276**:889–97.

13. Sandham JD, Hull RD, Brant RF, et al. A randomized, controlled trial of the use of pulmonary-artery catheters in high-risk surgical patients. *N Engl J Med* 2003;**348**:5–14.

14. Richard C, Warszawski J, Anguel N, et al. Early use of the pulmonary artery catheter and outcomes in patients with shock and acute respiratory distress syndrome: a randomized controlled trial. *JAMA* 2003;**290**:2713–20.

15. Harvey S, Harrison DA, Singer M, et al. Assessment of the clinical effectiveness of pulmonary artery catheters in management of patients in intensive care (PAC-Man): a randomised controlled trial. *Lancet* 2005;**366**:472–7.

16. Binanay C, Califf RM, Hasselblad V, et al. Evaluation study of congestive heart failure and pulmonary artery catheterization effectiveness: the ESCAPE trial. *JAMA* 2005;**294**:1625–33.

17. Shah MR, Hasselblad V, Stevenson LW, et al. Impact of the pulmonary artery catheter in critically ill patients: meta-analysis of randomized clinical trials. *JAMA* 2005;**294**:1664–70.

18. Harvey S, Young D, Brampton W, et al. Pulmonary artery catheters for adult patients in intensive care. *Cochrane Database of Systematic Reviews* 2006;CD003408.

19. Koo KK, Sun JC, Zhou Q, et al. Pulmonary artery catheters: evolving rates and reasons for use. *Crit Care Med* 2011;**39**:1613–18.

20. Rapoport J, Teres D, Steingrub J, et al. Patient characteristics and ICU organizational factors that influence frequency of pulmonary artery catheterization. *JAMA* 2000;**283**:2559–67.

21. Fein AM, Goldberg SK, Walkenstein MD, et al. Is pulmonary artery catheterization necessary for the diagnosis of pulmonary edema? *Am Rev Respir Dis* 1984;**129**:1006–9.

22. Hartung EJ, Ender J, Sgouropoulou S, et al. Severe air embolism caused by a pulmonary artery introducer sheath. *Anesthesiology* 1994;**80**:1402–3.

23. Bristow A, Batjer H, Chow V, et al. Air embolism via a pulmonary artery catheter introducer. *Anesthesiol* 1985;**63**:340–2.

24. Doblar DD, Hinkle JC, Fay ML, et al. Air embolism associated with pulmonary artery catheter introducer kit. *Anesthesiol* 1982;**56**:389–91.

25. Morris AH, Chapman RH, Gardner RM. Frequency of technical problems encountered in the measurement of pulmonary artery wedge pressure. *Crit Care Med* 1984;**12**:164–70.

26. Bridges EJ, Woods SL. Pulmonary artery pressure measurement: state of the art. *Heart Lung* 1993;**22**:99–111.

27. Brandstetter RD, Grant GR, Estilo M, et al. Swan–Ganz catheter: misconceptions, pitfalls, and incomplete user knowledge–an identified trilogy in need of correction. *Heart Lung* 1998;**27**:218–22.

28. Nadeau S, Noble WH. Misinterpretation of pressure measurements from the pulmonary artery catheter. *Canad Anaesth Soc J* 1986;**33**:352–63.

29. Booker KJ, Arnold JS. Respiratory-induced changes on the pulmonary capillary wedge pressure tracing. *Crit Care Nurse* 1993;**13**:80–8.

30. Fick A. Ueber die Messung des Blutquantums in den Herzventrikeln. *Sitzungsberichte der Physiologisch-Medizinosche Gesellschaft zu Wuerzburg* 1870;**2**:16.

31. Stewart GN. Researches on the circulation time and on the influences which affect it. IV. The output of the heart. *J Physiol* 1897;**22**:159–83.

32. Fegler G. Measurement of cardiac output in anesthetized animals by a thermodilution method. *Q J Exp Physiol* 1954;**39**:153–64.

33. Phillips RA, Hood SG, Jacobson BM, et al. Pulmonary artery catheter (PAC) accuracy and efficacy compared with flow probe

and transcutaneous Doppler (USCOM): an ovine cardiac output validation. *Crit Care Res Pract* 2012;**62**:1494.

34. Heerdt PM, Pond CG, Blessios GA, et al. Comparison of cardiac output measured by intrapulmonary artery Doppler, thermodilution, and electromagnetometry. *Ann Thorac Surg* 1992;**54**:959–66.

35. Heerdt PM, Blessios GA, Beach ML, et al. Flow dependency of error in thermodilution measurement of cardiac output during acute tricuspid regurgitation. *J Cardiothorac Vasc Anesth* 2001;**15**:183–7.

36. Bland JM, Altman DG. Statistical methods for assessing agreement between two methods of clinical measurement. *Lancet* 1986; **i**:307–10.

37. Critchley LA, Critchley JA. A meta-analysis of studies using bias and precision statistics to compare cardiac output measurement techniques. *J Clin Monitoring Comput* 1999;**15**:85–91.

38. Dhingra VK, Fenwick JC, Walley KR, et al. Lack of agreement between thermodilution and fick cardiac output in critically ill patients. *Chest* 2002;**122**:990–7.

39. Espersen K, Jensen EW, Rosenborg D, et al. Comparison of cardiac output measurement techniques: thermodilution, Doppler, CO_2-rebreathing and the direct Fick method. *Acta Anaesthesiol Scand* 1995;**39**:245–51.

40. Rich JD, Archer SL, Rich S. Evaluation of noninvasively measured cardiac output in patients with pulmonary hypertension [Abstract]. *Am J Respir Crit Care Med* 2011;**183**: A6440.

41. Reuter DA, Huang C, Edrich T, et al. Cardiac output monitoring using indicator-dilution techniques: basics, limits, and perspectives. *Anesth Analg* 2010;**110**:799–811.

42. Runciman WB, Ilsley AH, Roberts JG. An evaluation of thermodilution cardiac output measurement using the Swan–Ganz catheter. *Anaesthesia Intensive Care* 1981;**9**:208–20.

43. Kim ME, Lin YC. Determination of catheter wall heat transfer in cardiac output measurement by thermodilution. *Clin Exp Pharmacol Physiol* 1980;**7**:383–9.

44. Wong M, Skulsky A, Moon E. Loss of indicator in the thermodilution technique. *Cathet Cardiovasc Diagn* 1978;**4**:103–9.

45. Renner LE, Morton MJ, Sakuma GY. Indicator amount, temperature, and intrinsic cardiac output affect thermodilution cardiac output accuracy and reproducibility. *Crit Care Med* 1993;**21**:586–97.

46. Synder JV, Powner DJ. Effects of mechanical ventilation on the measurement of cardiac output by thermodilution. *Crit Care Med* 1982;**10**:677–82.

47. Stevens JH, Raffin TA, Mihm FG, et al. Thermodilution cardiac output measurement. Effects of the respiratory cycle on its reproducibility. *JAMA* 1985;**253**:2240–2.

48. Cigarroa RG, Lange RA, Williams RH, et al. Underestimation of cardiac output by thermodilution in patients with tricuspid regurgitation. *Am J Med* 1989;**86**:417–20.

49. Balik M, Pachl J, Hendl J. Effect of the degree of tricuspid regurgitation on cardiac output measurements by thermodilution. *Intens Care Med* 2002;**28**:1117–21.

50. Singh JP, Evans JC, Levy D, et al. Prevalence and clinical determinants of mitral, tricuspid, and aortic regurgitation (the Framingham Heart Study).

[Erratum in Am J Cardiol 1999;**84** (9):1143]. *Am J Cardiol* 1999;**83**:897–902.

51. Klein AL, Burstow DJ, Tajik AJ, et al. Age-related prevalence of valvular regurgitation in normal subjects: a comprehensive color flow examination of 118 volunteers. *J Am Soc Echocardiogr* 1990;**3**:54–63.

52. Fox ER, Wilson RS, Penman AD, et al. Epidemiology of pure valvular regurgitation in the large middle-aged African American cohort of the Atherosclerosis Risk in Communities study. *Am Heart J* 2007;**154**:1229–34.

53. Sherman SV, Wall MH, Kennedy DJ, et al. Do pulmonary artery catheters cause or increase tricuspid or pulmonic valvular regurgitation? *Anesth Analg* 2001;**92**:1117–22.

54. Marik PE, Baram M, Vahid B. Does the central venous pressure predict fluid responsiveness? A systematic review of the literature and the tale of seven mares. *Chest* 2008;**134**:172–8.

55. Calvin JE, Driedger AA, Sibbald WJ. Does the pulmonary capillary wedge pressure predict left ventricular preload in critically ill patients? *Crit Care Med* 1981;**9**:437–43.

56. Calvin JE, Driedger AA, Sibbald WJ. The hemodynamic effect of rapid fluid infusion in critically ill patients. *Surgery* 1981;**90**:61–76.

57. Hansen RM, Viquerat CE, Matthay MA, et al. Poor correlation between pulmonary artery wedge pressure and left ventricular end-diastolic volume after coronary artery bypass graft surgery. *Anesthesiology* 1986;**64**:764–70.

58. Oohashi S, Endoh H, Oohashi S, et al. Does central venous pressure or pulmonary capillary wedge pressure reflect the status of circulating blood volume in patients after extended

transsthoracic esophagectomy? *J Anesthesia* 2005;**19**:21–5.

59. Raper R, Sibbald WJ. Misled by the Wedge? The Swan–Ganz catheter and left ventricular preload. *Chest* 1986;**89**:427–34.

60. Baek SM, Makabaki GG, Bryan-Brown CW, et al. Plasma expansion in surgical patients with high central venous pressure (CVP); the relationship of blood volume to hematocrit, CVP, pulmonary wedge pressure, and cardiorespiratory changes. *Surgery* 1975;**78**:304–15.

61. Michard F, Teboul JL. Predicting fluid responsiveness in ICU patients: a critical analysis of the evidence. *Chest* 2002;**121**:2000–8.

62. Osman D, Ridel C, Ray P, et al. Cardiac filling pressures are not appropriate to predict hemodynamic response to volume challenge. *Crit Care Med* 2007;**35**:64–68.

63. Iberti TJ, Fischer EP, Leibowitz AB, et al. A multicenter study of physician's knowledge of the pulmonary artery catheter. Pulmonary Artery Study Group. *JAMA* 1990;**264**:2928–32.

64. Gnaegi A, Feihl F, Perret C. Intensive care physician's insufficient knowledge of right-heart catheterization at the bedside: time to act? *Crit Care Med* 1997;**25**:213–20.

65. Trottier SJ, Taylor RW. Physicians attitudes toward and knowledge of the pulmonary artery catheter: society of Critical care Medicine membership survey. *New Horiz* 1997;**5**:201–6.

66. Komadina KH, Schenk DA, La Veau P. Interobserver variability in the interpretation of pulmonary artery catheter pressure tracings. *Chest* 1991;**100**:1647–54.

67. Al-Kharrat T, Zarich S, Amoateng-Adjepong Y, et al. Analysis of observer variability in measurement of pulmonary artery occlusion pressures. *Am J Respir Crit Care Med* 1999;**160**:415–20.

68. Marik PE, Varon J, Heard SO. Interpretation of the pulmonary artery occlusion (wedge) pressure: physicians' knowledge *versus* the experts' knowledge. *Crit Care Med* 1998;**26**:1761–3.

69. Jacka MJ, Cohen MM, To T, et al. Pulmonary artery occlusion pressure estimation: how confident are anesthesiologists? *Crit Care Med* 2002;**30**:1197–203.

70. Ahrens TS. Is nursing education adequate for pulmonary artery catheter utilization? *New Horiz* 1997;**5**:281–6.

71. Johnston IG, Jane R, Fraser JF, et al. Survey of intensive care nurses' knowledge relating to the pulmonary artery catheter. *Anaesthesia Intensive Care* 2004;**32**:564–8.

72. Gattinoni L, Brazzi L, Pelosi P, et al. A trial of goal-oriented hemodynamic therapy in critically ill patients. *N Engl J Med* 1995;**333**:1025–32.

73. Hayes MA, Timmins AC, Yau E, et al. Elevation of systemic oxygen delivery in the treatment of critically ill patients. *N Engl J Med* 1994;**330**:1717–22.

74. Eisenberg PR, Jaffe AS, Schuster DP. Clinical evaluation compared to pulmonary artery catheterization in the hemodynamic assessment of critically ill patients. *Crit Care Med* 1984;**12**:549–53.

75. Quinn K, Quebbeman EJ. Pulmonary artery pressure monitoring in the surgical intensive care unit. Benefits vs difficulties. *Arch Surg* 1981;**116**:872–6.

76. Tuchschmidt J, Sharma OP. Impact of hemodynamic monitoring in a medical intensive care unit. *Crit Care Med* 1987;**15**:840–3.

77. Fellahi JL, Parienti JJ, Hanouz JL, et al. Perioperative use of dobutamine in cardiac surgery and adverse cardiac outcome: propensity-adjusted analyses. *Anesthesiology* 2008;**108**:979–87.

78. Sandison AJ, Wyncoll DL, Edmondson RC, et al. ICU protocol may affect the outcome of non-elective abdominal aortic aneurysm repair. *Eur J Vasc Endovasc Surg* 1998;**16**:356–61.

79. Gist RS, Stafford IP, Leibowitz AB, et al. Amniotic fluid embolism. *Anesth Analg* 2009;**108**:1599–602.

80. Rich JD, Shah SJ, Swamy RS, et al. Inaccuracy of Doppler echocardiographic estimates of pulmonary artery pressures in patients with pulmonary hypertension: implications for clinical practice. *Chest* 2011;**139**:988–93.

81. Fisher MR, Forfia PR, Chamera E, et al. Accuracy of Doppler echocardiography in the hemodynamic assessment of pulmonary hypertension. *Am J Respir Crit Care Med* 2009;**179**:615–21.

82. Rich JD. Counterpoint: can Doppler echocardiography estimates of pulmonary artery systolic pressures be relied upon to accurately make the diagnosis of pulmonary hypertension? No. *Chest* 2013;**143**:1536–9.

83. Galie N, Hoeper MM, Humbert M, et al. Guidelines for the diagnosis and treatment of pulmonary hypertension: the Task Force for the Diagnosis and Treatment of Pulmonary Hypertension of the European Society of Cardiology (ESC) and the European Respiratory Society (ERS), endorsed by the International Society of Heart and Lung Transplantation (ISHLT). [*Erratum in Eur Heart J.* 2011;32 (8):926]. *Eur Heart J* 2009;**30**:2493–537.

84. Saggar R, Sitbon O. Hemodynamics in pulmonary arterial hypertension: current and future perspectives. *Am J Cardiol* 2012;**110**:9S–15S.

85. McGlothlin D, Ivascu N, Heerdt PM. Anesthesia and pulmonary hypertension. *Progr Cardiovasc Dis* 2012;**55**:199–217.

86. Antonelli M, Levy M, Andrews PJ, et al. Hemodynamic monitoring in shock and implications for management. International Consensus Conference. *Intens Care Med* 2007;**33**:575–90.

87. Practice guidelines for pulmonary artery catheterization: an updated report by the American Society of Anesthesiologists Task Force on Pulmonary Artery Catheterization. *Anesthesiology* 2003;**99**:988–1014.

88. Hunt SA, Abraham WT, Chin MH, et al. 2009 focused update incorporated into the ACC/AHA 2005 Guidelines for the Diagnosis and Management of Heart Failure in Adults: a report of the American College of Cardiology Foundation/American Heart Association Task Force on Practice Guidelines: developed in collaboration with the International Society for Heart and Lung Transplantation. *Circulation* 2009;**119**:e391–e479.

89. McMurray JJ, Adamopoulos S, Anker SD, et al. ESC Guidelines for the diagnosis and treatment of acute and chronic heart failure 2012: The Task Force for the Diagnosis and Treatment of Acute and Chronic Heart Failure 2012 of the European Society of Cardiology. Developed in collaboration with the Heart Failure Association (HFA) of the ESC. *Eur Heart J* 2012;**33**:1787–847.

90. Ranucci M. Which cardiac surgical patients can benefit from placement of a pulmonary artery catheter? *Crit Care* 2006;**10 Suppl 3**:S6.

91. Handa F, Kyo SE, Miyao H. Reduction in the use of pulmonary artery catheter for cardiovascular surgery [Japanese]. *Masui – Jap J Anesthesiol* 2003;**52**:420–3.

92. Tuman KJ, McCarthy RJ, Spiess BD, et al. Effect of pulmonary artery catheterization on outcome in patients undergoing coronary artery surgery. *Anesthesiology* 1989;**70**:199–206.

93. Polonen P, Ruokonen E, Hippelainen M, et al. A prospective, randomized study of goal-oriented hemodynamic therapy in cardiac surgical patients. *Anesth Analg* 2000;**90**:1052–9.

94. Resano FG, Kapetanakis EI, Hill PC, et al. Clinical outcomes of low-risk patients undergoing beating-heart surgery with or without pulmonary artery catheterization. *J Cardiothorac Vasc Anesth* 2006;**20**:300–6.

95. Cowie BS, Cowie BS. Does the pulmonary artery catheter still have a role in the perioperative period? *Anaesth Intens Care* 2011;**39**:345–55.

96. Valentine RJ, Duke ML, Inman MH, et al. Effectiveness of pulmonary artery catheters in aortic surgery: a randomized trial. *J Vasc Surg* 1998;**27**:203–11.

97. Della Rocca G, Brondani A, Costa MG. Intraoperative hemodynamic monitoring during organ transplantation: what is new? *Curr Opin Organ Transplantation* 2009;**14**:291–6.

98. Lemson J, de Boode WP, Hopman JC et al. Validation of transpulmonary thermodilution cardiac output measurement in a pediatric animal model. *Pediat Crit Care Med* 2008;**9**:313–19.

99. Schiffmann H, Erdlenbruch B, Singer D, et al. Assessment of cardiac output, intravascular volume status, and extravascular lung water by transpulmonary indicator dilution in critically ill neonates and infants. *J Cardiothor Vasc Anesth* 2002;**16**:592–7.

100. Renner J, Broch O, Duetschke P, et al. Prediction of fluid responsiveness in infants and neonates undergoing congenital heart surgery. *Br J Anaesth* 2012;**108**:108–15.

101. Branski LK, Herndon DN, Byrd JF, et al. Transpulmonary thermodilution for hemodynamic measurements in severely burned children. *Crit Care* 2011;**15**:R118.

102. Lubrano R, Cecchetti C, Elli M et al. Prognostic value of extravascular lung water index in critically ill children with acute respiratory failure. *Intens Care Med* 2011;**37**:124–31.

103. Tibby SM, Hatherill M, Marsh MJ, et al. Clinical validation of cardiac output measurements using femoral artery thermodilution with direct Fick in ventilated children and infants. *Intens Care Med* 1997;**23**:987–91.

104. Pauli C, Fakler U, Genz T, et al. Cardiac output determination in children: equivalence of the transpulmonary thermodilution method to the direct Fick principle. *Intens Care Med* 2002;**28**:947–52.

105. Montenij LJ, de Waal EE, Buhre WF. Arterial waveform analysis in anesthesia and critical care. *Curr Opin Anaesthesiol* 2011;**24**:651–6.

106. Kiefer N, Hofer CK, Marx G, et al. Clinical validation of a new thermodilution system for the assessment of cardiac output and volumetric parameters. *Crit Care* 2012;**16**:R98.

107. Belda FJ, Aguilar G, Teboul JL, et al. Complications related to less-invasive haemodynamic monitoring. *Br J Anaesth* 2011;**106**:482–6.

108. Frezza EE, Mezghebe H. Indications and complications of arterial catheter use in surgical or

medical intensive care units: analysis of 4932 patients. *Am Surg* 1998;**64**:127–31.

109. Thomas F, Burke JP, Parker J, et al. The risk of infection related to radial vs femoral sites for arterial catheterization. *Crit Care Med* 1983;**11**:807–12.

110. Riker AI, Gamelli RL, Riker AI, et al. Vascular complications after femoral artery catheterization in burn patients. *J Trauma* 1996;**41**:904–5.

111. Galluccio ST, Chapman MJ, Finnis ME. Femoral-radial arterial pressure gradients in critically ill patients. *Crit Care Resusc* 2009;**11**:34–8.

112. Marik PE, Levitov A, Young A, et al. The use of NICOM (Bioreactance) and Carotid Doppler to determine volume responsiveness and blood flow redistribution following passive leg raising in hemodynamically unstable patients. *Chest* 2013;**143**:364–70.

113. Berkowitz DM, Danai PA, Eaton S, et al. Accurate characterization of extravascular lung water in acute respiratory distress syndrome. *Crit Care Med* 2008;**36**:1803–9.

114. Craig TR, Duffy MJ, Shyamsundar M, et al. Extravascular lung water indexed to predicted body weight is a novel predictor of intensive care unit mortality in patients with acute lung injury. *Crit Care Med* 2010;**38**:114–20.

115. Fernandez-Mondejar E, Rivera-Fernandez R, Garcia-Delgado M, et al. Small increases in extravascular lung water are accurately detected by transpulmonary thermodilution. *J Trauma* 2005;**59**:1420–3.

116. Tagami T, Kushimoto S, Yamamoto Y, et al. Validation of extravascular lung water measurement by single transpulmonary thermodilution:

human autopsy study. *Crit Care* 2010;**14**:R162.

117. Katzenelson R, Perel A, Berkenstadt H, et al. Accuracy of transpulmonary thermodilution versus gravimetric measurement of extravascular lung water. *Crit Care Med* 2004;**32**:1550–4.

118. Kushimoto S, Taira Y, Kitazawa Y, et al. The clinical usefulness of extravascular lung water and pulmonary vascular permeability index to diagnose and characterize pulmonary edema: a prospective multicenter study on the quantitative differential diagnostic definition for acute lung injury/acute respiratory distress syndrome. *Crit Care* 2012;**16**:R232.

119. Jozwiak M, Silva S, Persichini R, et al. Extravascular lung water is an independent prognostic factor in patients with acute respiratory distress syndrome. *Crit Care Med* 2013;**41**(2):472–80.

120. Tagami T, Sawabe M, Kushimoto S, et al. Quantative diagnosis of diffuse alveolar damage using extravascular lung water. *Crit Care Med* 2013;**41**:2234–5.

121. LeTourneau JL, Pinney J, Phillips CR. Extravascular lung water predicts progression to acute lung injury in patients with increased risk. *Crit Care Med* 2011;**2**:40.

122. Marik PE, Cavallazzi R, Vasu T, et al. Dynamic changes in arterial waveform derived variables and fluid responsiveness in mechanically ventilated patients. A systematic review of the literature. *Crit Care Med* 2009;**37**:2642–7.

123. Michard F, Alaya S, Zarka V, et al. Global end-diastolic volume as an indicator of cardiac preload in patients with septic shock. *Chest* 2003;**124**:1900–8.

124. Renner J, Gruenewald M, Brand P, et al. Global end-diastolic volume as a variable of fluid

responsiveness during acute changing loading conditions. *J Cardiothor Vasc Anesth* 2007;**21**:650–4.

125. Reuter DA, Felbinger TW, Moerstedt K, et al. Intrathoracic blood volume index measured by thermodilution for preload monitoring after cardiac surgery. *J Cardiothor Vasc Anesth* 2002;**16**:191–5.

126. Lichtwarck-Aschoff M, Zeravik J, Pfeiffer UJ. Intrathoracic blood volume accurately reflects circulatory volume status in critically ill patients with mechanical ventilation. *Intens Care Med* 1992;**18**:142–7.

127. Jabot J, Monnet X, Bouchra L, et al. Cardiac function index provided by transpulmonary thermodilution behaves as an indicator of left ventricular systolic function. *Crit Care Med* 2009;**37**:2913–18.

128. Mitchell JP, Schuller D, Calandrino FS, et al. Improved outcome based on fluid management in critically ill patients requiring pulmonary artery catheterization. *Am Rev Respir Dis* 1992;**145**:990–8.

129. Goepfert MS, Reuter DA, Akyol D, et al. Goal-directed fluid management reduces vasopressor and catecholamine use in cardiac surgery patients. *Intensive Care Med* 2007;**33**:96–103.

130. Mutoh T, Kazumata K, Ajiki M, et al. Goal-directed fluid management by bedside transpulmonary hemodynamic monitoring after subarachnoid hemorrhage. *Stroke* 2007;**38**:3218–24.

131. Mutoh T, Kazumata K, Ishikawa T, et al. Performance of bedside transpulmonary thermodilution monitoring for goal-directed hemodynamic management after subarachnoid hemorrhage. *Stroke* 2009;**40**:2368–74.

Chapter

16

Semi-invasive and non-invasive hemodynamic monitoring systems

Cédric Carrié, Mathieu Sèrié, and Matthieu Biais

Introduction

Hemodynamic monitoring systems in the critical care setting and in the perioperative period have been extensively studied for decades. We observed dramatic changes in hemodynamic monitoring, ranging from very invasive to mini-invasive and totally non-invasive technologies. Cardiac output (CO) monitoring in critically ill patients has been traditionally accomplished using the pulmonary artery catheter (PAC). But the value of PAC has been questioned because of its potential harmful invasiveness. Today, cardiac output and stroke volume can be assessed using various methods. Concomitantly, we have observed an increasing interest for functional and dynamic indices. Some of them are available alone at the bedside or coupled with cardiac output monitoring.

All these devices make sense only if they are paired with adapted treatment protocol.[1] Several protocols have been proposed according to the concept of hemodynamic optimization, ranging from complex algorithm using PAC and aiming at maximizing oxygen delivery, to simple one by minimizing dynamic indices thanks to a simple arterial line.

The aim of this chapter is to describe the technologies available for non- and semi-invasive hemodynamic monitoring and to discuss their principles, benefits, and limitations.

GENERAL OVERVIEW OF CURRENTLY AVAILABLE NON- AND SEMI-INVASIVE HEMODYNAMIC MONITORING DEVICES

(Table 16.1)

Cardiac output monitor

Non-invasive ultrasound devices

Esophageal Doppler

Esophageal Doppler (ED) measures blood flow velocity in the descending thoracic aorta using a transducer placed at the tip of a flexible probe. The diameter of the descending aorta is either estimated from normograms (CardioQ™, Deltex Medical Ltd, Chichester, UK) or measured by ultrasound M mode (Hemosonics™, Arrow, Reading, USA). Calculation of cardiac output is based on (i) aorta's diameter, (ii) distribution of cardiac output to the descending aorta, and (iii) the measured flow velocity of blood in the aorta.

Numerous validation studies have previously confirmed that ED was highly valuable to rapidly detect changes in CO.[2] The accuracy of this device is somewhat limited because it only provides an approximation of cardiac output. This limitation was recently demonstrated in a meta-analysis that found no significant bias (0.37 L/min) but large limits of agreement (−3.3 to 5 L/min) when CO obtained with ED is compared with pulmonary artery thermodilution.[3] Those results suggest that individual CO measurements obtained with ED may differ considerably from CO values obtained by thermodilution and consequently the two techniques are not interchangeable. Thus ED may be used as a trend monitor rather than as a device for exact measurement of CO. Moreover, probe position is crucial to obtain accurate measurements and requires frequent adjustments to optimize the signal in sedated, mechanically ventilated patients.[4] As an adequate training is required to become proficient in its use, some suggest that ED technique is operator-dependent.

Perioperative Hemodynamic Monitoring and Goal Directed Therapy, ed. Maxime Cannesson and Rupert Pearse. Published by Cambridge University Press. © Cambridge University Press 2014.

Table 16.1. Overview of cardiac output monitoring system

Technology	System	Invasiveness	Dynamic indices	Advantages	Limitations
Uncalibrated pulse contour analysis	FloTrac™	++	SVV	Mini-invasive Continuous CO monitoring Self-calibration system Positive Outcomes Studies	Not reliable for absolute value of CO measurement Sensitive to vasomotor tone and vasopressor administration
	Pulsioflex™	++	PPV/SVV	Mini-invasive Continuous CO monitoring Self-calibration system	Not enough validation studies
	LiDCO*rapid*™	++	PPV/SVV	Mini-invasive Continuous CO monitoring Self-calibration system	Not enough validation studies
	MostCare®	++	PPV/SVV	Mini-invasive Continuous CO monitoring Self-calibration system	Accuracy of cardiac output and SV has been debated
	NexFin™ HD	0	PPV/SVV	Non-invasive; Continuous CO monitoring Self-calibration system	Not enough validation studies Difficulties in keeping good quality signal in case of hypoperfusion
Doppler	Esophageal Doppler CardioQ™ Hemosonics™	+	ΔABF	Less invasive than arterial line Many positive outcome studies	Probe positioning Operator-dependent Training needed
	Suprasternal ultrasound USCOM™	0	-	Non-invasive CO measurement	Intermittent Operator-dependent Not enough validation studies
Partial CO₂ rebreathing system	NiCO™	+	-	Non-invasive CO measurement	Intermittent Discordant results Many limitations
Pulsed dye densitometry	DDG-330® analyzer	+	0	Non-invasive CO measurement	Intermittent Discordant results with many negative studies Not enough validation studies
Pulse wave transit time	esCCO™	0	PPV/SVV	Non-invasive; Continuous CO monitoring	Not enough validation studies Discordant results
Bioimpedance	BioZ® ECOM™	0	0	Non-invasive; Continuous CO monitoring	Many limitations Not enough validation studies Discordant results with many negative studies
Bioreactance	NICOM™	0	SVV	Non-invasive; Continuous CO monitoring	Not enough validation studies Many limitations

CO: cardiac output; deltaABF: respiratory variations in aortic blood flow; PPV: pulse pressure variations; SVV: stroke volume variations.

USCOM™

A completely non-invasive Doppler technology (USCOM™, USCOM, Sydney, Australia) allowing CO measurements by a suprasternal continuous Doppler probe has been recently developed. Its accuracy and precision in perioperative and critical care settings have been assessed with various results.[5,6] Recently, a meta-analysis pooled six studies to assess the accuracy and precision of this ultrasonic cardiac output monitor. The mean bias was -0.39 L/min (95% CI: -0.25 to -0.53 L/min), precision was 1.27 L/min, and percentage error was 42.7% (95% CI: 38.5–46.9%). The authors concluded that USCOM™ achieved similar agreement with bolus thermodilution to that of other minimally invasive methods of perioperative cardiac output monitoring.[7] This device might have a useful role for monitoring cardiac output, but its intermittent character limits any strategy of hemodynamic optimization in the perioperative period.

Pulse contour analysis

A growing number of calibrated and uncalibrated devices based on pulse contour analysis methods are currently available for assessing CO. This principle is based on the relation between blood pressure, stroke volume (SV), arterial compliance and systemic vascular resistance (SVR). SV can be continuously estimated by analyzing the arterial pressure waveform obtained from an arterial line if the arterial compliance and SVR are known. Systems using pulse contour analysis and requiring calibration (PiCCO™, Pulsion Medical Systems, Munich, Germany; VolumeView™, Edwards Life Sciences, Irvine, USA and LiDCO™ system, LiDCO, London, UK) are not detailed here. Principle, benefits and limitations of these invasive devices have been discussed in a previous chapter. Devices based on pulse contour analysis without external calibration, which have been extensively studied,[8,9] are the FloTrac system, the LiDCO rapid system, and the MostCare system. The recently commercialized Pulsioflex has not yet been studied. (No validation studies published nowadays.)

FloTrac system

The FloTrac system consists of the FloTrac sensor and the corresponding Vigileo Monitor. The system records hemodynamic variables performing its calculations on the most recent 20-s data. SV is calculated using arterial pulsatility (standard deviation of the pulse pressure over a 20-s interval), resistance, and compliance. CO is calculated as follows: CO = heart rate × SV. Stroke volume = K × pulsatility where K is a constant quantifying arterial compliance and vascular resistance, derived from a multivariate regression model including (i) Langewouter's aortic compliance assessed using biometric values (age, sex, height, and weight), (ii) mean arterial blood pressure (MAP), (iii) variance, (iv) skewness, and (v) kurtosis of the pressure curve. The rate of adjustment of K was done each minute. Pulsatility is proportional to the standard deviation of the arterial pressure wave over a 20-s interval.

Studies evaluating first-generation devices have revealed conflicting results and concluded in the inability of the devices to accurately measure an absolute value of cardiac output.[10–12] Second-generation devices showed good agreement with arterial or transpulmonary thermodilution in patients with normal SVR. However, the device was not able to monitor cardiac output in patients with low SVR (liver failure, sepsis), and several studies found a close correlation between bias and SVR.[13–16] Finally, the third-generation device was designed to correct this issue. Validation studies using this new algorithm demonstrated that it was able to correctly measure cardiac output even in the case of low SVR but was ineffective to assess abrupt changes in SVR (for example, induced by vasopressor).[17–19] However, the FloTrac system seems able to track changes in cardiac output induced by volume expansion, passive leg raising and positive end-expiratory pressure.[20–22]

MostCare

The MostCare™ (*Vytech* Health, Padova, Italy) uses a pressure recording analytic method (PRAM) that does not require adjustments to demographic variables. Briefly, PRAM is based on the analysis of the whole arterial pressure wave morphology (both systole and diastole) for each heart beat by sampling of 1000 Hz and automatic detection of all significant curve points: systolic and diastolic points, dicrotic notch, and points of instability. These points and the wave contour are evaluated and weighted according to the application of the physical theory of perturbations to obtain the systemic impedance and hemodynamic parameters. CO is evaluated as the ratio of the area under the pressure curve in systole (both the pulsatile and the continuous components) to the systemic impedance evaluated from both the systolic and diastolic phases. So far, there have been limited studies that have evaluated the accuracy of this system to monitor absolute values of CO and its ability to track changes in CO, with discordant results. A team investigated the device in various states (unstable, septic, and cardiac surgery patients) and found positive results.[23–26] However, other groups have recently published negative results with this device.[27–29]

LiDCO™ rapid

LiDCO™ rapid system uses a pulse pressure algorithm named PulseCO™ to track changes in SV. This algorithm is based on the assumption that the net power change in the system in a heartbeat is the difference between the amount of blood entering the system (SV) and the amount of blood flowing out peripherally. It uses the principle of conservation of mass (power) and assumes that following correction for compliance there is a linear relationship between netpower and netflow. Whereas LiDCO™ plus requires calibration using transpulmonary lithium indicator dilution technique, LiDCO™ rapid uses nomograms for cardiac output estimation. LiDCO™ rapid is able to monitor cardiac output with accuracy as long as no major hemodynamic changes are observed.[30,31]

Finally, the main advantages of pulse contour devices without need of external calibration are their simplicity to use (plug and play), no operator-dependent measure, and their ability to track changes in CO induced by volume expansion. However, they suffer from several limits. Such devices are based on assumptions, arterial compliance is estimated, and they are sensitive to vasomotor changes and vasopressor administration.

These devices should be considered as "trending cardiac output" rather than real CO monitors.

Non-invasive hemodynamic system using finger cuff technology

The Nexfin device continuously records the arterial pressure curve and computes CO by pulse contour analysis. This analysis consists in estimating SV by dividing the area under the systolic part of the arterial pressure curve by the aortic impedance.[32] Aortic impedance is determined from a three-element Windkessel model that incorporates the influence of nonlinear effects of arterial pressure, patient's age, height, weight and gender on aortic mechanical properties.[33] The Nexfin method was developed on a database including invasive and non-invasive finger arterial pressures together with thermodilution cardiac output values obtained during cardiac surgery,[32,34] in healthy subjects during passive head-up tilt,[35] and with low arterial pressure and treatment with catecholamines in severe septic shock.[36]

So far, only a few studies have shown a relevant interest of this device compared to transpulmonary dilution or esophageal Doppler in steady-state conditions.[37,38] However, recent studies have found very discordant results for detecting rapid changes in cardiac index following fluid challenge and to predict fluid responsiveness after cardiac surgery.[39,40] In hemodynamically unstable conditions, the device was not reliable to estimate absolute values of CO and for tracking changes in CO after volume expansion, with high percentage error and a poor correlation compared to transpulmonary thermodilution.[41] Moreover, the NexFin™ could not record the arterial curve due to finger hypoperfusion in 15% of patients.

The main advantages of this device are that it provides continuous measurements of arterial pressure and totally non-invasive cardiac output measurement, and is very easy to use and plug in and play. However, more clinical validation studies (especially in operating room) are needed.

Carbon dioxide rebreathing system (NiCO™)

NiCO™ (Novametrix, Medical Systems, Wallingford, USA) measures CO based on the Fick principle using CO_2 as an indicator, according to the formula: $CO = \mathring{V}_{CO_2}/(Cv_{CO_2} - Ca_{CO_2})$ where $\mathring{V}_{CO_2}$ is CO_2 elimination, Ca_{CO_2} the arterial CO_2 content, and Cv_{CO_2} the mixed venous CO_2 content. $\mathring{V}_{CO_2}$ is calculated from minute ventilation, and Ca_{CO_2} estimated from end-tidal CO_2. Instead of measuring directly Cv_{CO_2}, cardiac output can be calculated by the differential CO_2 partial rebreathing method with the help of a disposable rebreathing loop. Partial rebreathing reduces CO_2 elimination and increases $etCO_2$, assuming that the mixed venous CO_2 concentration remains constant. Measurements of $\mathring{V}_{CO_2}$ and $etCO_2$ are thus made during a first period of non-rebreathing and a subsequent rebreathing period using the modified Fick equation: $CO = \Delta\mathring{V}_{CO_2}/\Delta Ca_{CO_2}$. A limitation of the rebreathing CO_2 cardiac output method is that it only measures the nonshunted portion of the cardiac output. The NiCO™ system thus estimates Qs/Qt using a shunt correction algorithm, which uses oxygen saturation from pulse oxymetry and the fractional concentration of inspired oxygen.

Several studies have investigated the accuracy of the partial-rebreathing system to determinate CO. Overall, the CO_2 rebreathing system has shown significant bias (range: -0.58 to -1.73 L/min) in patients undergoing cardiac surgery or in hemodynamically stable ICU patients.[42] Moreover, it suffers from a lack of agreement in spontaneously breathing patients, when minute ventilation is low or shunt fractions are high. Moreover, an elevated CO decreases the accuracy of the cardiac output determinations.[43,44] Another drawback to the partial-rebreathing system is that it can only measure CO, but is unable to monitor intravascular volume status or fluid responsiveness. To date, there have been no reports on the device demonstrating outcome benefit when used in hemodynamically unstable patients.

Thoracic electrical bioreactance and bioimpedance

Bioreactance and bioimpedance are based on the principle that the frequency of changes in aortic volume during the cardiac cycle can be detected by alternating electrical signals across the thorax. These techniques are totally non-invasive but are based on several assumptions which might result in erroneous determinations of the CO in hemodynamically unstable patients.[42]

Thoracic bioimpedance (BioZ™, CardioDynamics, San Diego, USA) measures the electrical resistance to high-frequency, low-magnitude alternating current transmitted by electrodes placed across the chest. TEB have been shown to be reliable in healthy volunteers, but results are discordant in critically ill or surgical patients. Although newer generation devices have shown marked improvement in correlation and precision, bioimpedance stroke volume calculations were not reliable compared to thermodilution measurements, making the degree of agreement unacceptable for clinical practice.[45] Moreover, its clinical application in perioperative settings appears limited by artifacts related to ventilation, electrocautery, and many cardiorespiratory conditions.[46] The precise positioning of the electrodes – essential to the reliability of the measurement – can cause problems in certain types of surgery. Thoracotomy or laparotomy also invalidates the relationship between impedance

and intrathoracic blood volume on which the measurement of cardiac output is based.

To overcome those limitations, the ECOM™ (Conmed Corp, Utica, USA) uses a novel approach to detect the bioimpedance signal by placing the electrodes on the distal end of an endotracheal tube. However, recent validation studies comparing the tracheal impedance device and pulmonary artery thermodilution found wide limits of agreement and high percentage error, meaning that tracheal impedance cannot be an acceptable alternative to thermodilution in cardiac surgical patients.[47,48] However, SVV given by ECOM have been validated to predict fluid responsiveness with good accuracy and discrimination.[49]

Another newly marketed bioreactance device is the NICOM™ (Cheetah Medical, Portland, OR), which measures changes in the frequency of the electrical currents traversing the chest, rather than changes in impedance, potentially making it less sensitive to noise.[50,51] However, early reports of the NICOM's performance against thermodilution or esophageal Doppler do not support a greater accuracy compared with thermodilution, bias and limits of agreement still above the clinically acceptable limits.[52]

CO monitoring derived from pulse oximetry
Pulsed dye densitometry

The DDG-330® analyzer (Nihon Kohden, Tokyo, Japan) allows intermittent cardiac output measurement based on transpulmonary dye dilution with transcutaneous signal detection adapted from pulse oximetry. The arterial blood concentration of indocyanine green is estimated by optical absorbance measurements after its venous injection. Unfortunately a variety of factors, such as vasoconstriction, interstitial edema, movements, or ambient light artifacts, severely impaired the intermittent cardiac output assessment.[53]

Pulse wave transit time (esCCO™)

The esCCO™ device (Nihon Kohden, Tokyo, Japan) is a new non-invasive method of monitoring cardiac output which derives from pulse wave transit time (PWTT). The algorithm calculates esCCO stroke volume continuously using the negative correlation between SV and PWTT. Very easy to use (plug and play), it requires no additional connection than the ECG and the plethysmographic wave. Early studies have shown a strong correlation but the device required thermodilution calibration limiting its clinical applications for routine circulatory monitoring.[54] Since then, the software has been updated and calibration has been replaced by adjustment to morphometric parameters. Unfortunately, validation studies failed to show a significant correlation compared to thermodilution or echocardiography.[55,56]

Functional hemodynamic monitoring

This part will only focus on different functional hemodynamic parameters available on different monitors. Fluid responsiveness assessment is detailed in another chapter.

In order to be used at the bedside by the physician, dynamic parameters have to be automatically and continuously monitored and if possible, non-invasively.[57,58]

Semi-invasive devices

Respiratory variations of stroke volume (SVV) or arterial pulse pressure (PPV) are the most accurate predictors of fluid responsiveness in mechanically ventilated patients.[59] These dynamic parameters must be continuously calculated and available on bedside monitor or on cardiac output monitor.

- *Pulse contour analysis*: dynamic indices obtained with FloTrac system, LiDCO™ plus system and PiCCO have been validated to predict fluid responsiveness.[20,60,61] However, results concerning SVV obtained with PRAM are disappointing.[27]

- *Automated algorithm for PPV monitoring*: some automated algorithms for PPV monitoring are proposed alone, such as the one implemented on Philips Intellivue MP 70 monitors (Philips, Suresnes, France) by Aboy et al. It has been validated in the clinical setting.[62] Other algorithms are more confidential, invasive and/or partially validated such as Auler's and Pestel's algorithms.[63,64]

Non-invasive devices for fluid responsiveness assessment

- *Esophageal Doppler:* aortic flow respiratory variations shown on the monitor are able to predict fluid responsiveness in mechanically ventilated patients.[65]

- *Finger cuff* :
  - CNAP system: this device does not allow CO monitoring by itself, but PPV obtained manually with this device has been shown to be highly predictable of fluid responsiveness in the operating room.[66,67] Automated algorithm for PPV monitoring using this device remains to be evaluated.
  - Nexfin device: only one study evaluated the ability of PPV and SVV obtained with this device to predict fluid responsiveness with negative results.[40]

- *Pleth variability index (PVI)*: this is an automated and continuous calculation of respiratory variations in the perfusion index. PVI can predict fluid responsiveness in mechanically ventilated patients in the operating room and ICU.[68,69] However, in addition to the traditional limits of cardiorespiratory interactions, indices from the plethysmography can only be used in cases of deep sedation, absence of peripheral vasoconstriction or use of vasopressor use.[70,71]

HOW TO CHOOSE THE MOST APPROPRIATE HEMODYNAMIC MONITORING SYSTEM

Hemodynamic monitoring devices and treatment protocols

It seems important to remember that none of the hemodynamic monitoring techniques can improve outcome by themselves unless they are paired with a therapeutic protocol.[1] Thus, despite the lack of precision of most CO monitoring systems, numerous positive outcome studies have demonstrated that perioperative strategies of hemodynamic monitoring coupled with treatment protocol have been shown to reduce surgical mortality and morbidity.[72]

Perioperative CO optimization

The principle of hemodynamic optimization strategy evolved during the past decade. Initial treatment protocols were very complex and were elaborated to reach supraphysiologic oxygen delivery values, using very aggressive therapeutic (blood transfusion, vasopressor, inotrope, vasodilator) and invasive monitoring (pulmonary arterial catheter). Progressively, treatments protocols, monitoring, and therapeutic goals were simplified. Thus, a strategy based on fluid titration to maximize SV (until it reaches the plateau of the Frank–Starling relationship) using a non-invasive CO monitor such as esophageal Doppler was able to decrease postoperative morbidity.[73] Such a strategy is now strongly recommended by the National Health Service in the UK and the French Society of Anesthesiology for perioperative hemodynamic optimization in high-risk surgical patients.[74,75] Other published studies demonstrated that a perioperative hemodynamic optimization using a mini-invasive tool is possible and of benefit to patients.[76–78]

For this purpose, the esophageal Doppler system has the most evidence regarding improvement of outcome in patients undergoing high-risk surgery and therefore should be strongly considered in such a setting.[73]

Functional hemodynamic parameters

Theoretically, maximizing cardiac output may be done using dynamic parameters. Minimizing these indices (PPV, SPV, SVV) could lead to an increase in CO and oxygen delivery, and thus could be used as a therapeutic goal.[79] In this way, several authors have explored the effects of such a strategy in major surgery on patient outcome. Two recent studies tested the hypothesis that minimizing PPV or SVV may be used as a therapeutic goal with positive results.[80,81] Another approach consists of integrating dynamic parameters into therapeutic protocols in addition to other parameters such as cardiac output. These strategies seem also to have given positive results.[76,78]

Even if these results are very encouraging, the level of evidence concerning this approach is relatively low because these studies are still not numerous and they included few patients. Further studies are required to better define how these parameters can be implemented in clinical protocols for perioperative fluid management.

How to choose the most appropriate monitoring device

Adaptation to patient

Considering the inherent limitations of the different cardiac output monitoring devices, it is obvious that no single hemodynamic monitoring system can fit with all clinical situations.[82] Therefore, different devices may be used in an integrative concept along a typical clinical patient pathway, as recently described by Alhashemi et al. and detailed in another chapter.[82] Whenever accurate measurement of cardiac output or pulmonary artery pressures are necessary, as in cardiac surgery, it is still highly recommended to have a pulmonary arterial catheter available. In non-cardiac surgery, there is no justification in using invasive lines when their risks outweigh their benefits. However, because currently available non-invasive systems are not as reliable as invasive ones, using an inappropriate monitoring device in challenging situations could lead to inappropriate therapeutics. The final choice of a hemodynamic monitoring system depends on both patient and pathology.[81] Thus semi-invasive and reliable monitoring systems should still be preferred during major surgery in high-risk patients, and operators must always be aware of the limitations of devices in order to adapt the therapeutic protocol to the patient's condition.

Despite quality and design heterogeneity in trial, a meta-analysis stratified the effect of goal directed therapy based on the predicted mortality risk. It suggested that, although mortality benefit was greatest among patients in the extremely high-risk subgroup, the reduction of complication rates was seen in all subgroups of GDT patients.[83]

Institutional decision

Implementation of a monitoring device must depend on the institutional constraints and the acceptance of potential users, the only prerequisite for a widespread use of perioperative hemodynamic optimization protocol. Furthermore, patient management is a continuum of care and it is essential to maintain compatibility among hemodynamic monitoring technologies between different departments (ward, emergency department, operating room, and ICU) within the institution. An interesting method of management is the recent development of technological platforms allowing movement from a totally non-invasive hemodynamic monitoring system to a mini-invasive one and then to an invasive one. This new approach permits flexible monitoring.

Conclusions

Today, large panels of mini-invasive and totally non-invasive hemodynamic monitoring systems have been developed for monitoring CO and dynamic parameters of fluid responsiveness. Despite valuable technological improvements, none of the currently available hemodynamic monitoring devices responds to all of the validation criteria compared to the gold standard. Yet, these systems have still been tested in clinical outcome studies and numerous studies have demonstrated their usefulness in decreasing postoperative morbidity when they are coupled with clearly defined and generally adopted protocols. Finally, choosing the most appropriate hemodynamic monitor depends on institutional approach within different departments, the preoperative risk of the patient and/or type of surgery in an integrative approach.

References

1. Pinsky MR, Payen D. Functional hemodynamic monitoring. *Crit Care* 2005;**9**:566–72.

2. Dark PM, Singer M. The validity of trans-esophageal Doppler ultrasonography as a measure of cardiac output in critically ill adults. *Intensive Care Med* 2004;**30**:2060–6.

3. Schober P, Loer SA, Schwarte LA. Perioperative hemodynamic monitoring with transesophageal Doppler technology. *Anesth Analg* 2009;**109**:340–53.

4. Lefrant JY, Bruelle P, Aya AG, et al. Training is required to improve the reliability of esophageal Doppler to measure cardiac output in critically ill patients. *Intens Care Med* 1998;**24**:347–52.

5. Tan HL, Pinder M, Parsons R, et al. Clinical evaluation of USCOM ultrasonic cardiac output monitor in cardiac surgical patients in intensive care unit. *Br J Anaesth* 2005; **94**:287–91.

6. Chand R, Mehta Y, Trehan N. Cardiac output estimation with a new Doppler device after off-pump coronary artery bypass surgery. *J Cardiothorac Vasc Anesth* 2006;**20**:315–19.

7. Chong SW, Peyton PJ. A meta-analysis of the accuracy and precision of the ultrasonic cardiac output monitor (USCOM). *Anaesthesia* 2012; **67**:1266–71.

8. Marik PE. Noninvasive cardiac output monitors: a state-of the-art review. *J Cardiothorac Vasc Anesth* 2013;**27**:121–34.

9. Mayer J, Suttner S. Cardiac output derived from arterial pressure waveform. *Curr Opin Anaes* 2009;**22**:804–8.

10. de Waal EE, Kalkman CJ, Rex S, et al. Validation of a new arterial pulse contour-based cardiac output device. *Crit Care Med* 2007;**35**:1904–9.

11. Monnet X, Anguel N, Naudin B, et al. Arterial pressure-based cardiac output in septic patients: different accuracy of pulse contour and uncalibrated pressure waveform devices. *Crit Care* 2010;**14**:R109.

12. Zimmermann A, Kufner C, Hofbauer S, et al. The accuracy of the Vigileo/FloTrac continuous cardiac output monitor. *J Cardiothorac Vasc Anesth* 2008;**22**:388–93.

13. Biais M, Nouette-Gaulain K, Cottenceau V, et al. Cardiac output measurement in patients undergoing liver transplantation: pulmonary artery catheter versus uncalibrated arterial pressure waveform analysis. *Anesth Analg* 2008;**106**:1480–6.

14. Biancofiore G, Critchley LA, Lee A, et al. Evaluation of an uncalibrated arterial pulse contour cardiac output monitoring system in cirrhotic patients undergoing liver surgery. *Br J Anaesth* 2009; **102**:47–54.

15. Chatti R, de Rudniki S, Marque S, et al. Comparison of two versions of the Vigileo-FloTrac system (1.03 and 1.07) for stroke volume estimation: a multicentre, blinded comparison with oesophageal Doppler measurements. *Br J Anaesth* 2009;**102**:463–9.

16. Hadian M, Kim HK, Severyn DA, et al. Cross-comparison of cardiac output trending accuracy of LiDCO, PiCCO, FloTrac and pulmonary artery catheters. *Crit Care* 2010;**14**:R212.

17. De Backer D, Marx G, Tan A, et al. Arterial pressure-based cardiac output monitoring: a multicenter validation of the third-generation software in septic patients. *Intensive Care Med* 2011;**37**:233–40.

18. Meng L, Tran NP, Alexander BS, et al. The impact of phenylephrine, ephedrine, and increased preload on third-generation Vigileo-FloTrac and esophageal doppler cardiac output measurements. *Anesth Analg* 2011;**113**:751–7.

19. Monnet X, Anguel N, Jozwiak M, et al. Third-generation FloTrac/ Vigileo does not reliably track changes in cardiac output induced by norepinephrine in critically ill patients. *Br J Anaesth* 2012;**108**:615–22.

20. Biais M, Nouette-Gaulain K, Cottenceau V, et al. Uncalibrated pulse contour-derived stroke volume variation predicts fluid responsiveness in mechanically ventilated patients undergoing liver transplantation. *Br J Anaesth* 2008;**101**:761–8.

21. Biais M, Nouette-Gaulain K, Quinart A, et al. Uncalibrated stroke volume variations are able to predict the hemodynamic

effects of positive end-expiratory pressure in patients with acute lung injury or acute respiratory distress syndrome after liver transplantation. *Anesthesiology* 2009;**111**:855–62.

22. Biais M, Vidil L, Sarrabay P, et al. Changes in stroke volume induced by passive leg raising in spontaneously breathing patients: comparison between echocardiography and Vigileo/FloTrac device. *Crit Care* 2009; **13**:R195.

23. Franchi F, Silvestri R, Cubattoli L, et al. Comparison between an uncalibrated pulse contour method and thermodilution technique for cardiac output estimation in septic patients. *Br J Anaesth* 2011;**107**:202–8.

24. Giomarelli P, Biagioli B, Scolletta S. Cardiac output monitoring by pressure recording analytical method in cardiac surgery. *Eur J Cardiothoracic Surg* 2004;**26**:515–20.

25. Romano SM, Pistolesi M. Assessment of cardiac output from systemic arterial pressure in humans. *Crit Care Med* 2002;**30**:1834–41.

26. Scolletta S, Romano SM, Biagioli B, et al. Pressure recording analytical method (PRAM) for measurement of cardiac output during various haemodynamic states. *Br J Anaesth* 2005; **95**:159–65.

27. Biais M, Cottenceau V, Jean M, et al. Evaluation of stroke volume variations obtained with the pressure recording analytic method. *Crit Care Med* 2012;**40**:369–71.

28. Maj G, Monaco F, Landoni G, et al. Cardiac index assessment by the pressure recording analytic method in unstable patients with atrial fibrillation. *J Cardiothorac Vasc Anesth* 2011;**25**:476–80.

29. Paarmann H, Groesdonk HV, Sedemund-Adib B, et al. Lack of agreement between pulmonary arterial thermodilution cardiac output and the pressure recording analytical method in postoperative cardiac surgery patients. *Br J Anaesth* 2011;**106**:475–81.

30. Cecconi M, Dawson D, Grounds RM, et al. Lithium dilution cardiac output measurement in the critically ill patient: determination of precision of the technique. *Intensive Care Med* 2009;**35**:498–504.

31. Cecconi M, Fawcett J, Grounds RM, et al. A prospective study to evaluate the accuracy of pulse power analysis to monitor cardiac output in critically ill patients. *BMC Anesthesiol* 2008;**8**:3.

32. Wesseling KH, Jansen JR, Settels JJ, et al. Computation of aortic flow from pressure in humans using a nonlinear, three-element model. *J Appl Physiol* 1993;**74**:2566–73.

33. Westerhof N, Elzinga G, Sipkema P. An artificial arterial system for pumping hearts. *J Appl Physiol* 1971;**31**:776–81.

34. Jansen JR, Schreuder JJ, Mulier JP, et al. A comparison of cardiac output derived from the arterial pressure wave against thermodilution in cardiac surgery patients. *Br J Anaesth* 2001;**87**:212–22.

35. Harms MP, Wesseling KH, Pott F, et al. Continuous stroke volume monitoring by modelling flow from non-invasive measurement of arterial pressure in humans under orthostatic stress. *Clin Sci* 1999;**97**:291–301.

36. Jellema WT, Wesseling KH, Groeneveld AB, et al. Continuous cardiac output in septic shock by simulating a model of the aortic input impedance: a comparison with bolus injection thermodilution. *Anesthesiology* 1999;**90**:1317–28.

37. Broch O, Renner J, Gruenewald M, et al. A comparison of the Nexfin(R) and transcardiopulmonary thermodilution to estimate cardiac output during coronary artery surgery. *Anaesthesia* 2012;**67**:377–83.

38. Martina JR, Westerhof BE, van Goudoever J, et al. Noninvasive continuous arterial blood pressure monitoring with Nexfin(R). *Anesthesiology* 2012; **116**:1092–103.

39. Bubenek-Turconi SI, Craciun M, Miclea I, et al. Noninvasive continuous cardiac output by the Nexfin before and After preload-modifying maneuvers: a comparison with intermittent thermodilution cardiac output. *Anesth Analg* 2013;**117**:366–72.

40. Fischer MO, Coucoravas J, Truong J, et al. Assessment of changes in cardiac index and fluid responsiveness: a comparison of Nexfin and transpulmonary thermodilution. *Acta Anaesthesiol Scand* 2013;**57**:704–12.

41. Monnet X, Picard F, Lidzborski E, et al. The estimation of cardiac output by the Nexfin device is of poor reliability for tracking the effects of a fluid challenge. *Crit Care* 2012;**16**:R212.

42. Funk DJ, Moretti EW, Gan TJ. Minimally invasive cardiac output monitoring in the perioperative setting. *Anesth Analg* 2009;**108**:887–97.

43. Rocco M, Spadetta G, Morelli A, et al. A comparative evaluation of thermodilution and partial CO_2 rebreathing techniques for cardiac output assessment in critically ill patients during assisted ventilation. *Intens Care Med* 2004;**30**:82–7.

44. Tachibana K, Imanaka H, Takeuchi M, et al. Effects of reduced rebreathing time, in spontaneously breathing patients, on respiratory effort and accuracy in cardiac output measurement when using a partial carbon dioxide rebreathing technique: a prospective observational study. *Crit Care* 2005;**9**:R569–74.

45. de Waal EE, Konings MK, Kalkman CJ, et al. Assessment of stroke volume index with three different bioimpedance algorithms: lack of agreement compared to thermodilution. *Intens Care Med* 2008;**34**:735–9.

46. Marik PE, Pendelton JE, Smith R. A comparison of hemodynamic parameters derived from transthoracic electrical bioimpedance with those parameters obtained by thermodilution and ventricular angiography. *Crit Care Med* 1997;**25**:1545–50.

47. Maus TM, Reber B, Banks DA, et al. Cardiac output determination from endotracheally measured impedance cardiography: clinical evaluation of endotracheal cardiac output monitor. *J Cardiothorac Vasc Anesth* 2011;**25**:770–5.

48. van der Kleij SC, Koolen BB, Newhall DA, et al. Clinical evaluation of a new tracheal impedance cardiography method. *Anaesthesia* 2012;**67**:729–33.

49. Fellahi JL, Fischer MO, Rebet O, et al. A comparison of endotracheal bioimpedance cardiography and transpulmonary thermodilution in cardiac surgery patients. *J Cardiothorac Vasc Anesth* 2012;**26**:217–22.

50. Benomar B, Ouattara A, Estagnasie P, et al. Fluid responsiveness predicted by noninvasive bioreactance-based passive leg raise test. *Intens Care Med* 2010;**36**:1875–81.

51. Squara P, Denjean D, Estagnasie P, et al. Noninvasive cardiac output monitoring (NICOM): a clinical validation. *Intens Care Med* 2007;**33**:1191–4.

52. Conway DH, Hussain OA, Gall I. A comparison of noninvasive bioreactance with oesophageal Doppler estimation of stroke volume during open abdominal surgery: an observational study. *Eur J Anaesthesiol* 2013;**30**:501–8.

53. Hofer CK, Buhlmann S, Klaghofer R, et al. Pulsed dye densitometry with two different sensor types for cardiac output measurement after cardiac surgery: a comparison with the thermodilution technique. *Acta Anaesthesiol Scand* 2004;**48**:653–7.

54. Ishihara H, Okawa H, Tanabe K, et al. A new non-invasive continuous cardiac output trend solely utilizing routine cardiovascular monitors. *J Clin Monitor Comp* 2004;**18**:313–20.

55. Bataille B, Bertuit M, Mora M, et al. Comparison of esCCO and transthoracic echocardiography for non-invasive measurement of cardiac output intensive care. *Br J Anaesth* 2012;**109**:879–86.

56. Ishihara H, Sugo Y, Tsutsui M, et al. The ability of a new continuous cardiac output monitor to measure trends in cardiac output following implementation of a patient information calibration and an automated exclusion algorithm. *J Clin Monitor Comp* 2012;**26**:465–71.

57. Biais M, Ouattara A, Janvier G, et al. Case scenario: respiratory variations in arterial pressure for guiding fluid management in mechanically ventilated patients. *Anesthesiology* 2012;**116**:1354–61.

58. Cannesson M. Arterial pressure variation and goal-directed fluid therapy. *J Cardiothorac Vasc Anesth* 2010;**24**:487–97.

59. Marik PE, Cavallazzi R, Vasu T, et al. Dynamic changes in arterial waveform derived variables and fluid responsiveness in mechanically ventilated patients: A systematic review of the literature. *Crit Care Med* 2009;**37**:2642–7.

60. Berkenstadt H, Margalit N, Hadani M, et al. Stroke volume variation as a predictor of fluid responsiveness in patients undergoing brain surgery. *Anesth Analg* 2001;**92**:984–9.

61. Cecconi M, Monti G, Hamilton MA, et al. Efficacy of functional hemodynamic parameters in predicting fluid responsiveness with pulse power analysis in surgical patients. *Minerva anestesiologica* 2012;**78**:527–33.

62. Cannesson M, Slieker J, Desebbe O, et al. The ability of a novel algorithm for automatic estimation of the respiratory variations in arterial pulse pressure to monitor fluid responsiveness in the operating room. *Anesth Analg* 2008;**106**:1195–200.

63. Auler JO, Jr., Galas F, Hajjar L, et al. Online monitoring of pulse pressure variation to guide fluid therapy after cardiac surgery. *Anesth Analg* 2008;**106**:1201–6.

64. Pestel G, Fukui K, Hartwich V, et al. Automatic algorithm for monitoring systolic pressure variation and difference in pulse pressure. *Anesth Analg* 2009;**108**:1823–9.

65. Monnet X, Rienzo M, Osman D, et al. Esophageal Doppler monitoring predicts fluid responsiveness in critically ill ventilated patients. *Intensive Care Med* 2005;**31**:1195–201.

66. Biais M, Stecken L, Ottolenghi L, et al. The ability of pulse pressure variations obtained with CNAP device to predict fluid responsiveness in the operating room. *Anesth Analg* 2011;**113**:523–8.

67. Monnet X, Dres M, Ferre A, et al. Prediction of fluid responsiveness by a continuous non-invasive assessment of arterial pressure in critically ill patients: comparison with four other dynamic indices. *Br J Anaesth* 2012;**109**:330–8.

68. Cannesson M, Attof Y, Rosamel P, et al. Respiratory variations in pulse oximetry plethysmographic waveform amplitude to predict fluid responsiveness in the operating room. *Anesthesiology* 2007;**106**:1105–11.

69. Desebbe O, Cannesson M. Using ventilation-induced plethysmographic variations to optimize patient fluid status. *Curr Opin Anaesthesiol* 2008;**21**:772–8.

70. Biais M, Cottenceau V, Petit L, et al. Impact of norepinephrine on the relationship between pleth variability index and pulse pressure variations in ICU adult patients. *Crit Care* 2011;**15**:R168.

71. Monnet X, Guerin L, Jozwiak M, et al. Pleth variability index is a weak predictor of fluid responsiveness in patients receiving norepinephrine. *Br J Anaesth* 2013;**110**:207–13.

72. Hamilton MA, Cecconi M, Rhodes A. A systematic review and meta-analysis on the use of preemptive hemodynamic intervention to improve postoperative outcomes in moderate and high-risk surgical patients. *Anesth Analg* 2011;**112**:1392–402.

73. Phan TD, Ismail H, Heriot AG, et al. Improving perioperative outcomes: fluid optimization with the esophageal Doppler monitor, a metaanalysis and review. *J Am Coll Surg* 2008;**207**:935–41.

74. NICE Draft Guidance on Cardiac Output Monitoring Device Published for Consultation. In http://www.nice.org.uk/newsroom/pressreleases/DraftGuidanceOnCardiacOutputMonitoringDevice.jsp, editor.

75. Vallet B, Blanloeil Y, Cholley B, et al. Guidelines for perioperative haemodynamic optimization. *Annales francaises d'anesthesie et de reanimation* 2013;**32**:454–62.

76. Benes J, Chytra I, Altmann P, et al. Intraoperative fluid optimization using stroke volume variation in high risk surgical patients: results of prospective randomized study. *Crit Care* 2010;**14**:R118.

77. Cecconi M, Fasano N, Langiano N, et al. Goal-directed haemodynamic therapy during elective total hip arthroplasty under regional anaesthesia. *Crit Care* 2011;**15**:R132.

78. Mayer J, Boldt J, Mengistu AM, et al. Goal-directed intraoperative therapy based on autocalibrated arterial pressure waveform analysis reduces hospital stay in high-risk surgical patients: a randomized, controlled trial. *Crit Care* 2010;**14**:R18.

79. Biais M. Stroke volume variation: just a fancy tool or a therapeutic goal? *Crit Care Med* 2012;**40**:335–6.

80. Lopes MR, Oliveira MA, Pereira VO, et al. Goal-directed fluid management based on pulse pressure variation monitoring during high-risk surgery: a pilot randomized controlled trial. *Crit Care* 2007;**11**:R100.

81. Ramsingh DS, Sanghvi C, Gamboa J, et al. Outcome impact of goal directed fluid therapy during high risk abdominal surgery in low to moderate risk patients: a randomized controlled trial. *J Clini monit Comput* 2013;**27**:24–57.

82. Alhashemi JA, Cecconi M, Hofer CK. Cardiac output monitoring: an integrative perspective. *Crit Care* 2011;**15**:214.

83. Cecconi M, Corredor C, Arulkumaran N, et al. Clinical review: goal-directed therapy – what is the evidence in surgical patients? The effect on different risk groups. *Crit Care* 2013;**17**:209.

Chapter

17

Mean systemic pressure monitoring

Michael R. Pinsky

Introduction

Accurate assessment of cardiovascular state in the critically ill is difficult because easily measured hemodynamic parameters, such as blood pressure and cardiac output (CO) can co-exist with different levels of ventricular pump function and effective circulating blood volume. Presumably, by adding measures of ventricular function and effective circulating blood volume to the assessment, the bedside clinician can now define accurately cardiovascular state and predict accurately response to specific interventions or insults. As discussed above, measures of dynamic arterial pulse pressure or left ventricular (LV) stroke volume variation (PPV and SVV, respectively) identify threshold levels above which patients are highly likely to be volume responsive. However, instead of using PPV or SVV to define volume responsiveness, if one uses them as a surrogate for ventricular responsiveness or performance, then one can use the absolute levels of PPV and SVV as indirect measures of ventricular performance. Accordingly, the only parameter missing from an analysis of cardiovascular state is the estimation of effective circulating blood volume. Furthermore, although fluid resuscitation therapy is important in the management of unstable patients, excessive fluid resuscitation can be harmful in acute lung injury,[1] head injury,[2] and postoperative patients.[3] Thus, a measure of effective volume status is useful to avoid volume overload since even volume overloaded patients may remain volume responsive.

As described earlier in this volume (Chapter 5), the effective circulating blood volume in the systemic circulation can be estimated as mean systemic pressure (Pms).[4] Pms is a functional measure of effective intravascular volume status. Conceptually,

it is defined as the pressure anywhere in the circulation during circulatory arrest. Importantly, the pressure gradient between right atrial pressure (Pra) and Pms defines the driving pressure for venous return, and together with the resistance to venous return defines CO (Figure 17.1). Accordingly, by knowing Pms, Pra, and CO, one can also calculate the resistance to venous return as the inverse slope of the flow to the pressure difference. This chapter will explore methods of measuring Pms and their clinical applications.

Stop-flow measures of Pms

The fundamental method of measuring Pms is to induce circulatory arrest and to rapidly equilibrate the pressures in the arterial and venous vascular beds by opening a large a–v fistula.[5] These initial studies first in dogs and then in man reported Pms valves between 8 and 12 mmHg. In support of this finding, Jellinek et al.[6] estimated Pms in highly anesthetized non-volume resuscitated patients during episodes of apnea and ventricular fibrillation and found a Pms value of 10.2 and 12 mmHg, respectively. Importantly, these values reflect Pms under conditions of deep anesthesia and without volume resuscitation. As we shall see, in recent studies values of Pms often range from 18–30 mmHg. Although the stop-flow technique can be used in the perioperative environment, it is limited to subjects experiencing ventricular fibrillation or circulatory arrest during cardiopulmonary bypass. Furthermore, the measures of Pms are independent of the prior measure of Pra and make the calculation of the resistance to venous return questionable. Still, this approach reflects the gold standard for measuring Pms and was used by previous workers to validate their newer techniques.

Perioperative Hemodynamic Monitoring and Goal Directed Therapy, ed. Maxime Cannesson and Rupert Pearse.
Published by CAMBRIDGE UNIVERSITY PRESS. © Cambridge University Press 2014.

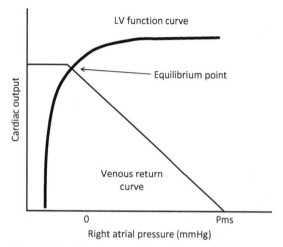

Figure 17.1. Relation between cardiac output and right atrial pressure when the right atrial pressure (Pra) is independently varied defines two separate curves. The LV function curve is also displayed in Figure 17.1, but with cardiac output and not stroke volume as the flow unit; and the venous return curve. The intersection of the two curves defines steady-state cardiac output and is referred to as the equilibrium point. The zero cardiac output Pra intercept of the venous return curve is the mean systemic pressure (Pms); the slope of the cardiac output to Pra line is inversely proportional to the resistance to venous return.

Instantaneous venous return curves

Pinsky[8] reasoned that, if Pra was slowly increased by positive-pressure inspiration owing to the associated increase in intrathoracic pressure, then only Pra would increase, as Pms would be unaffected by the small tidal volume associated increase in lung volume causing diaphragmatic descent. Assuming that right ventricular (RV) stroke volume changes followed RV filling changes, then the resultant RV stroke volume to Pra relation with Pra on the *x*-axis should have a negative slope inversely proportional to the resistance to venous return and a positive pressure zero RV stroke volume intercept approximating Pms. Since Pms is a function of circulating blood volume and the blood flow distribution among various vascular beds, Pms can vary quickly if vasomotor tone increases or if blood flow distribution switches from different types of vascular beds with different proportions of stressed to unstressed volume and differing degrees of resistance to venous return. For example, the splanchnic circulation has a large amount of unstressed volume present before adding further volume creates a measurable distending pressure. Thus if much of the cardiac output is going to the gut, as often occurs in a postprandial state, then a large amount of blood will be allocated to that circulation and not be available to the rest of the circulation. However, if sympathetic tone were to increase, then splanchnic arterial resistance and overall splanchnic vasomotor tone would increase, decreasing inflow into the splanchnic circulation and decreasing unstressed volume, resulting in an autotransfusion of blood into the systemic circulation. Pinsky and Matuschak[9] examined these interactions in a canine model of acute endotoxic shock and compared it to baseline conditions. Using their previously validated instantaneous venous return curve analysis, they examined the effect of intravascular volume loading and removal on the slope and zero flow intercept of the instantaneous venous return curves (Figure 17.2). They demonstrated that acute endotoxemia increased whole body unstressed volume, but did not change systemic vascular compliance. Although these findings are interesting and potentially explain many of the observed cardiovascular characteristics seen in human sepsis, this approach is not feasible for clinical practice. First, measures of RV stroke volume using 2-D echocardiography during positive pressure ventilation, though possible are not practical. Second, the integration of beat-to-beat RV stroke volume values with their respective Pra values measured at the R wave are prone to measurement errors in Pra values as they fluctuate widely. Thus, this technique is excellent for validating other techniques in animals and humans but is of little clinical utility.

Inspiratory hold maneuver construction of venous return curves

Since venous return and cardiac output in the steady state must be equal, if the increase in Pra was slight and held constant until LV stroke volume stabilized, which usually takes about 4–6 heart beats, then one could plot steady-state Pra and CO measures as Pra was varied. Vesprille and Jansen[10] studied the relation between steady-state cardiac output, measured by an arterial pulse contour algorithm derived estimate of LV stroke volume, and Pra during a series of steady-state end-inspiratory pauses of 5, 7.5, 10, 12.5 and 15 cm H_2O and compared their estimates of Pms to those measured immediately before by the instantaneous venous return technique in pigs. They demonstrated that both techniques gave similar estimates of Pms and its change in response to intravascular volume loading. Subsequently, Maas et al. demonstrated that this inspiratory-hold technique could also be used to measure Pms in ventilator-dependent patients[11–12] (Figure 17.3) and that the calculated Pms accurately

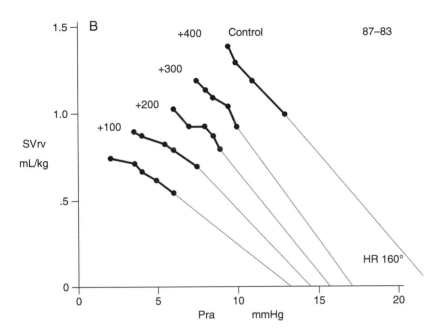

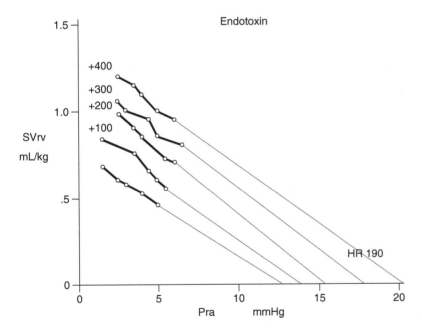

Figure 17.2. The summary right ventricular stroke volume (SVrv) and right atrial pressure (Pra) data pairs for a series of volume loading steps and their extrapolated linear regression lines to zero SVrv for one animal during control and acute endotoxin infusion states. Heart rate, HR. Note that, during endotoxin, the HR is higher and the venous return slopes less steep (increased resistance) than control. Reproduced, with permission, from reference 9.

followed changes in intravascular volume. Thus, this approach should allow for analysis of the determinants of cardiovascular response to pharmacological manipulations in appropriately selected patients.

Importantly, two recent studies used the inspiratory-hold technique to define the cardiovascular effect of varying norepinephrine infusion rates of cardiac output. Maas et al.[13] studied the effect of increasing mean arterial pressure by 20 mmHg in 16 post-coronary artery bypass surgery patients. In all, Pms increased (21.4 to 27.6 mmHg) and Pra increased (7.6 to 8.6 mmHg), the resistance to venous return increased and SVV decreased in all, reflecting the expected response to increased LV afterload on preload responsiveness. However, cardiac output decreased in ten patients (4.46 to 3.96 L/min) while it increased in six other

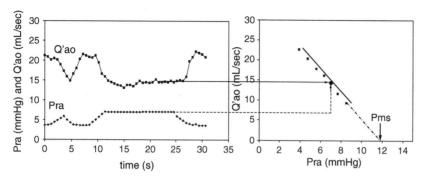

Figure 17.3. Trend recording of estimated aortic flow (Q'ao) using arterial pressure contour analysis and right atrial pressure (Pra) during a transient inspiratory-hold maneuver (left) and the associated data point on the subsequent venous return curve construction. The zero Q'ao intercept is taken to reflect mean systemic pressure (Pms). Reproduced, with permission, from reference 11.

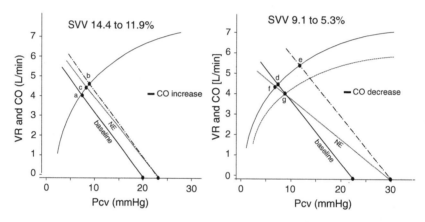

Figure 17.4. Schematic diagram of the effects of norepinephrine (NE). Venous return (VR) curve and cardiac output (CO) curve constructed from average values of central venous pressure (Pcv), mean systemic pressure and CO for patient who increased CO (left) and decreased CO (right) after NE dose increase. "a" indicates the working point of the circulation during baseline; "b" volume effect of generalized venoconstriction on CO by NE; "c" additional effect of venoconstriction on resistance to venous return (RVR); "d" indicates the working point of the circulation during baseline; "e" volume effect of generalized venoconstriction on CO by NE; "f" additional effect of venoconstriction on RVR; "g" effect of decreased heart function. Reproduced with permission from reference 13.

patients (4.06 to 4.31 mL/min). It turned out that the deciding factor as to whether cardiac output increased or decreased in these patients was their baseline LV reserve as estimated by their initial SVV. Those patients with a decrease in cardiac output had a lower initial SVV that decreased further (9.1 to 5.3%), whereas the increased cardiac output group had a good initial SVV that, though decreasing, remained in the preload responsive range during norepinephrine infusion (14.4% to 11.9%) (Figure 17.4). These data underscore the importance of baseline ventricular reserve when determining the expected response to vasopressor drug therapy. Indeed, one way to document poor LV functional reserve is to increase mean arterial pressure and document a fall in cardiac output. In a similar study Persichini et al.[14] examined the effect of lowering

norepinephrine levels in septic patients deemed no longer to require their initial level of vasopressor support. They demonstrated that reducing norepinephrine causes a minimal decrease in cardiac output because, although the reduced dose of norepinephrine resulted in the expected decrease in Pms (33 to 26 mmHg), the slope of the venous return curve increased, minimizing the effect of the decreasing Pms on cardiac output.

These recent studies are exciting because they demonstrate that measures of Pms at the bedside can be made and interpreted in a physiological fashion, explaining desperate responses to defined pharmacologic challenges. Although a major step forward, unfortunately this inspiratory-hold technique requires a sedated and ventilated patient, requires repeated measures at different end-inspiratory pressures, and plotting of those data off-line to estimate Pms. This is not the sort of approach that will be easily applied even in the patients in whom it can be used. What is needed is a more simplified approach applicable to all patients.

Vascular peripheral stop-flow estimates of mean systemic pressure

Our group studied two simpler bedside methods for determining Pms, as previously suggested by Anderson.[15] The first technique examines the stop-flow vascular pressure in a peripheral artery or vein as an approximation of Pms. Anderson hypothesized that the circulation of the arm behaves similarly to total systemic circulation during steady-state conditions, with venous flow behaving as if its upstream pressure is Pms. Thus, although all vascular beds will have their own equilibrium pressure in the isolated state, when lumped together they drain as if their upstream pressures were similar (Figure 17.5). The second approach by Parkin and Leaning proposed to estimate effective circulatory volume based on an electrical analog simplification of Guytonian circulatory physiology[16] estimating mean circulatory pressure (Pmsa) from directly measured Pra, mean arterial pressure, and CO. To assess this assumption, Maas et al. measured transient stop-flow forearm arterial and venous equilibrium pressure, referred to as arm equilibrium pressure (Parm) and compared that to the estimated Pms using the inspiratory hold maneuver technique in postoperative surgical patients. They varied effective circulating blood volume by a head-up tilt maneuver to decrease effective circulating blood volume and by a bolus infusion of fluid to increase effective circulating blood volume. They showed that Parm faithfully tracked Pms, whereas Pmsa displayed a systemic bias, which could be accounted for by dividing Pmsa by 0.7.

These data demonstrate that estimates of Pms measured Pa 30 seconds after stop-flow (Parm) are interchangeable with Pms calculated using inspiratory hold maneuvers in mechanically ventilated postoperative cardiac surgery patients. Furthermore, changes in volume status by head-up tilt and volume infusion maneuvers were similarly tracked by Pms, Parm, and Pmsa. These data support the hypothesis formulated by Anderson that, during steady-state flow conditions, the arm is representative of the entire circulation, such that a rapid vascular occlusion will result in its stop-flow Pa approximating Pms. Thus, both inspiratory hold Pms and stop-flow Parm can be used at the bedside to measure effective circulating blood volume. Furthermore, Pmsa can reliably track changes in effective circulating blood volume status.

The use of both Parm and Pmsa have practical advantages over the previously validated inspiratory hold maneuver Pms approach. Neither require positive-pressure breathing or multiple simultaneous measures of Pra and cardiac output during inspiratory hold maneuvers and both can be rapidly and repeatedly measured sequentially as treatment or time progresses. Parm requires only the peripheral arterial catheter. Pmsa requires both central venous and peripheral arterial catheters. Thus, these two novel approaches markedly increase the applicability of assessment of effective circulating blood volume to a broader patient population. Cecconi et al.[17] calculated Pmsa and its change in response of 111 bolus fluid challenges (250 mL) in

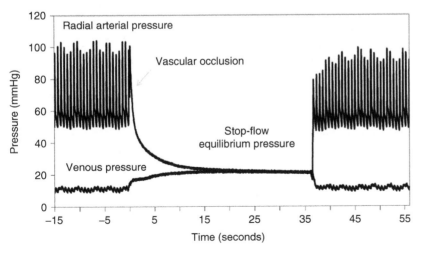

Figure 17.5. Representative registration of radial artery pressure and venous pressure before (−15 to 0 seconds), during (0 to 35 seconds) and after the occlusion of the upper arm of a patient. Arm vascular occlusion equilibrium pressure (Parm) is taken as the arterial pressure 30 seconds after stop-flow. Note the influence of mechanical ventilation on arterial and venous pressure before and after occlusion. Reproduced with permission from Maas JJ, Pinsky MR, Geerts BF, et al. Estimation of mean systemic filling pressure in postoperative cardiac surgery patients with three methods. *Intens Care Med* 2012;**38**:1452–60.

39 postoperative surgical patients. They saw that, in all patients, Pmsa increased (3.1±1.8 mmHg), whereas in those patients whose cardiac output increased by >10% (referred to as responders) the Pmsa–Pra gradient (referred to as the pressure gradient for venous return or dVR) increased more in responders than in non-responders (1.16±0.8 vs. 0.2±1, P<0.001) because Pra increased more in non-responders than in responders. These data demonstrate that one can not only measure Pms at the bedside, but that it follows predicted fashions to known challenges.

Recently, Lee et al. compared Pmsa to Pms measured by the instantaneous venous return technique described above wherein RV stroke volume and Pra are plotted over a positive pressure breath to estimate the zero RV stroke volume intercept at Pms. They compared the ability of Pmsa to track Pms during volume loading and removal before and after the induction of acute endotoxic shock in a canine model.[18] They demonstrated that Pmsa closely tracked Pms under both conditions. These data collectively support the use of both Parm and Pmsa as simple bedside measures of Pms. Hopefully, the subsequent use of these measures will supplement present bedside monitoring and allow us to understand better a given patient's cardiovascular state and predict response to therapy or insult before they occur.

Conflicts of interest

Consultant: Edwards LifeSciences, Inc; LiDCO Ltd.

Research support: NIH, DoD, Edwards Life-Sciences, Inc.

References

1. Wiedemann HP, Wheeler AP, Bernard GR, et al. Comparison of two fluid-management strategies in acute lung injury. *N Engl J Med* 2006;**354**:2564–75.

2. Huang SJ, Hong WC, Han YY, et al. Clinical outcome of severe head injury using three different ICP and CPP protocol-driven therapies. *J Clin Neurosci* 2006;**13**:818–22.

3. Brandstrup B, Tonnesen H, Beier-Holgersen R, et al. Effects of intravenous fluid restriction on postoperative complications: comparison of two perioperative fluid regimens: a randomized assessor-blinded multicenter trial. *Ann Surg* 2003;**238**:641–8.

4. Guyton AC, Lindsey AW, Abernathy B, Richardson T. Venous return at various right atrial pressures and the normal venous return curve. *Am J Physiol* 1957;**189**:609–15.

5. Guyton AC, Polizo D, Armstrong GG. Mean circulatory filling pressure measured immediately after cessation of heart pumping. *Am J Physiol* 1954;**179**:261–7.

6. Jellinek H, Krenn H, Oczenski W, et al. Influence of positive airway pressure on the pressure gradient for venous return in humans. *J Appl Physiol* 2000;**88**:926–32.

7. Schipke JD, Heusch G, Sanii AP, Gams E, Winter J. Static filling pressure in patients during induced ventricular fibrillation. *Am J Physiol* 2003;**285**:H2510–15.

8. Pinsky MR. Instantaneous venous return curves in an intact canine preparation. *J Appl Physiol* 1984;**56**:765–71.

9. Pinsky MR, Matuschak GM. Cardiovascular determinants of the hemodynamic response to acute endotoxemia in the dog. *J Crit Care* 1986;**1**:18–31.

10. Versprille A, Jansen JR. Mean systemic filling pressure as a characteristic pressure for venous return. *Pflugers Arch* 1985; **405**:226–33.

11. Maas JJ, Geerts BF, van den Berg PC, Pinsky MR, Jansen JR. Assessment of venous return curve and mean systemic filling pressure in postoperative cardiac surgery patients. *Crit Care Med* 2009;**37**:912–18.

12. Jansen JR, Maas JJ, Pinsky MR. Bedside assessment of mean systemic filling pressure. *Curr Opin Crit Care* 2010; **16**:231–6.

13. Maas JJ, Pinsky MR, de Wilde RB, de Jonge E, Jansen JR. Cardiac output response to norepinephrine in postoperative cardiac surgery patients: interpretation with venous return and cardiac function curves. *Crit Care Med* 2013;**41** (1):143–50.

14. Persichini R, Silva S, Teboul JL, et al. Effects of norepinephrine on mean systemic pressure and venous return in human septic shock. *Crit Care Med* 2012;**40** (12):3146–53.

15. Anderson RM. *The Gross Physiology of the Cardiovascular System.* Tucson: Racquet Press, 1993.

16. Parkin WG, Leaning MS. Therapeutic control of the circulation. *J Clin Monit Comput* 1993;**22**:391–400.

17. Cecconi M, Ayes HD, Geison M, et al. Change in mean systemic filling pressure during fluid challenge in postsurgical intensive care patients. *Intens Care Med* 2013;**39**:1299–305.

18. Lee JM, Ogundele O, Pike F, Pinsky MR. Effect of acute endotoxemia on analogue estimates of mean systemic pressure. *J Crit Care* 2013;**28** (5):880.e9–15.

Chapter

18

Fluid responsiveness assessment

Xavier Monnet and Jean-Louis Teboul

Introduction

In patients with an acute circulatory failure, the primary goal of volume expansion is to increase cardiac output. However, this expected effect is inconstant, so that in many instances, fluid administration does not result in any hemodynamic benefit. In such cases, fluid could only exert some deleterious effects. It is now well demonstrated that excessive fluid administration is harmful, especially during acute respiratory distress syndrome (ARDS)[1] and in sepsis or septic shock.[2] This is the reason why some indices have been developed in order to assess "fluid responsiveness" before deciding to perform volume expansion. While preload markers have been used for many years for this purpose, they have been repeatedly shown to be unreliable, mainly due to physiological issues. As alternatives, "dynamic" indices have been introduced. These indices are based upon the changes in cardiac output or stroke volume resulting from various changes in preload conditions, induced by heart–lung interactions, postural maneuvers, or by the infusion of small amounts of fluids. The hemodynamic effects and the reliability of these "dynamic" indices of fluid responsiveness are now well described. From their respective advantages and limitations, it is also possible to describe their clinical interest and the clinical setting where they are applicable.

Fluid responsiveness: physiology and concept

Fluid responsiveness corresponds to the ability of the heart to "respond" to fluid infusion by a significant increase in cardiac output. It implies two conditions. The first is that fluid administration induces a sufficient increase in cardiac preload. The second is that

both ventricles are preload-dependent. According to the Frank–Starling relationship (Figure 18.1), the changes in cardiac output in response to changes in cardiac preload depend on the slope of the curve.[3] In the case of preload responsiveness of the right ventricle, the fluid-induced increase in preload results in an increase in right ventricular stroke volume. In the case of preload responsiveness of the left ventricle, this eventually increases the left ventricular stroke volume and cardiac output.

A "significant" response of cardiac output to volume expansion is commonly defined by an increase by 10%–15% of stroke volume or cardiac output.[3] These cutoffs are reasonable, since they correspond to clinically significant changes. Moreover, they are in keeping with the least significant change of cardiac output and stroke volume provided by many monitoring devices, including pulmonary and transpulmonary thermodilution devices.[4]

The importance of the concept of fluid responsiveness for clinical practice is supported by two pieces of evidence. First, if no criterion is used to predict the response to fluid infusion, volume expansion in patients with circulatory failure will result in a significant increase in cardiac output in only one-half of the patients.[5] Second, excessive administration of fluid increases mortality, as is now clearly demonstrated in patients with sepsis or septic shock[2] and in the case of ARDS.[1] Thus, predicting fluid responsiveness has become an important clinical challenge, and different tools have been investigated for this purpose.

Static indices of preload

For many years, prediction of fluid responsiveness was based upon the estimation of cardiac preload, a low preload indicating volume expansion and a high

Perioperative Hemodynamic Monitoring and Goal Directed Therapy, ed. Maxime Cannesson and Rupert Pearse.
Published by Cambridge University Press. © Cambridge University Press 2014.

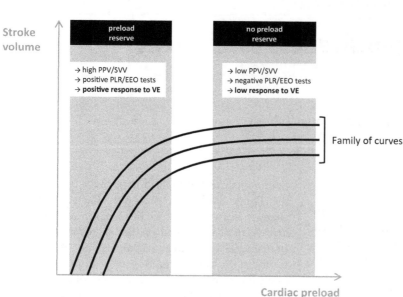

Figure 18.1. *Frank–Starling relationship.* Once the ventricle is functioning on the steep part of the Frank–Starling curve, there is a preload reserve. Volume expansion (VE) induces a significant increase in stroke volume. The pulse pressure (PPV) and stroke volume (SVV) variations are marked, and the passive leg raising (PLR) and end-expiratory occlusion (EEO) tests are positive. By contrast, once the ventricle is operating near the flat part of the curve, there is no preload reserve and fluid infusion has little effect on the stroke volume. There is a family of Frank–Starling curves depending upon the ventricular contractility.

preload preventing fluid administration. The central venous pressure and the pulmonary artery occlusion pressure have been used extensively for this purpose. However, today it is very clear that this approach is not reliable, as has been shown by several studies and emphasized by extensive meta-analyses.[7,8]

The main reason is physiological. As displayed in Figure 18.1, the slope of the Frank–Starling curve depends on the ventricular function. This explains why a similar level of a "static" preload marker could be associated with a significant or a negligible fluid-induced increase in cardiac output. Except for extremely low or high values, such indices should no longer be used to predict fluid responsiveness.[8]

Another reason for the lack of reliability of static markers of preload might reside in errors in their measurement. This is particularly true for the pressure markers of preload. For instance, assessing left ventricular end-diastolic pressure through the pulmonary artery occlusion pressure might be subject to many pitfalls and misinterpretations.[9] Similarly, the measurement of central venous pressure requires precise positioning of the pressure transducer in relation to the right atrium and must be measured at end-expiration, two conditions that are far from being systematically fulfilled in clinical practice.

For these reasons, alternative indices have been developed, which are all based on the same principle. The concept of "functional hemodynamic monitoring" is to induce a change in cardiac preload, whatever the mean, and to observe the resultant change of cardiac output or stroke volume.[4]

Respiratory variation of hemodynamic signals

Hemodynamic effects and prediction of fluid responsiveness

Mechanical ventilation in the assist control mode induces cyclic changes in intrathoracic and transpulmonary pressures. In the case of preload dependence of both ventricles, these changes result in an increase in left ventricular stroke volume at the end of inspiration and a decrease in left ventricular stroke volume at the end of inspiration.[10]

These respiratory changes in stroke volume can be assessed at the bedside by different measures. First, they are reflected by changes in the arterial pulse pressure, so that preload dependence is associated with pulse pressure variation (PPV) during mechanical ventilation.[10] Provided that arterial compliance does not change, arterial pulse pressure is physiologically proportional to stroke volume.[11] PPV has been the first dynamic index of preload responsiveness that has been demonstrated to predict fluid responsiveness. Today there is a large amount of evidence that a PPV higher than 13%[12] predicts fluid responsiveness with a good accuracy. This is particularly emphasized by a large meta-analysis of almost 700 patients in total.[13]

As for any test, there is not one precise cutoff of PPV that discriminates between patients with and without preload dependence. The higher the PPV is above 13%, the more fluid responsiveness is likely. The lower the PPV is below 9%, the more it is unlikely.[12] When PPV is within the "gray zone" between 9 and 13%, PPV should be used cautiously to predict fluid responsiveness.[12]

Other surrogates of stroke volume have been demonstrated to predict fluid responsiveness through their respiratory variations, such as stroke volume derived from pulse contour analysis, peak velocity of the subaortic blood flow measured with echocardiography, and descending aortic blood flow assessed with esophageal Doppler.[4] An interesting technique might be to assess PPV from an arterial waveform obtained from the non-invasive volume-clamp method, which only requires a pneumatic ring wrapped around a finger.[14,15]

The respiratory variation of the amplitude of the plethysmography signal has been suggested as an indirect surrogate of PPV.[16] While it has been shown to be reliable by some studies,[16,17] some others found worse results.[18] This discrepancy might come from the setting in which the studies were conducted, the negative ones including critically ill patients in intensive care units. Compared to patients in the operating or perioperating context, such patients are more likely subject to factors altering the relationship between PPV and the plethysmography variation, such as administration of vasopressors.[19,20]

Advantages and limitations

The strongest advantage of the indices based on the respiratory variation of stroke volume, in particular of PPV, is that they rely on a very solid evidence base.[13] PPV is now automatically measured by several monitors available on the market.

The circumstances where PPV, as well as all the other respiratory variations indices, cannot be used for predicting fluid responsiveness must be kept in mind for proper use at the bedside. Cardiac arrhythmias obviously exaggerate the variations of stroke volume from one cardiac cycle to the other, irrespective of preload dependence. Similarly, spontaneous breathing activity, even under mechanical ventilation, induces inhomogeneous variations of intrathoracic and transpulmonary pressures from

one cycle to the other, increasing the respiratory variation of stroke volume and pulse pressure.[21,22] ARDS is associated with low lung compliance and requires ventilation with low tidal volumes. A low tidal volume[23,24] and a low lung compliance[25] both contribute to reducing the changes in intravascular and intracardiac pressures created by ventilation, which eventually leads to some false-negative cases. Open-chest surgery also reduces the influence of ventilation on the cardiovascular system.[26] Ventilation with a high respiratory rate may be another limitation. If the ratio of heart rate over respiratory rate is low, i.e., if respiratory rate is elevated, the number of cardiac cycles per respiratory cycle might be too low to allow respiratory stroke volume variation to occur.[27] Nevertheless, this occurs for respiratory rates as high as 40 breaths/min.[27] Finally, the presence of an increased abdominal pressure may also reduce the predictive ability of the respiratory variation indices of fluid responsiveness.[28] In such a case, a higher PPV cutoff value must be considered to predict fluid responsiveness.[28]

Respiratory variation of vena cava

Another way to use heart–lung interactions for predicting fluid responsiveness is to measure the respiratory variation of the diameter of vena cava. The principle is that hypovolemia is associated with a high compliance of the veins. Thus, the increase in intrathoracic pressure during ventilation is more likely to reduce the vena cava diameter in the case of hypovolemia than in the case of normo/hypervolemia.

The respiratory variation of the inferior vena cava diameter[29] and the collapsibility of the superior vena cava[30] have been found to predict fluid responsiveness with a good reliability. The limitations of these methods are in the skills in echocardiography that are mandatory, especially for the superior vena cava collapsibility, which can only be assessed with transesophageal echocardiography. Also, the presence of some spontaneous breathing activity, with irregular variations in intrathoracic pressure, prevents such tests from being used. Low lung compliance and mechanical ventilation with a low tidal volume should, as for PPV, minimize the effect of ventilation on the vena cava diameter and thus invalidate the method.

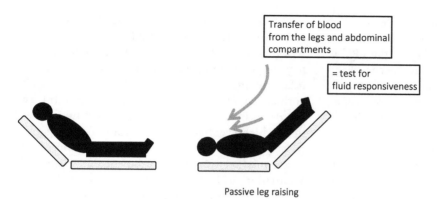

Transfer of blood
from the legs and abdominal
compartments

= test for
fluid responsiveness

Passive leg raising

Figure 18.2. *Passive leg raising*. The passive leg raising test consists of measuring the hemodynamic effects of a leg elevation up to 45°. A simple way to perform the postural maneuver is to transfer the patient from the semi-recumbent posture to the passive leg raising position by using the automatic motion of the bed.

Passive leg raising

Hemodynamic effects

The passive leg raising test (PLR) test is based upon the principle that a large part of blood volume is contained in the venous compartment. Moving a patient from the semi-recumbent position to a position with legs elevated at 45° and trunk horizontal induces a transfer of venous blood from the lower part of the body toward the cardiac chambers (Figure 18.2).[31] The resultant augmentation of right and left cardiac preload eventually increases cardiac output in case of preload-dependence and not in the alternative case.[22] PLR is a "self-volume challenge", which has the advantage of being reversible.[31]

Prediction of fluid responsiveness

The ability of the PLR test to predict fluid responsiveness has been demonstrated by a number of studies, some of them being included in a meta-analysis.[32] These studies show that a PLR-induced increase in cardiac output induced by PLR predicts the response to the ensuing volume expansion with good sensitivity and specificity.[32]

Technical considerations and limitations

It is important to consider the way PLR is performed. PLR should be started from the semi-recumbent rather than from the horizontal position.[31] This allows mobilization not only of the venous blood from the inferior limbs, but also from the large splanchnic reservoir (Figure 18.2), which significantly increases the sensitivity of the test.[33] Also, the PLR maneuver should ideally be performed by using the automatic motion of an electrical bed. This prevents the need to grab the patient's feet, which could be painful and induce a confusing sympathetic simulation. A demonstrative movie is available in a review published about this topic.[31]

Another important technical aspect is that the PLR test cannot be assessed through simple changes in arterial pressure, but rather requires a more direct estimation of cardiac output. It has repeatedly been shown that the PLR-induced changes in arterial pulse pressure are less reliable than the simultaneous changes in cardiac output for predicting fluid responsiveness.[32] This might be due to the fact that PLR alters the physiological relationship between stroke volume and arterial pulse pressure. Accordingly, the PLR test has been described with esophageal Doppler, and the changes in aortic blood flow, with pulse-contour analysis, and the changes in cardiac output, cardiac output measured by bioreactance and endotracheal bioimpedance cardiography, sub-aortic blood velocity measured by echocardiography and ascending aortic velocity measured by suprasternal Doppler. Interestingly, it has been shown that, in patients under mechanical ventilation, with stable ventilatory settings, the changes in end-tidal carbon dioxide could be used to assess the PLR effects, as they reflect the changes in cardiac output.[34] This would allow use of the PLR test with a simple, non-expansive and non-invasive device. Nevertheless, the fact that the PLR test could not be used by simply measuring arterial pressure actually represents a limitation.

Another limitation is that PLR requires the patient to remain quiet during the body motion and that it cannot be performed during surgical interventions. Finally, the reliability of the PLR test has been questioned in the particular condition of intra-abdominal hypertension. The reason might be that an elevated intra-abdominal pressure could prevent the flow of venous blood from the lower to the upper part of the body. Supporting this idea, one study found a low predictive value of the test in patients with intra-abdominal pressure higher than 16 mmHg.[35] A limitation of this single study is that the intra-abdominal pressure was not measured during the PLR maneuver in these patients, while it is very plausible that PLR increases the abdominal compliance and reduces intra-abdominal pressure. Thus, the reason why intra-abdominal hypertension would limit the reliability of the test becomes less obvious. This important question is still pending.

End-expiratory occlusion test

Hemodynamic effects

The end-expiratory occlusion (EEO) test is based upon the fact that mechanical ventilation induces a cyclic reduction of cardiac preload, due to the cyclic increase in intrathoracic pressure at inspiration. Interrupting mechanical ventilation at end-expiration for a few seconds, as it is regularly performed for measuring the intrinsic positive end-expiratory pressure, interrupts this cyclic reduction of preload, acting like a brief volume challenge (Figure 18.3). It has been demonstrated that an increase in pulse contour analysis-derived cardiac output by more than 5% during a 15-second end-expiratory occlusion predicts the positive response of cardiac output to an ensuing fluid loading with a good reliability.[25,36]

Advantages and limitations

The great advantage of the test is that it is very easy to perform. Also, it can be used in case of cardiac arrhythmias, as the effects cover several cardiac cycles.[36] However, certain conditions must be fulfilled to ensure the test reliability. First and obviously, it requires that the patient is intubated. Second, the EEO test requires a 15-second interruption of ventilation, since shorter interruptions would not allow its hemodynamic effects to develop, especially due to the long lung transit time. The patient must be able to sustain a 15-second EEO without interrupting it. Third, it is much easier to assess the EEO-test effects with a real-time measurement of cardiac output. Even if the increase in arterial pulse pressure during EEO is also indicative of fluid responsiveness,[36] this requires a display of the arterial pressure trace with a high resolution scale (see the figure in[36]), which is not possible on standard bedside monitors. Another limitation of the EEO test is that it requires a ventilator that allows automatic occlusion of the respiratory circuit at end-expiration, which is still not possible in some machines used in the operating room.

The question has been raised whether the predictive ability of the EEO test could depend upon the PEEP level. This was not the case in a study in which the EEO test was conducted under PEEP at 5 cmH$_2$O or 13 cmH$_2$O. Increasing the PEEP level may recruit some lung volume, so that the reduction in intrathoracic pressure during the EEO is similar to that induced at a lower PEEP level.[37]

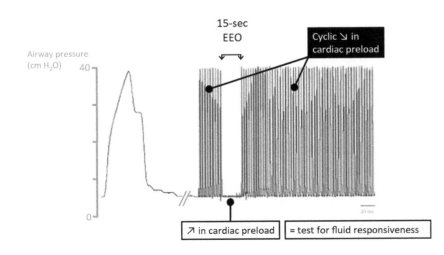

Figure 18.3. *End-expiratory occlusion test.* The end-expiratory occlusion (EEO) test consists of interrupting mechanical ventilation at the end of expiration during 15 seconds. This suppresses the cyclic decrease in cardiac preload, which normally occurs at each mechanical insufflation. Therefore, this brief procedure should increase cardiac preload and can serve as a test to assess preload responsiveness and hence to predict the response to a subsequent fluid infusion.

Fluid challenge

In order to challenge preload dependence, administering fluid intravenously is obviously the best way to ensure that cardiac preload actually increased. The "classical" fluid challenge consists in rapidly injecting 500 mL of fluid intravenously and in observing its hemodynamic effect in order to decide whether or not to administer more fluid. This technique has been used for years, especially when the above-cited tests were not already developed. While it is obviously reliable, the "classical" fluid challenge may be problematic in patients at risk of fluid overload, i.e., in case of ARDS and septic shock. In the case where the fluid challenge does not increase cardiac output, the volume of fluid that was administered during the challenge contributes to deleteriously increasing the positive cumulative fluid balance.

In this regard, it has been proposed to replace the "classical" by a "mini-fluid challenge," with administration of only 100 mL of fluid.[37] The method is obviously seducing. However, the technique used to measure the changes in cardiac output resulting from so small an amount of fluid must be very precise. Echocardiography has been proposed for this purpose.[37] Whether easier to use and more precise methods, such as pulse contour analysis, are also suitable for assessing the effects of the test is an interesting question for future research.

Using predictors of fluid responsiveness in practice: utility and choice depending on the setting

Prediction of fluid responsiveness should be considered differently, depending upon the clinical setting. First, one must remember that preload dependence is a physiological condition. Thus, positive predictors of fluid responsiveness should lead to volume expansion only in the case of circulatory failure. Second, in the initial phase of an obvious hypovolemic or septic shock, detecting preload dependence is useless, since fluid responsiveness is constant under such conditions. The operating theatre might be particularly adapted for the respiratory variation of stroke volume or surrogates in anesthetized patients, except if low tidal volumes are used for mechanical ventilation. In addition, such indices can be assessed by means of a simple arterial catheter or by non-invasive hemodynamic monitoring devices, which are suitable for this setting. The EEO test might also be useful, provided that the ventilator allows interruption of ventilation at end-expiration for 15 seconds.

In critically ill patients, the frequent presence of cardiac arrhythmias, low lung compliance and ventilation with low tidal volumes associated with ARDS, the presence of some spontaneous breathing and of low lung compliance often prevents the use of PPV and related indices. The respiratory variation of vena cava can be used as an alternative in the case of cardiac arrhythmias. The EEO and PLR tests are often suitable, provided their conditions of application are fulfilled.

The use of predictors of fluid responsiveness may also depend upon the context in which they are used. In the perioperating setting, prediction of fluid responsiveness might be part of the pre-emptive hemodynamic treatment that has been shown to reduce the rate of postoperative complications and the hospital length-of-stay in different categories of surgical patients.[38,39] In the context of intensive care units, indicators of preload dependence may be particularly useful for detecting fluid unresponsiveness.[40] Such a condition should refrain from volume expansion. This would contribute to avoiding excessive fluid administration, which is associated with poor prognosis in the case of septic shock and ARDS.

Conclusions

Several tools are available today that allow clinicians to assess volume responsiveness using dynamic procedures. These tools allow fluid to be administered with the assurance that it will lead to the expected increase in cardiac output. In particular, this should be included in protocols guiding the hemodynamic treatment in the operating room setting. In the intensive care unit, these tools may be particularly useful in order to refrain from volume expansion and should reduce the risk of overzealous fluid administration.

Conflicts of interest

Professors Monnet and Teboul are members of the Medical Advisory Board of Pulsion Medical Systems.

References

1. Jozwiak M, Silva S, Persichini R, et al. Extravascular lung water is an independent prognostic factor in patients with acute respiratory distress syndrome. *Crit Care Med* 2013;**41**:472–80.

2. Vincent JL, Sakr Y, Sprung CL, et al. Sepsis in European intensive care units: results of the SOAP study. *Crit Care Med* 2006;**34**:344–53.

3. Marik PE, Monnet X, Teboul JL. Hemodynamic parameters to guide fluid therapy. *Ann Intens Care* 2011;**1**:1.

4. Monnet X, Persichini R, Ktari M, Jozwiak M, Richard C, Teboul JL. Precision of the transpulmonary thermodilution measurements. *Crit Care* 2011;**15**:R204.

5. Michard F, Teboul JL. Predicting fluid responsiveness in ICU patients: a critical analysis of the evidence. *Chest* 2002;**121**: 2000–8.

6. Marik PE, Baram M, Vahid B. Does central venous pressure predict fluid responsiveness? A systematic review of the literature and the tale of seven mares. *Chest* 2008;**134**:172–8.

7. Marik PE, Cavallazzi R. Does the central venous pressure predict fluid responsiveness? An updated meta-analysis and a plea for some common sense. *Crit Care Med* 2013;**41**:1774–81.

8. Richard C, Monnet X, Teboul JL. Pulmonary artery catheter monitoring in 2011. *Curr Opin Crit Care* 2011;**17**:296–302.

9. Michard F, Teboul JL. Using heart–lung interactions to assess fluid responsiveness during mechanical ventilation. *Crit Care* 2000;**4**:282–9.

10. Chemla D, Hebert JL, Coirault C. Total arterial compliance estimated by stroke volume-to-aortic pulse pressure ratio in humans. *Am J Physiol* 1998;**274**: H500–5.

11. Cannesson M, Le Manach Y, Hofer CK, et al. Assessing the diagnostic accuracy of pulse pressure variations for the prediction of fluid responsiveness: a "gray zone" approach. *Anesthesiology* 2011;**115**:231–41.

12. Marik PE, Cavallazzi R, Vasu T, Hirani A. Dynamic changes in arterial waveform derived variables and fluid responsiveness in mechanically ventilated patients: a systematic review of the literature. *Crit Care Med* 2009;**37**:2642–7.

13. Monnet X, Dres M, Ferre A, et al. Prediction of fluid responsiveness by a continuous non-invasive assessment of arterial pressure in critically ill patients: comparison with four other dynamic indices. *Br J Anaesth* 2012;**109**:330–8.

14. Solus-Biguenet H, Fleyfel M, Tavernier B, et al. Non-invasive prediction of fluid responsiveness during major hepatic surgery. *Br J Anaesth* 2006;**97**:808–16.

15. Cannesson M, Attof Y, Rosamel P, et al. Respiratory variations in pulse oximetry plethysmographic waveform amplitude to predict fluid responsiveness in the operating room. *Anesthesiology* 2007;**106**:1105–11.

16. Cannesson M, Desebbe O, Rosamel P, et al. Pleth variability index to monitor the respiratory variations in the pulse oximeter plethysmographic waveform amplitude and predict fluid responsiveness in the operating theatre. *Br J Anaesth* 2008;**101**:200–6.

17. Monnet X, Guerin L, Jozwiak M, et al. Pleth variability index is a weak predictor of fluid responsiveness in patients receiving norepinephrine. *Br J Anaesth* 2013;**110**:207–13.

18. Monnet X, Lamia B, Teboul JL. Pulse oximeter as a sensor of fluid responsiveness: do we have our finger on the best solution? *Crit Care* 2005;**9**:429–30.

19. Biais M, Cottenceau V, Petit L, Masson F, Cochard JF, Sztark F. Impact of norepinephrine on the relationship between pleth variability index and pulse pressure variations in ICU adult patients. *Crit Care* 2011;**15**:R168.

20. Heenen S, De Backer D, Vincent JL. How can the response to volume expansion in patients with spontaneous respiratory movements be predicted? *Crit Care* 2006;**10**:R102.

21. Monnet X, Rienzo M, Osman D, et al. Passive leg raising predicts fluid responsiveness in the critically ill. *Crit Care Med* 2006;**34**:1402–7.

22. De Backer D, Heenen S, Piagnerelli M, Koch M, Vincent JL. Pulse pressure variations to predict fluid responsiveness: influence of tidal volume. *Intens Care Med* 2005;**31**:517–23.

23. Muller L, Louart G, Bousquet PJ, et al. The influence of the airway driving pressure on pulsed pressure variation as a predictor of fluid responsiveness. *Intens Care Med* 2010;**36**:496–503.

24. Monnet X, Bleibtreu A, Ferré A, et al. Passive leg raising and end-expiratory occlusion tests perform better than pulse pressure variation in patients with low respiratory system compliance. *Crit Care Med* 2012;**40**:152–7.

25. de Waal EE, Rex S, Kruitwagen CL, Kalkman CJ, Buhre WF. Dynamic preload indicators fail to predict fluid responsiveness in open-chest conditions. *Crit Care Med* 2009;**37**:510–15.

26. De Backer D, Taccone FS, Holsten R, Ibrahimi F, Vincent JL. Influence of respiratory rate on stroke volume variation in mechanically ventilated patients. *Anesthesiology* 2009;**110**:1092–7.

27. Jacques D, Bendjelid K, Dunerret S, Colling J, Piriou V, Viale JP. Pulse pressure variation and stroke volume variation during increased intra-abdominal

pressure: an experimental study. *Crit Care* 2011;**15**:R33.

28. Feissel M, Michard F, Faller JP, Teboul JL. The respiratory variation in inferior vena cava diameter as a guide to fluid therapy. *Intens Care Med* 2004;**30**:1834–7.

29. Vieillard-Baron A, Chergui K, Rabiller A, et al. Superior vena caval collapsibility as a gauge of volume status in ventilated septic patients. *Intens Care Med* 2004;**30**:1734–9.

30. Monnet X, Teboul JL. Passive leg raising. *Intens Care Med* 2008;**34**:659–63.

31. Cavallaro F, Sandroni C, Marano C, et al. Diagnostic accuracy of passive leg raising for prediction of fluid responsiveness in adults: systematic review and meta-analysis of clinical studies. *Intens Care Med* 2010;**36**:1475–1483.

32. Jabot J, Teboul JL, Richard C, Monnet X. Passive leg raising for predicting fluid responsiveness: importance of the postural change. *Intens Care Med* 2009;**35**:85–90.

33. Monnet X, Bataille A, Magalhaes E, et al. End-tidal carbon dioxide is better than arterial pressure for predicting volume responsiveness by the passive leg raising test. *Intens Care Med* 2013;**39**:93–100.

34. Mahjoub Y, Touzeau J, Airapetian N, et al. The passive leg-raising maneuver cannot accurately predict fluid responsiveness in patients with intra-abdominal hypertension. *Crit Care Med* 2010;**38**:1824–9.

35. Monnet X, Osman D, Ridel C, Lamia B, Richard C, Teboul JL. Predicting volume responsiveness by using the end-expiratory occlusion in mechanically ventilated intensive care unit patients. *Crit Care Med* 2009;**37**:951–6.

36. Silva S, Jozwiak M, Teboul JL, Persichini R, Richard C, Monnet X. End-expiratory occlusion test predicts preload responsiveness independently of positive end-expiratory pressure during acute respiratory distress syndrome. *Crit Care Med* 2013;**41**:1692–701.

37. Muller L, Toumi M, Bousquet PJ, et al. An increase in aortic blood flow after an infusion of 100 ml colloid over 1 minute can predict fluid responsiveness: the mini-fluid challenge study. *Anesthesiology* 2011;**115**:541–7.

38. Cecconi M, Corredor C, Arulkumaran N, et al. Clinical review: goal-directed therapy-what is the evidence in surgical patients? The effect on different risk groups. *Crit Care* 2013;**17**:209.

39. Hamilton MA, Cecconi M, Rhodes A. A systematic review and meta-analysis on the use of preemptive hemodynamic intervention to improve postoperative outcomes in moderate and high-risk surgical patients. *Anesth Analg* 2011;**112**:1392–402.

40. Teboul JL, Monnet X. Detecting volume responsiveness and unresponsiveness in intensive care unit patients: two different problems, only one solution. *Crit Care* 2009;**13**:175.

Chapter

19

Non-invasive and continuous arterial pressure monitoring

Berthold Bein and Christoph Ilies

Introduction

ECG registration, pulse oximetry, and intermittent oscillometric blood pressure measurements represent the minimum requirements for perioperative monitoring. Arterial cannulation and intravascular measurement represent the clinical gold standard for precise arterial pressure monitoring and blood gas analysis. This procedure in contrast to oscillometric methods requires experienced and skilled personnel, suitable equipment, is more costly, and is associated with several potentially harmful side effects for the patient. Infections, impaired peripheral circulation leading to necrosis in severe cases, and blood loss due to undetected disconnection are only some of them.[1] There is no doubt that, in several clinical scenarios, the benefit outweighs the risk. This is, for instance, the case in high-risk patients where most accurate arterial pressure readings as well as arterial blood gas sampling are necessary for guiding adequate and goal directed therapy.

Nevertheless, there are several scenarios where reliable and close meshed arterial pressure monitoring is desirable, but arterial cannulation might not be adequate or not possible due to missing equipment or lack of trained staff. This may be the case in intermediate care units, emergency departments, during semi-invasive procedures under sedation in elderly patients (e.g., colonoscopy, bronchoscopy, transesophageal echocardiography) as well as during surgical procedures under anesthesia with rapid and pronounced changes of arterial pressure (e.g., cesarean section, electroconvulsive therapy). In these cases, discontinuous oscillometric pressure readings may be either too imprecise or a rapidly changing blood pressure could be missed by the standard measurement cycle of 5 minutes.[2]

Over the past few years non-invasive continuous arterial pressure measurement techniques have been newly developed or substantially improved and many clinical studies have addressed their performance in different clinical settings. At present, algorithms for cardiac output measurement or calculation of dynamic preload variables are implemented on these monitors. Because in many cases arterial blood sampling is not mandatory, continuous, non-invasive monitors may be an acceptable alternative in daily clinical practice.

The "real" blood pressure

For every assessment of a new measurement technique or monitor, a comparison with the actual blood pressure is needed. But what is the actual blood pressure? In humans, blood pressure shows minimal changes with every heart beat and differs depending on the measuring site. A well-known phenomenon is the peripheral pulse amplification. Caused by arterial stiffness and reflection of early pressure waves from the arterial wall, systolic pressure is higher and diastolic lower in more distally located arteries, such as the brachial artery and radial artery compared with the aorta. The mean arterial pressure is more constant throughout the arterial tree. This effect is age related and reflects patients' specific cardiovascular risk, which is dependent on central aortic absolute pressures.[3,4] Although long-term cardiovascular outcome is not an important issue during perioperative hemodynamic monitoring, we must be aware that distinct differences in arterial pressure occur between different measuring sites, which cannot be estimated from age or individual patient factors.[5] For practical reasons, the blood pressure obtained in the radial or femoral artery is considered to be the "gold standard" in perioperative arterial pressure monitoring.

Another point deals with the accuracy of oscillometric arterial pressure monitoring systems,

Perioperative Hemodynamic Monitoring and Goal Directed Therapy, ed. Maxime Cannesson and Rupert Pearse.
Published by Cambridge University Press. © Cambridge University Press 2014.

representing the non-invasive gold standard compared with invasive measurements. When evaluating a new non-invasive continuous technique, accuracy at least as good as for non-invasive discontinuous measurements is a prerequisite. Larger studies showed marked differences between invasive and oscillometric measurements. In 852 patients treated on an intensive care unit, oscillometric systolic pressures overestimated invasive measurements in the hypotensive and underestimated it in the hypertensive range.[6] The difference between the two measurements was pressure dependent and partially above 10 mmHg, with 95% limits of agreement up to −15.32 to +35.42 mmHg. For mean arterial pressure, the difference was lower with a bias of 3.90 mmHg and 95% limits of agreement from −9.72 to 17.52.

Due to the overestimation of systolic pressure in the hypotensive range, there was a correlation between oscillometric measurements below 70 mmHg and acute renal failure and mortality compared with invasive measurements, i.e., hypotensive measurements despite overestimation in fact were severely hypotensive values. This correlation was not present for oscillometric mean arterial pressure, indicating a better agreement with invasive pressure. Therefore, only mean oscillometric arterial pressure should be used for therapy decisions and control. These discrepancies were confirmed by another report on patients in shock showing that 18.9% of systolic oscillometric readings differed by at least 20 mmHg, and 29.1% of diastolic readings differed by more than 10 mmHg from invasive measurements.[7]

Validation of continuous non-invasive methods

While the validation protocol for automated sphygmomanometers is widely accepted, there is no actual or applicable standard for comparison of continuous non-invasive devices. The cutoff values published by the Association for the Advancement of Medical Instrumentation (AAMI), namely a mean difference below 5 mmHg with a standard deviation below 8 mmHg compared with invasive measurements, were developed for automated sphygmomanometers and are probably not adequate for non-invasive continuous devices and actually excluded by the standard. Validation should be performed against the clinical gold standard, intravascular measurements. There is some debate concerning the adequate statistical approach. It is widely accepted that correlation statistics are not meaningful for analysis. At present, method comparison is mostly performed by Bland–Altman analysis with correction for multiple measurements calculating mean pressure difference (bias) and the standard deviation of the mean pressure difference (precision; two standard deviations are referred to as limits of agreement). Nevertheless, there are no explicit cutoff values regarding Bland–Altman analysis except the AAMI criteria. The percentage error (PE) can be used to compare the precision of the new monitor with the gold standard. It is calculated by dividing twice the standard deviation of the bias by the average of both measurement methods. In a recent study, cutoff values for the so-called "interchangeability" of monitors for arterial pressure measurement were calculated.[8] Two monitors can be used interchangeably when the PE is lower than 14.7% for systolic, 17.5% for diastolic, and 18.7% for mean arterial pressure. The percentage of values within a certain range of mean arterial pressure difference is also often used to describe accuracy.

We have to be aware that a weak accuracy of the analyzed monitor may depend on many reasons. Morbid obesity, patient movement, and low peripheral perfusion are only some patient-related issues. Others include differences in arterial pressure readings depending on the site of measurement or on the actual calibration technique. As mentioned above, central pressure in the aorta is different from the periphery due to peripheral amplification and different arterial wall stiffness of smaller vessels. As some devices are calibrated against oscillometric non-invasive intermittent blood pressure (NIBP), this may also contribute to an error. Nevertheless, in daily clinical practice, at least in the perioperative setting, we also rely on NIBP measurements, and therefore the absolute difference is probably not as important as the adequate detection of blood pressure changes. According to the above-mentioned studies we should also base our therapeutic decisions on mean arterial pressure, which normally differs less between methods, and best represents organ perfusion pressure.

Measurement techniques

Arterial tonometry

Arterial tonometry uses a technique similar to applanation tonometry, known for the assessment of intraocular pressure. A device containing several pressure sensors is attached above the radial artery and compresses it against the underlying tissue and bone.

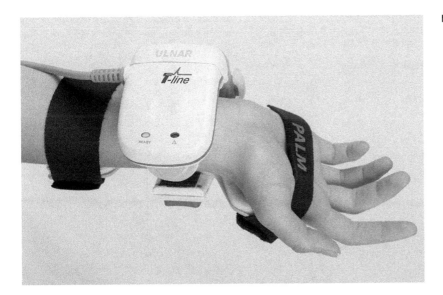

Figure 19.1. The T-line device.

The arterial wall is therefore flattened and discharged from hemodynamic forces. The pulse pressure is then directly applied to the attached sensors and can be transformed to a beat-to-beat pressure curve corresponding to the arterial pressure. The maximal pressure amplitude corresponds to mean arterial pressure. Using Fast Fourier transformation, the obtained pressure curve corresponds well to central pressures without the peripheral pulse pressure amplification that usually occurs in peripheral arteries.[9] Central pressure obtained by tonometry, either from the carotid or from the radial artery, is claimed to better predict cardiovascular events than peripheral pressures obtained by oscillometric or invasive measurements.[4,10,11] Apart from devices for research purposes, two monitors were commercially available, namely the Colin tonometer and the T-Line. The Colin tonometer was evaluated in only a few studies with varying results.[12–15] Overall accuracy was weak and the monitor is no longer available. The best evaluated monitor using tonometry so far is the T-Line, which will be presented later on.

Vascular unloading technique

The vascular unloading or volume clamp method was described in 1975 by Peňáz.[16,17] Finger blood flow can be measured by photoplethysmography. Absorption of the emitted light is linear to blood flow. Using a pneumatic finger cuff, the blood flow can be kept constant using servo control loops. The arterial wall is unloaded, meaning that the intravascular pressure is transmitted directly to the pressure cuff. For example, during systole the pressure emitted by the systolic increase in wall tension equals the pressure needed to keep the flow constant. Using specific algorithms, the pressure changes of the cuff are used to create an arterial pressure curve similar to an invasive one. Depending on the manufacturer, waveforms are either reconstructed to be similar to brachial artery waveforms, or an oscillometric measurement is used for calibration. The first monitor using the vascular unloading technique in the 1990s was the FINAPRES (FINger Arterial PRESsure). Monitors available for clinical use today (Nexfin and CNAP) are presented below.

Non-invasive continuous arterial pressure monitors

T-Line

The T-Line device (Tensys Medical, San Diego, CA, USA) contains a wrist splint and a bracelet where a disposable sensor pad is attached (Figure 19.1). The bracelet keeps the wrist slightly extended, whereas the bracelet is positioned above the radial artery. The Tensys technology uses an automatic scanning procedure for detection of the best quality for the arterial pressure signal. The pressure signal obtained after applanation of the radial artery corresponds to mean arterial pressure. An algorithm is used to adapt the signal to the patient's body mass index, to calculate systolic and diastolic pressures and to construct

Table 19.1. Results of the Bland–Altman analysis from selected validation studies for the different devices. LOA: 95% limits of agreement, PE: percentage error, * met criteria for interchangeability regarding PE, ° met AAMI criteria; OT: operation theatre; ICU: intensive care unit. [1]: results only from 50 patients with version 3.5

Device	Study	Setting	Patients, n	Pressure	Bias (±SD), mmHg	LOA, mmHg	PE,%
T-line (TL-200)	Dueck, 2012[18]	OT	19	SAP	2.3 (7.8)°	−13 – 7.7	-
				DAP	1.7 (6.2)°	−10.6 – 14	-
				MAP	2.3 (5.9)°	−9.4 – 14	-
T-line (TL-200)	Saugel, 2012[19]	ICU	28	SAP	−9 (14.5)	−37.5 – 19.5	23
				DAP	5.2 (9.6)	−13.5 – 23.9	31
				MAP	0.5 (8.7)	−16.5 – 17.5	21
T-line (TL-200pro)	Saugel, 2013[20]	ICU	34	SAP	−1.4 (8.9)	−18.7 – 16	14*
				DAP	4.4 (6.6)°	−8.7 – 17.4	21
				MAP	0.7 (5.2)°	−9.4 – 10.8	12*
Nexfin	Broch, 2013[24]	OT	50	SAP	6.5 (17.5)	−27.8 – 40.9	29
				DAP	9.3 (15.8)	−21.6 – 40.2	55
				MAP	6.2 (11.7)	−16.7 – 29.2	29
Nexfin	Fischer, 2012[26]	ICU	50	SAP	5.7 (—)	−22.5 – 34	-
				DAP	−8.9 (—)	−22.6 – 4.7	-
				MAP	−4.6 (6.5)°	−17.3 – 8.1	-
Nexfin	Martina, 2012[25]	OT	50	SAP	0.5 (6.7)°	-	-
				DAP	2.8 (6.4)°	-	-
				MAP	2.2 (6.4)°	-	-
Nexfin	Hohn, 2013[27]	ICU	25	SAP	−9 (25)	−58 – 48	-
				DAP	-	-	-
				MAP	6 (12)	−18 – 30	-
Nexfin	Garnier, 2012[29]	ICU/OT Children	41	SAP	13.5 (13.4)	−39.7 – 12.8	-
				DAP	0.2 (6.6)°	−12.8 – 13.2	-
				MAP	−2.6 (7.7)°	−17.7 – 12.5	-
CNAP	Jeleazcov, 2010[31]	OT	88	SAP	6.7 (13.9)	not comparable	-
				DAP	−5.6 (11.4)		-
				MAP	−1.6 (11)		-
CNAP	Hahn, 2012[32]	OT	100 [1]	SAP	0.9 (13.2)	−24.9 – 26.8	-
				DAP	−2.8 (8.6)	−19.7 – 14.1	-
				MAP	−3.1 (9.5)	−21.6 – 15.4	-
CNAP	Ilies, 2012[8]	OT	85	SAP	4.2 (10)	−27 – 35	16.6
				DAP	−5.8 (6)	−23 – 12	18
				MAP	−4.3 (6.8)°	−24 – 15	15.8*
CNAP	Jagadeesh, 2012[33]	ICU	30	SAP	−10.4 (5.8)	−4.6 – 25.4	-
				DAP	5.3 (3)°	−13.4 – 2.7	-
				MAP	−0.04 (2.5)°	−6 – 6	-

the waveform. Servo control loops are used to track arterial pressure changes. The system needs approximately 90 seconds after start-up to display a calibrated continuous blood pressure curve and needs no external calibration.

Apart from satisfactory results regarding older versions, there are at present only few clinical studies validating the latest T-Line system. Statistical results of all studies are shown in Table 19.1. The third-generation device, the TL-200, was recently compared with invasive measurements at the opposite radial artery in 19 patients undergoing different surgical procedures under general anesthesia.[18] The authors concluded a high correlation and good agreement of the TL-200 with A-Line values over a wide dynamic range of BP. Another study reported on 28 unselected critically ill patients, where invasive femoral artery pressures were compared with the TL-200.[19] The authors concluded that, apart from high limits of agreement especially for systolic and diastolic pressures, the TL-200 was basically feasible in unselected medical ICU patients, but drew attention to the possible bias regarding invasive measurements obtained at the femoral artery compared with radial ones. The same authors actually report on the newest version, the TL-200pro with an improved disposable pressure sensor. This was compared with femoral invasive measurements in 34 critically ill patients.[20] The authors concluded that the TL-200pro provides measurements with high agreement and precision especially for mean arterial pressure.

One of the main disadvantages of the applanation technique is the dependency of an optimal signal obtained exactly above the artery. Therefore, patient movement may cause erroneous readings. In the TL-200, only moderate movement leads to a delay of 15 seconds until the system recovers, whereas severe movement leads to a complete restart requiring 35 seconds until an uncalibrated, and even 90 seconds until a calibrated, pressure reading is again displayed continuously.[18]

Summary

First reports of the new generation tonometry monitors are promising. From the reported investigations, the monitor can be used for arterial pressure monitoring in perioperative and intensive care. Compared with other monitors, systolic pressure shows a good agreement with invasive pressures. At the moment, data on tracking fast blood pressure changes, effects of volume loss, vasoactive medication, or cardiac dysrhythmia are still lacking. Data from pediatric patients are also not available at present.

Finapres/Nexfin

The Finapres monitor (Finapres Medical Systems, Amsterdam, the Netherlands) is based on the Peñáz principle and has been established more than 20 years. There are over 300 studies from different medical fields proving its ability to monitor blood pressure. The Nexfin (Edwards Life Sciences, Irvine, CA, USA) is based on the Finapres technique, but has been miniaturized and further developed for the perioperative setting. The Nexfin stand-alone monitor measures blood pressure using an inflatable finger cuff, available in four sizes, which is attached to the middle phalanx of the middle, index, or ring finger. A pressure transducer is mounted on the forearm. Compensation of vertical movement of the extremity using the so-called "heart reference system" can be performed by using a second sensor measuring the height of the transducer compared with heart level. The Nexfin system uses an algorithm for brachial reconstruction, which improved agreement of non-invasive continuous measurements with invasive readings at the brachial or radial site.[21,22] The system uses an autocalibration technique, the so-called "Physiocal" algorithm, in order to adapt to changes of vascular tone.[23] After initial calibration of the system of about 2 minutes duration, the Physiocal leads to periodical interruptions of pressure readings of about 70 beats.[23] Besides blood pressure, the monitor displays cardiac output, stroke volume, vascular resistance, and a contractility index based on the non-invasive pressure.

Broch and co-workers recently evaluated the Nexfin in 50 patients both before and after cardiopulmonary bypass (CPB) against femoral and radial invasive measurements.[24] The Nexfin correlated better with femoral than with radial pressures. Correlation was lower after CPB, probably due to changes in vascular resistance of the peripheral vasculature. Acute changes of arterial pressure following passive leg raising before and after CPB could be detected with moderate accuracy. Martina et al. also evaluated the Nexfin system in 53 patients undergoing cardiothoracic surgery and found better agreement shown by the lowest reported bias and standard deviation and a low within-subject variability compared with radial artery invasive measurements.[25] Their data showed a significant improvement of the agreement of the raw pressure curve using the finger to brachial reconstruction algorithm. The authors concluded that Nexfin adequately follows pressure changes and is comparable to invasive monitoring. Fischer reported on 50 patients after cardiac surgery at admission to the intensive care unit. Bias and precision of mean arterial pressure fulfilled the aforementioned AAMI criteria. He therefore concluded that the Nexfin device is convenient, safe, and reliable in measuring continuous non-invasive arterial pressure.[26] Hohn recently compared the Nexfin with invasive radial measurements in 25 ICU patients and investigated the effects of catecholamines and peripheral edema.[27] The study suffered some limitations, as only single beat femoral and radial invasive measurements were used for comparison. Nevertheless, the accuracy and precision of the Nexfin was low and the limits of agreement were rather wide in this mixed intensive care population. Norepinephrine administration, as well as peripheral edema, had a negative impact on the accuracy of the Nexfin and the authors did not support the use of Nexfin in this population due to its reduced accuracy.

Nexfin also provides a small finger cuff for children. In a validation study of a prototype, Hofhuizen and co-workers compared the Nexfin with invasive measurements at the radial, brachial, or femoral site in 13 children with a median age of 11 months undergoing cardiac surgery.[28] In addition to problems obtaining an adequate plethysmographic signal in a considerable number of patients, the system according to the authors was able to accurately reflect blood pressure and track pressure changes. In a larger study, Garnier et al. validated the Nexfin particularly with the XS and S cuff sizes against invasive measurements at the radial, brachial, or femoral site in 41 patients with a median age of 9 years undergoing surgery or treatment on the ICU.[29] The authors concluded that Nexfin is feasible in pediatric patients with a good agreement, especially regarding mean and diastolic intra-arterial pressures. Data received during interventional electrophysiology also suggest that the system is feasible to detect sudden hypotension during tachyarrhythmia, although signal calibration increased from 4% to 19% of measuring time during tachycardia.[30]

Summary

The development of the Nexfin is based on more than 20 years of experience from the Finapres monitor. Different technical algorithms have improved its accuracy compared with invasive measurements during perioperative and ICU care in adult and pediatric patients.

Measurement is discontinued during the physical autocalibration up to 19% of measuring time during arrhythmia. Based on the most recent validation studies, the system works well in an optimal setting, whereas there are also studies reporting greater differences to the gold standard, especially in ICU

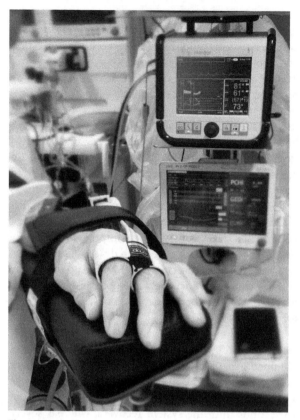

Figure 19.2. The CNAP monitor.

patients. Mean arterial pressure seems the most reliable. Vasopressors and peripheral edema impact on the accuracy of the system.

CNAP

The CNAP (**C**ontinuous **N**on-invasive **A**rterial **P**ressure Monitor 500, CNSystems, Graz, Austria) is the most recent monitor based on the Peňáz principle (Figure 19.2). Pressure is obtained by a double finger cuff, which allows a switch of the measured finger. A pressure transducer is mounted at the forearm. After initial calibration lasting approximately 2–3 minutes, calibration is performed using a standard oscillometric blood pressure cuff at user predefined intervals, automatically at pressure changes of more than 25mmHg for more than 45 seconds or manually at any time. The continuous pressure curve is only discontinued during ipsilateral oscillometric measurements or when changing measurement from one to another finger cuff during complete recalibration. A so-called VERIFI algorithm was recently implemented in order to eliminate effects of vascular tone on the accuracy of the system. The CNAP is available as a stand-alone monitor or as an OEM module for host monitors. As well as the already implemented calculation of pulse pressure variation, an algorithm for cardiac output is currently under clinical investigation and is expected to be released soon.

The first large validation study against radial invasive measurements in 88 patients undergoing different types of surgery was published in 2010.[31] The authors concluded CNAP to be a useful alternative to invasive measurements with comparable precision and acceptable accuracy. CNAP was able to detect intraoperative hypotension and fast changes of arterial pressure. A study from 2012 evaluated the monitor with two different software versions in 100 patients undergoing orthopedic surgery.[32] The accuracy of the system improved with the software update, but was too low according to the AAMI criteria used by the authors. Nevertheless, they concluded that CNAP provided valuable measurements for daily clinical practice. Our group investigated the accuracy of the CNAP during induction and maintenance of general anesthesia in 85 patients.[8] Whereas mean pressure was interchangeable with invasive measurements during maintenance of anesthesia, accuracy deteriorated during induction and hypotensive periods, probably due to changes in vascular tone. Gayat reported on CNAP measurements during induction of anesthesia and tracheal intubation in 52 patients. While changes of blood pressure were detected with a delay of between 7.5 seconds for the highest and 10 seconds for the lowest value, the authors rated the precision of the CNAP as not satisfactory. It remains unclear if changes of vascular tone were responsible for these disappointing results. In all these cited studies the VERIFI algorithm was not yet implemented into the monitor.

Jagadeesh and co-workers validated the CNAP compared with radial invasive measurements in 30 cardiac surgical ICU patients.[33] The authors concluded that CNAP values are comparable to invasive ones and that CNAP can be used as an alternative. CNAP also accurately and quickly measured changes of blood pressure during rapid ventricular pacing.[34]

Data comparing CNAP with NIBP during cesarean section under spinal anesthesia showed inconsistent results. Whereas our group reported on the significantly increased detection of hypotensive episodes and the lower absolute blood pressures detected with the CNAP monitor,[35] McCarthy considered the OEM module system as disadvantageous compared with NIBP.[36] While reliability of NIBP and CNAP were similar, CNAP often missed values due to the recalibration procedure. A reason may be the predefined automated calibration interval used in this study. Finally, data from pediatric patients also showed acceptable agreement, whereas it was postulated that improvement of the finger cuffs in small sizes probably would be beneficial.[37,38]

Summary

The CNAP is the most recent monitor based on the Peñáz principle. With implementation of updated software algorithms, its accuracy and agreement with invasive measurements improved during general anesthesia in adults and children, on the ICU, and with some limitations also for cesarean section under spinal anesthesia. In comparison with other systems, calibration is performed against a NIBP measurement, which also has an error compared with invasive measurements. There is no evidence regarding the optimal calibration interval, although the system should be recalibrated after changes of vascular tone such as induction of anesthesia. Like in other systems, mean arterial pressure is most accurate. From our own experience, vasopressors in moderate doses do not affect accuracy whereas marked peripheral edema does.

Conclusions

Non-invasive continuous arterial pressure monitors independent of the underlying system significantly improved their accuracy as a result of advancing technical improvement. Beneath system specific limitations, accuracy and agreement with invasive measurements of the Peñáz or applanation tonometry-based monitors seems similar. Mean arterial pressure should be used for therapy decisions for all three monitors. In the near future we expect further improvements and implications of better algorithms for cardiac output or fluid responsiveness. The next step from measuring blood pressure is to monitor and consequently improve cardiac output and thus oxygen delivery. This could be made available for a larger proportion of patients without the need for invasive monitoring limited to tertiary care centers or intensive care units.

References

1. Brzezinski M, Luisetti T, London MJ. Radial artery cannulation: a comprehensive review of recent anatomic and physiologic investigations. *Anesth Analg* 2009;**109**(6):1763–81.

2. American_Society_of_Anesthesiologists. Standards of the American Society of Anesthesiologists: Standards for Basic Anesthetic Monitoring. 2011; Available from: http://www.asahq.org/For-Members/~/media/For%20Members/documents/Standards%20Guidelines%20Stmts/Basic%20Anesthetic%20Monitoring%202011.ashx

3. Wilkinson IB, Franklin SS, Hall IR, Tyrrell S, Cockcroft JR. Pressure amplification explains why pulse pressure is unrelated to risk in young subjects. *Hypertension* 2001;**38**(6):1461–6.

4. Roman MJ, Devereux RB, Kizer JR, et al. Central pressure more strongly relates to vascular disease and outcome than does brachial pressure: the Strong Heart Study. *Hypertension* 2007;**50**(1):197–203.

5. Choi CU, Kim EJ, Kim SH, et al. Differing effects of aging on central and peripheral blood pressures and pulse wave velocity: a direct intraarterial study. *J Hypertens* 2010;**28**(6):1252–60.

6. Lehman LW, Saeed M, Talmor D, Mark R, Malhotra A. Methods of blood pressure measurement in the ICU. *Crit Care Med* 2013;**41**(1):34–40.

7. Horowitz D, Amoateng-Adjepong Y, Zarich S, Garland A, Manthous CA. Arterial line or cuff BP? *Chest* 2013;**143**(1):270–1.

8. Ilies C, Bauer M, Berg P, et al. Investigation of the agreement of a continuous non-invasive arterial pressure device in comparison with invasive radial artery measurement. *Br J Anaesth* 2012;**108**(2):202–10.

9. Nelson MR, Stepanek J, Cevette M, et al. Noninvasive measurement of central vascular pressures with arterial tonometry: clinical revival of the pulse pressure waveform? *Mayo Clin Proc* 2010;**85**(5):460–72.

10. London GM, Blacher J, Pannier B, et al. Arterial wave reflections and survival in end-stage renal failure. *Hypertension* 2001;**38**(3):434–8.

11. Safar ME, Blacher J, Pannier B, et al. Central pulse pressure and mortality in end-stage renal disease. *Hypertension* 2002;**39**(3):735–8.

12. Hansen S, Staber M. Oscillometric blood pressure measurement used for calibration of the arterial tonometry method contributes significantly to error. *Eur J Anaesthesiol* 2006;**23**(9):781–7.

13. Steiner LA, Johnston AJ, Salvador R, Czosnyka M, Menon DK. Validation of a tonometric noninvasive arterial blood pressure monitor in the intensive care setting. *Anaesthesia* 2003;**58**(5):448–54.

14. Normand H, Lemarchand E, Arbeille P, et al. Beat-to-beat agreement of noninvasive tonometric and intra-radial arterial blood pressure during microgravity and hypergravity generated by parabolic flights. *Blood Press Monit* 2007;**12**(6):357–62.

15. Weiss BM, Spahn DR, Rahmig H, Rohling R, Pasch T. Radial artery tonometry: moderately accurate but unpredictable technique of continuous non-invasive arterial pressure measurement. *Br J Anaesth* 1996;**76**(3):405–11.

16. Penaz J. [Current photoelectric recording of blood flow through the finger]. *Cesk Fysiol* 1975;**24**(4):349–52.

17. Penaz J, Voigt A, Teichmann W. [Contribution to the continuous indirect blood pressure measurement]. *Z Gesamte Inn Med* 1976;**31**(24):1030–3.

18. Dueck R, Goedje O, Clopton P. Noninvasive continuous beat-to-beat radial artery pressure via TL-200 applanation tonometry. *J Clin Monit Comput* 2012;**26**(2):75–83.

19. Saugel B, Fassio F, Hapfelmeier A, et al. The T-Line TL-200 system for continuous non-invasive blood pressure measurement in medical intensive care unit patients. *Intens Care Med* 2012;**38**(9):1471–7.

20. Saugel B, Meidert AS, Hapfelmeier A, et al. W. Non-invasive continuous arterial pressure measurement based on radial artery tonometry in the intensive care unit: a method comparison study using the T-Line TL-200pro device. *Br J Anaesth* 2013;**111**(2):185–90.

21. Guelen I, Westerhof BE, van der Sar GL, et al. Validation of brachial artery pressure reconstruction from finger arterial pressure. *J Hypertens* 2008;**26**(7):1321–7.

22. Bos WJ, van Goudoever J, van Montfrans GA, van den Meiracker AH, Wesseling KH. Reconstruction of brachial artery pressure from noninvasive finger pressure measurements. *Circulation* 1996;**94**(8):1870–5.

23. Imholz BP, Wieling W, van Montfrans GA, Wesseling KH. Fifteen years experience with finger arterial pressure monitoring: assessment of the technology. *Cardiovasc Res* 1998;**38**(3):605–16.

24. Broch O, Bein B, Gruenewald M, et al. A comparison of continous non-invasive arterial pressure with invasive radial and femoral pressure in patients undergoing cardiac surgery. *Minerva Anestesiol* 2013;**79**(3):248–56.

25. Martina JR, Westerhof BE, van Goudoever J, et al. Noninvasive continuous arterial blood pressure monitoring with Nexfin(R).

Anesthesiology 2012;**116** (5):1092–103.

26. Fischer MO, Avram R, Carjaliu I, et al. Non-invasive continuous arterial pressure and cardiac index monitoring with Nexfin after cardiac surgery. *Br J Anaesth* 2012;**109**(4):514–21.

27. Hohn A, Defosse JM, Becker S, et al. Non-invasive continuous arterial pressure monitoring with Nexfin(R) does not sufficiently replace invasive measurements in critically ill patients. *Br J Anaesth* 2013;**111**(2):178–84.

28. Hofhuizen CM, Lemson J, Hemelaar AE, et al. Continuous non-invasive finger arterial pressure monitoring reflects intra-arterial pressure changes in children undergoing cardiac surgery. *Br J Anaesth* 2010;**105** (4):493–500.

29. Garnier RP, van der Spoel AG, Sibarani-Ponsen R, Markhorst DG, Boer C. Level of agreement between Nexfin non-invasive arterial pressure with invasive arterial pressure measurements in children. *Br J Anaesth* 2012;**109** (4):609–15.

30. Maggi R, Viscardi V, Furukawa T, Brignole M. Non-invasive continuous blood pressure monitoring of tachycardic episodes during interventional electrophysiology. *Europace* 2010;**12**(11):1616–22.

31. Jeleazcov C, Krajinovic L, Munster T, et al. Precision and accuracy of a new device (CNAPTM) for continuous non-invasive arterial pressure monitoring: assessment during general anaesthesia. *Br J Anaesth* 2010;**105**(3):264–72.

32. Hahn R, Rinosl H, Neuner M, Kettner SC. Clinical validation of a continuous non-invasive haemodynamic monitor (CNAP™ 500) during general anaesthesia. *Br J Anaesth* 2012;**108**(4):581–5.

33. Jagadeesh AM, Singh NG, Mahankali S. A comparison of a continuous noninvasive arterial pressure (CNAP) monitor with an invasive arterial blood pressure monitor in the cardiac surgical ICU. *Ann Card Anaesth* 2012;**15** (3):180–4.

34. Schramm C, Huber A, Plaschke K. The accuracy and responsiveness of continuous noninvasive arterial pressure during rapid ventricular pacing for transcatheter aortic valve replacement. *Anesth Analg* 2013;**117**(1):76–82.

35. Ilies C, Kiskalt H, Siedenhans D, et al. Detection of hypotension during Caesarean section with continuous non-invasive arterial pressure device or intermittent oscillometric arterial pressure measurement. *Br J Anaesth* 2012;**109**(3):413–19.

36. McCarthy T, Telec N, Dennis A, Griffiths J, Buettner A. Ability of non-invasive intermittent blood pressure monitoring and a continuous non-invasive arterial pressure monitor (CNAP) to provide new readings in each 1-min interval during elective caesarean section under spinal anaesthesia. *Anaesthesia* 2012;**67** (3):274–9.

37. Dewhirst E, Corridore M, Klamar J, et al. Accuracy of the CNAP monitor, a noninvasive continuous blood pressure device, in providing beat-to-beat blood pressure readings in the prone position. *J Clin Anesth* 2013;**25**(4):309–13.

38. Kako H, Corridore M, Rice J, Tobias JD. Accuracy of the CNAP monitor, a noninvasive continuous blood pressure device, in providing beat-to-beat blood pressure readings in pediatric patients weighing 20–40 kilograms. *Paediatr Anaesth* 2013;**23**(11):989–93.

Chapter

20

Monitoring the microcirculation

Daniel De Backer and Katia Donadello

Introduction

Optimization of tissue perfusion is one of the primary goals of perioperative optimization and resuscitation of the critically ill. Adequacy of tissue perfusion is often assumed from systemic measures including blood pressure, cardiac output, and venous oxygen saturation. However, microcirculatory alterations may occur even when global hemodynamic variables are within targets. Alterations in microcirculatory blood flow have been identified in several disease processes[1,2] and are associated with outcome.[3,4] Microcirculatory alterations also occur in the perioperative period.[5–7] In patients submitted to high-risk surgery, the severity of the alterations was associated with development of perioperative complications.[7] Assessment of the microcirculation may thus be desirable.

The incidence and relevance of microcirculatory alterations have been reviewed in detail in Chapter 8. The characteristics of these microvascular alterations have profound implications for monitoring. These are characterized by a decrease in capillary density, but also and more importantly, by heterogeneity in perfusion, with perfused capillaries in close vicinity of non-perfused capillaries.[1,2,8]

It is thus crucial that the technique used to evaluate the microcirculation can take into account its heterogeneous aspect. A heterogeneous perfusion leads to more severe alterations in tissue oxygenation than a homogenously decreased perfusion.[9,10] Heterogeneity of perfusion leads to altered oxygen extraction capabilities[9–13] and is associated with heterogeneity in oxygenation.[14] In patients with sepsis, heterogeneity but not blood flow velocity is associated with outcome.[15] The heterogeneity of perfusion is thus critical and the spatial resolution of the monitoring device should be sharp enough to disclose this heterogeneity in tissue perfusion and oxygenation. In this chapter, we will discuss the advantages and limitations of the techniques used to assess the microcirculation at the bedside.

Clinical examination and biomarkers

Clinical examination is unfortunately not appropriate for detecting microcirculatory alterations. If skin mottling is associated with impairment of skin microcirculation, skin perfusion is unfortunately often dissociated from more central beds, as skin vasoconstriction often occurs in shock states, in response to decrease in temperature, or in response to administration to vasopressor agents. Accordingly, evaluation of skin perfusion by central to toe temperature difference cannot track central microcirculatory perfusion.[16]

Lactate would theoretically be a good surrogate for assessing the microcirculation. Unfortunately, this relation even when found is relatively loose,[17,18] perhaps because lactate levels are affected not only by an increased production in hypoxic conditions, but also by aerobic lactate production under influence of inflammatory mediators and adrenergic stimulation, and by decreased lactate clearance. Interestingly, dynamic changes in lactate may better correlate with dynamic changes in microvascular perfusion than with absolute values.[19]

Techniques used to evaluate the microcirculation

Several techniques can be used to evaluate the microcirculation. Some of these directly measure microvascular perfusion, while others use indirect indices of tissue oxygenation.

Perioperative Hemodynamic Monitoring and Goal Directed Therapy, ed. Maxime Cannesson and Rupert Pearse.
Published by Cambridge University Press. © Cambridge University Press 2014.

Of note, whatever the device used, it would investigate the microcirculation only in the microvascular bed in which it is implemented. The ability of that specific window to represent other beds depends on the mechanisms implicated in microvascular disease (generalized, diffuse but somewhat heterogeneous or localized), on organ microvascular architecture, and on local factors (local vasoconstriction/pressure). Hence the area being investigated should be considered as a window that reflects alterations that are likely to be observed in other areas, provided that local factors do not exacerbate the lesion in the investigated area. Some areas may be more relevant than others. During the surgical intervention, various organs can be investigated. In the intact patient, the sublingual area is of particular clinical relevance, given the relationship between alterations in the microcirculation in the sublingual area and organ dysfunction[7] and outcome.[3,4] When it can be mounted on endoscopes, gastric or duodenal areas will be of interest.

Laser Doppler techniques

Laser Doppler can be used to evaluate the microcirculation. It provides blood flow measurements in relative units (mV), and relative changes to baseline values can only be assessed. The flow measured by current laser Doppler devices represents the aggregate flow in several vessels of variable size (including arterioles, capillaries, and venules) and different directions comprising the sampling volume, which is a volume of tissue comprised between 0.5 to 1 mm³. The heterogenous aspect of microvascular alterations can thus not be detected. Nevertheless, microvascular reactivity can be assessed during vascular occlusion tests, as discussed later.

In speckle laser Doppler technology a very thin laser beam is generated and scans a piece of tissue, allowing measurement of flow in single vessels and generating flow perfusion histograms. In experimental conditions, these techniques have demonstrated their ability to disclose sepsis-induced heterogeneity in perfusion.[14] In critically ill patients this technique can nowadays only be applied to the skin with all limitations discussed above, but in future it is likely that these would be mounted on endoscopes.

Videomicroscopic techniques

Application of small microscopes to tissues allows the direct visualization of microvessels. The main difficulty resides in the illumination of the depth of

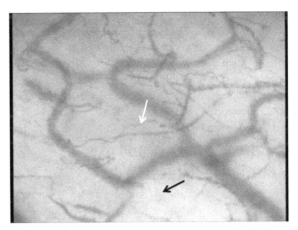

Figure 20.1. Sublingual microcirculation in septic shock. Photograph of the sublingual microcirculation in a patient with septic shock using a sidestream dark field (SDF) imaging device. Red blood cells are identified as gray bodies. The white arrow shows a perfused capillary, the black arrow identifies a stopped flow capillary.

tissue and in the method used to discard the light reflected at the surface of the tissue.

Orthogonal polarization spectral (OPS) and sidestream dark field (SDF) imaging techniques rely on the principle that, when applied on the surface of an organ, light diffuses into it and is reflected by the deeper layer of the tissues making it translucent.[20] At the wavelength used (530 nm), light is absorbed by hemoglobin, independently of its oxygenation state, allowing visualization of microvascular vessels. In the OPS imaging technique,[21] polarized light is applied to the tissue. The light reflected near the surface of the tissue retains its original characteristics and is discarded by a polarization filter, while the light entering in the depth of the tissue hits many cells and loses its polarized nature and is not stopped by the filter. In the SDF technique, the inner image-conducting core is isolated from the multiple light-emitting diodes positioned at the outer surface of the objective so that the light reflected by the outer surface cannot enter the image conducting core.[22]

Both devices can be used to study tissues protected by a thin epithelial layer, such as mucosal surfaces. In experimental settings and in the operative field, it can be applied at the surface of most organs, including brain, gut, and liver. In critically ill patients, the sublingual area is the most easily accessible mucosal surface, but ileostomies and colostomies, rectal and vaginal mucosa can also be investigated. Tissue perfusion can be characterized in individual capillaries and venules, but arterioles, located in deeper layers, are usually not visualized (Figure 20.1).

Red blood cells are identified as black bodies, while white blood cells and platelets can sometimes be seen as refringent bodies. Tissue perfusion is still best evaluated using semi-quantitative assessment.[1,23,24] as software for flow measurement require manual interventions to ensure adequate vessel detection or flow characterization.[24]

Measurement of PO_2 and oxygen saturation in tissues

Measurements of tissue PO_2 are based on Clarke-type electrodes. These electrodes measure the average PO_2 in a large sampling volume. PO_2 electrodes are not able to disclose PO_2 heterogeneity as these are sensitive to the highest PO_2 comprising the sampling volume. PO_2 histograms can be generated, but each of the individual PO_2 measurements represents the highest PO_2 of a large sampling volume and thus zones of low PO_2 may be missed, leading to erroneous conclusions.

Near-infrared spectroscopy (NIRS) uses near-infrared light to measure oxy- and deoxyhemoglobin in tissues. Several devices have been developed. In humans it is mostly applied on muscle, but brain is also a topic of interest. These devices measure the hemoglobin oxygen saturation and the hemoglobin content in a given sampling volume that depends on the quality of the used light, and its depth depends on the distance separating the emitting and receiving optodes. Oxygen saturation (SO_2) is measured in vessels and should not be interpreted as measurements of tissue oxygen saturation even though a modest absorption of light occurs in the tissues. As most of the blood in tissues is venous blood, NIRS SO_2 measurements are mostly influenced by local venous hemoglobin oxygen saturation.

Both techniques are not suitable for investigating the microcirculation in conditions of heterogeneous blood flow, such as in sepsis, but can detect global decreases in flow or in oxygenation. However, these techniques are interesting for assessing microvascular reactivity, when combined with a transient vascular occlusion test.

A place for occlusion tests?

Occlusion tests can be conducted with laser Doppler and NIRS devices to evaluate the microvascular and tissular response to hypoxia. After transient ischemia obtained by arterial occlusion with a cuff placed around the arm, the speed at which flow or SO_2 recovers is mostly determined by endothelial reactivity and by the capacity to recruit arterioles and capillaries, hence reflecting the integrity of the microcirculation. Other factors such as tissular O_2 consumption and microvascular hemoglobin content also play a role (Figure 20.2).

Multiple studies reported that endothelial vasoreactivity is altered in patients with sepsis[25-31] and is related to outcome.[27] It should be noted that vascular occlusion tests and video-microscopic evaluation of

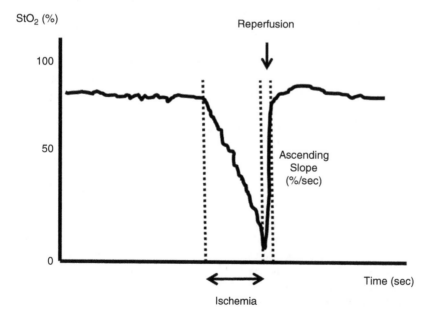

Figure 20.2. Vascular occlusion test. Evolution of StO_2 at the level of the thenar eminence (measured by near infrared spectroscopy) during a vascular occlusion test.

the microcirculation do not fully evaluate the same components of the microcirculation. Occlusion tests evaluate the capacity of maximal recruitment of the microcirculation, while video-microscopic techniques evaluate the actual state of the microcirculation. Both are related, but may differ somewhat. One may make the analogy with a car: the occlusion test reflects the maximal speed that the car can reach, while video-microscopic techniques reflect the actual speed of the car in the traffic.

Indirect measurements: tissue and venous CO_2 measurements

Measurements of PCO_2 in the tissues provide indirect information on tissue perfusion. Tissue CO_2 content represents the balance between CO_2 production and flow to the tissue. It is influenced by arterial CO_2 content, reflected by $PaCO_2$, so that the tissue to arterial gradient, or PCO_2 gap, is usually calculated as tissue PCO_2 – $PaCO_2$. PCO_2 gap reflects the adequacy for metabolic needs more than tissue hypoxia, unless very large values of PCO_2 gap are reached.[32] PCO_2 in tissues can be measured by electrodes, by tonometry, or transcutaneously. Even though the sampling volume is large, and heterogeneity can thus not be assessed, the measured value is mostly influenced by the most abnormal (highest) value in the sampled volume, so that this measurement is able to detect zones of impaired perfusion and/or tissue hypoxia. Gastric tonometry was initially used, but this technique is no longer used, mostly because of technical problems such as duodenal reflux and interference of feeding with PCO_2 measurements. Recently, sublingual and buccal PCO_2 monitoring have been developed.[33] Sublingual PCO_2 tracks microvascular blood flow, as the sublingual PCO_2 gap is inversely related to the proportion of perfused capillaries.[34] Sublingual PCO_2 is altered in sepsis, and non-survivors present more severe alterations.[35] Tissue PCO_2 can also be measured at earlobe, using transcutaneous PCO_2 electrodes. For this purpose, the skin of the patient should not be locally heated, to prevent local vasodilation. Although promising, limited evidence supports the use of this technique. In one trial, the ear to arterial PCO_2 gap was increased in patients with septic shock, and especially in non-survivors.[36] Given this limited experience, technical limitations and applicability are not well defined.

Do venous to arterial PCO_2 gradients reflect alterations in tissue perfusion? In patients with circulatory failure, venous to arterial PCO_2 gradient is increased in patients with a poor outcome.[37,38] However, it is difficult to ascertain whether this is due to microcirculatory dysfunction or to global hypoperfusion and cannot be sorted out at this stage.

Conclusions

Several techniques can now be used to investigate microcirculation at the bedside. Video-microscopic devices are best for evaluating microcirculation, taking into account its heterogeneous aspect. However, their use is not always easy, especially in spontaneously breathing patients, and continuous monitoring is not feasible. Tissue CO_2 monitoring and maybe venous to arterial CO_2 gradients appear promising, but require further validation. None of these is yet ready for routine clinical practice as microcirculatory endpoints for resuscitation, and the impact of therapeutic interventions have not yet been well defined.

References

1. De Backer D, Creteur J, Preiser JC, et al. Microvascular blood flow is altered in patients with sepsis. *Am J Respir Crit Care Med* 2002;**166**:98–104.

2. De Backer D, Creteur J, Dubois MJ, et al. Microvascular alterations in patients with acute severe heart failure and cardiogenic shock. *Am Heart J* 2004;**147**:91–9.

3. Sakr Y, Dubois MJ, De Backer D, et al. Persistent microvasculatory alterations are associated with organ failure and death in patients with septic shock. *Crit Care Med* 2004;**32**:1825–31.

4. den Uil CA, Lagrand WK, van der Ent M, et al. Impaired microcirculation predicts poor outcome of patients with acute myocardial infarction complicated by cardiogenic shock. *Eur Heart J* 2010;**31**:3032–9.

5. De Backer D, Dubois MJ, Schmartz D, et al. Microcirculatory alterations in cardiac surgery: effects of cardiopulmonary bypass and anesthesia. *Ann Thorac Surg* 2009;**88**:1396–403.

6. Atasever B, Boer C, Goedhart P, et al. Distinct alterations in sublingual microcirculatory blood flow and hemoglobin oxygenation in on-pump and off-pump coronary artery bypass graft surgery. *J Cardiothorac Vasc Anesth* 2011;**25**(**5**):784–90.

7. Jhanji S, Lee C, Watson D, et al. Microvascular flow and tissue

oxygenation after major abdominal surgery: association with post-operative complications. *Intens Care Med* 2009;**35**:671–7.

8. De Backer D, Donadello K, Taccone FS, et al. Microcirculatory alterations: potential mechanisms and implications for therapy. *Ann Intens Care* 2011;**1**:27.

9. Goldman D, Bateman RM, Ellis CG. Effect of decreased O_2 supply on skeletal muscle oxygenation and O_2 consumption during sepsis: role of heterogeneous capillary spacing and blood flow. *Am J Physiol Heart Circ Physiol* 2006;**290**:H2277–85.

10. Walley KR. Heterogeneity of oxygen delivery impairs oxygen extraction by peripheral tissues: theory. *J Appl Physiol* 1996;**81**:885–94.

11. Farquhar I, Martin CM, Lam C, et al. Decreased capillary density in vivo in bowel mucosa of rats with normotensive sepsis. *J Surg Res* 1996;**61**:190–6.

12. Ellis CG, Bateman RM, Sharpe MD, et al. Effect of a maldistribution of microvascular blood flow on capillary O_2 extraction in sepsis. *Am J Physiol* 2002;**282**:H156–64.

13. Humer MF, Phang PT, Friesen BP, et al. Heterogeneity of gut capillary transit times and impaired gut oxygen extraction in endotoxemic pigs. *J Appl Physiol* 1996;**81**:895–904.

14. Legrand M, Bezemer R, Kandil A, et al. The role of renal hypoperfusion in development of renal microcirculatory dysfunction in endotoxemic rats. *Intensive Care Med* 2011;**37**:1534–42.

15. Edul VS, Enrico C, Laviolle B, et al. Quantitative assessment of the microcirculation in healthy volunteers and in patients with septic shock. *Crit Care Med* 2012;**40**:1443–8.

16. Boerma EC, Kuiper MA, Kingma WP, et al. Disparity between skin perfusion and sublingual microcirculatory alterations in severe sepsis and septic shock: a prospective observational study. *Intens Care Med* 2008;**34**:1294–8.

17. Hernandez G, Boerma EC, Dubin A, et al. Severe abnormalities in microvascular perfused vessel density are associated to organ dysfunctions and mortality and can be predicted by hyperlactatemia and norepinephrine requirements in septic shock patients. *J Crit Care* 2013;**28**:538–14.

18. De Backer D, Donadello K, Sakr Y, et al. Microcirculatory alterations in patients with severe sepsis: impact of time of assessment and relationship with outcome. *Crit Care Med* 2013;**41**:791–9.

19. De Backer D, Creteur J, Dubois MJ, et al. The effects of dobutamine on microcirculatory alterations in patients with septic shock are independent of its systemic effects. *Crit Care Med* 2006;**34**:403–8.

20. Slaaf DW, Tangelder GJ, Reneman RS, et al. A versatile incident illuminator for intravital microscopy. *Int J Microcirc Clin Exp* 1987;**6**:391–7.

21. Groner W, Winkelman JW, Harris AG, et al. Orthogonal polarization spectral imaging: a new method for study of the microcirculation. *Nat Med* 1999;**5**:1209–12.

22. Goedhart P, Khalilzada M, Bezemer R, et al. Sidestream Dark Field (SDF) imaging: a novel stroboscopic LED ring-based imaging modality for clinical assessment of the microcirculation. *Optics Express* 2007;**15**:15101–14.

23. Boerma EC, Mathura KR, van der Voort PH, et al. Quantifying bedside-derived imaging of microcirculatory abnormalities in septic patients: a prospective validation study. *Crit Care* 2005;**9**:R601–6.

24. De Backer D, Hollenberg S, Boerma C, et al. How to evaluate the microcirculation: report of a round table conference. *Crit Care* 2007;**11**:R101.

25. Pareznik R, Knezevic R, Voga G, et al. Changes in muscle tissue oxygenation during stagnant ischemia in septic patients. *Intens Care Med* 2006;**32**:87–92.

26. De Blasi RA, Palmisani S, Alampi D, et al. Microvascular dysfunction and skeletal muscle oxygenation assessed by phase-modulation near-infrared spectroscopy in patients with septic shock. *Intens Care Med* 2005;**31**:1661–8.

27. Creteur J, Carollo T, Soldati G, et al. The prognostic value of muscle StO(2) in septic patients. *Intens Care Med* 2007;**33**:1549–56.

28. Girardis M, Rinaldi L, Busani S, et al. Muscle perfusion and oxygen consumption by near-infrared spectroscopy in septic-shock and non-septic-shock patients. *Intens Care Med* 2003;**29**:1173–6.

29. Skarda DE, Mulier KE, Myers DE, et al. Dynamic near-infrared spectroscopy measurements in patients with severe sepsis. *Shock* 2007;**27**:348–53.

30. Doerschug KC, Delsing AS, Schmidt GA, et al. Impairments in microvascular reactivity are related to organ failure in human sepsis. *Am J Physiol Heart Circ Physiol* 2007;**293**:H1065–71.

31. Nevière R, Mathieu D, Chagnon JL, et al. Skeletal muscle microvascular blood flow and oxygen transport in patients with severe sepsis. *Am J Respir Crit Care Med* 1996;**153**:191–5.

32. Schlichtig R, Bowles SA. Distinguishing between aerobic and anaerobic appearance of dissolved CO_2 in intestine during low flow. *J Appl Physiol* 1994;**76**:2443–51.

33. Weil MH, Nakagawa Y, Tang W, et al. Sublingual capnometry: a new noninvasive measurement for diagnosis and quantitation of severity of circulatory shock. *Crit Care Med* 1999;**27**:1225–9.

34. Creteur J, De Backer D, Sakr Y, et al. Sublingual capnometry tracks microcirculatory changes in septic patients. *Intens Care Med* 2006;**32**:516–23.

35. Marik PE. Sublingual capnography: a clinical validation study. *Chest* 2001;**120**:923–7.

36. Vallee F, Mateo J, Dubreuil G, et al. Cutaneous ear lobe PCO_2 at 37 °C to evaluate micro perfusion in septic patients. *Chest* 2010;**138**:1062–70.

37. Vallee F, Vallet B, Mathe O, et al. Central venous-to-arterial carbon dioxide difference: an additional target for goal-directed therapy in septic shock? *Intens Care Med* 2008;**34**:2218–25.

38. Futier E, Robin E, Jabaudon M, et al. Central venous O saturation and venous-to-arterial CO difference as complementary tools for goal-directed therapy during high-risk surgery. *Crit Care* 2010;**14**:R193.

Chapter

21

ScvO$_2$ monitoring

Alice Carter and Rupert Pearse

Background

Central and mixed venous saturations have been used in assessing the adequacy of global oxygen perfusion in critically ill patients for many years.[1] Central venous oxygen saturation (ScvO$_2$) refers to the hemoglobin oxygen saturation of blood in the superior vena cava.[2] This compares with mixed venous oxygen saturation (SvO$_2$), which refers to blood sampled from the proximal pulmonary artery.[2]

The measurement of ScvO$_2$ predates the measurement of SvO$_2$ and has been proposed as a surrogate for SvO$_2$ to determine the relationship between oxygen delivery (DO$_2$) and demand (VO$_2$).[3] This remains controversial, though recent studies have shown that there is a good correlation in the trend of SvO$_2$ and ScvO$_2$.[4] However, the relationship is much more complex and the two variables should not be confused or used interchangeably.[5] In general, both provide a good reflection of tissue perfusion, but are complicated by an inability to allow for regional and microcirculatory variations.[1]

The advent of the pulmonary artery (PA) catheter enabled the measurement of SvO$_2$. The increased use of ScvO$_2$ over SvO$_2$ is partly because of the potential complications and controversies surrounding the pulmonary catheter and the subsequent decline in its use.[5] In addition, the common use of central venous catheters in critical care patients for other reasons has facilitated the routine sampling of ScvO$_2$ and led to its use as a therapeutic endpoint in various trials across a number of clinical settings.[1] In the first trials there was no difference demonstrated, but more recent trials have shown improvements in outcome using ScvO$_2$ as a therapeutic endpoint.[6]

Physiology

Changes in central venous oxygen saturation may reflect both physiological and pathological responses. Interpretation therefore requires understanding of how ScvO$_2$ is determined. ScvO$_2$ reflects the adequacy of tissue oxygenation by balancing global oxygen delivery (DO$_2$) and global tissue oxygen consumption (VO$_2$) in blood from the head, neck, and upper limbs.[7] The normal value remains unknown and there is little published data describing the "normal" in healthy individuals. Many interventional studies are based on critically unwell patients, but values are often quoted around 70%.[8] Given the uncertainty, it may be more accurate to describe a normal range, as values as low as 65% have been described in healthy hospital inpatients.[9]

By applying the principles of the Fick equation, venous oxygen content can be calculated by oxygen consumption (VO$_2$), arterial oxygen content (CaO$_2$), and cardiac output (CO)[1] (see Figure 21.1).

$$VO_2 = CO \times CaO_2 - CO \times CvO_2$$
$$CaO_2 = (SaO_2 \times Hb \times 1.34) + (0.02 \times PaO_2)$$

If the factors determining oxygen content and oxygen consumption remain constant, ScvO$_2$ is directly proportional to cardiac output. This has also been demonstrated in a study of healthy volunteers using orthostatic hypotension as a model for hypovolemia. A decreased cardiac output from 4.3 to 2.7 L min^{-1} resulted in a reduced ScvO$_2$ baseline of 75% to 60% over the same time period.[10]

$$CO = \frac{VO_2}{CaO_2 - CvO_2}$$

Figure 21.1. Rearrangement of Fick equation.

Perioperative Hemodynamic Monitoring and Goal Directed Therapy, ed. Maxime Cannesson and Rupert Pearse.
Published by Cambridge University Press. © Cambridge University Press 2014.

Oxygen content is determined by oxygen hemoglobin saturation and by oxygen dissolved in blood. At standard atmospheric pressure, the latter is small and it is often accepted practice to measure oxygen hemoglobin saturation alone. However, changes in inspired oxygen concentration will alter the oxygen content of blood and thus the ScvO$_2$ value. Taking into account the hemoglobin saturation curve, at high partial pressures of oxygen only a small change in saturation will occur. At lower partial pressures, like those recorded in venous blood and in the steeper part of the curve, a small change in partial pressure will dramatically alter the saturation value.[11] In addition to this, clinical studies have shown that supplemental oxygen results in a further increase in venous saturation relative to arterial saturation.[11] This rise may mask any hemodynamic changes when ScvO$_2$ is used as a monitor, and thus changes in inspired oxygen fraction must be noted when using ScvO$_2$ as a therapeutic endpoint.

As ScvO$_2$ is dependent on functional cardiovascular and respiratory systems, changes in value may reflect not only altered tissue perfusion, but may also indicate a variety of other physiological or pathological states. Pathological conditions to consider are impaired oxygen uptake or factors downstream in the oxygen cascade. It is therefore important to remember that ScvO$_2$ is a marker of global tissue perfusion and will fail to identify regional abnormalities.

Throughout the perioperative period, large fluctuations in ScvO$_2$ are often observed.[12] These can be attributed to both changes in oxygen delivery and oxygen consumption. Often the latter is overlooked but considerable. Increases in oxygen consumption as a result of anxiety, pain, and shivering may all reduce venous saturation. Oxygen consumption can be reduced by analgesia, sedation, and by both general and regional anesthetic techniques, this decrease being achieved by reduced motor activity, reduced work of breathing, and reduced core body temperature. Intravenous hypnotic agents such as benzodiazepines and propofol reduce metabolic demand by blunting the sympathetic neurohumoral response.[13] In addition, some volatile anesthetic agents may reduce sympathetic tone with reduced cardiac output at higher doses.[13] Decreased neuronal oxygen consumption has been associated with the administration of barbiturates, benzodiazepines, propofol, and volatile anesthetic gases.[13] It is therefore imperative that interpretation during the perioperative

period takes into account other factors that may also influence the absolute ScvO$_2$ value.

As mentioned above, ScvO$_2$ is sometimes used as a surrogate for SvO$_2$. The relationship between the two values is complex and reflects the difference between oxygen delivery and consumption in different parts of the body in health and disease.[5] Regional variations result in different values in the superior vena cava and inferior vena cava with ScvO$_2$ usually slightly lower than SvO$_2$ in healthy patients.[2] Increased oxygen extraction will reduce the venous oxygen content and, similarly, reduced oxygen uptake will increase it. For example, venous saturation of coronary venous blood is 30% compared with 90% from the renal vein. This reflects the higher oxygen extraction of myocardial tissue versus the homeostatic role of the kidney. As the latter receives a greater proportion of cardiac output, sampling from the inferior vena cava will reveal higher oxygen content.[2] Changes here in values may not be pathological, but reflect physiological responses. However, the values reverse in states of shock and it has been reported that ScvO$_2$ is higher than SvO$_2$. Cardiac output may be preferentially diverted to coronary and cerebral circulations rather than to the splanchnic and renal beds, resulting in lower oxygen content of blood in the inferior vena cava. This highlights how it is important that the catheter tip is positioned in the superior vena cava at all times.

Measurement

ScvO$_2$ monitoring is relatively simple and less invasive than some alternative methods of cardiac output monitoring. It requires the placement of a central venous catheter with the tip placed in the superior vena cava (SVC).[4] As mentioned earlier, sampling site can greatly affect the ScvO$_2$ value and, for this reason, a femoral central catheter is not recommended. Inadvertent placement of a central venous catheter into the right atrium may also produce significantly lower ScvO$_2$ values than SVC placement due to drainage of myocardial venous blood directly into the right atrium. ScvO$_2$ can then be measured either by intermittent sampling or by continuous measurement using a fiberoptic catheter. There is no evidence to suggest one method is preferable especially in the perioperative patient.

Intermittent sampling is a comparatively cheap, reliable method providing "snapshot" values.[1] Samples of blood are analyzed in widely available blood gas analyzers, which utilize co-oximetry to measure hemoglobin saturation. The different light absorption wavelengths of oxygenated and deoxygenated hemoglobin are used to calculate the respective concentrations. Co-oximetry also enables the identification of other forms of hemoglobin such as carboxyhemoglobin and methemoglobin. However, this method does not allow the clinician to observe "spikes" in $ScvO_2$, for example, if a patient coughs and then settles. In addition, optimal frequency of sampling remains unknown, there may be a time-lag from sampling to $ScvO_2$ value, and specific errors may occur as a result of diluted or unhomogenized blood samples.[13]

Fiberoptic catheters enable continuous measurement using spectrophotometry.[1] This "real-time" monitoring has clear advantages. However, this method is more expensive and subject to signal drift, though this can be corrected by frequent calibration. Artifact may also arise if the fiberoptic catheter abuts the vessel wall. Previously, optically active compounds such as bilirubin and carboxyhemoglobin interfered with results, but this is no longer a problem. It is a relatively new technique, and the initial lack of success with $ScvO_2$ monitoring may be due in part to the inadequacies of the old ways of monitoring. Its use has increased since its utilization as an endpoint to guide fluid, and hemodynamic therapy in patients admitted to hospital with severe sepsis or septic shock improved in-hospital mortality in this cohort of patients[6].

Validation

Although the initial trials using $ScvO_2$ did not demonstrate any improvement in outcomes, the evidence base supporting $ScvO_2$ as a therapeutic target has grown recently.[6] Observational studies have demonstrated an association between a low $ScvO_2$ and a poor prognosis in heart failure,[14] trauma,[15] and sepsis.[6] There is also an increasing body of literature describing changes in $ScvO_2$ during the perioperative period.[1] Low $ScvO_2$ values have been shown to correlate with increased postoperative complications following major surgery.[4]

The first clinical application of $ScvO_2$ was in the assessment of cardiogenic shock in patients admitted to hospital with acute coronary events. Derangements of $ScvO_2$ correlated with the degree of myocardial dysfunction and a threshold of 60% highlighted a number of patients with heart failure.[15]

Clinical studies have suggested the use of $ScvO_2$ in assessing traumatic shock. In one series of 26 major trauma victims, an $ScvO_2$ less than 65% was not only a marker of blood loss, but was also found to be more reliable than traditional observations such as blood pressure, CVP, pulse.[15] So far, no trials using $ScvO_2$ as an endpoint to guide therapeutic interventions in trauma patients have yet been conducted.

One of the first successful trials to use continuous $ScvO_2$ monitoring to target therapy was in the early management of severe sepsis and septic shock.[6] In septic shock, $ScvO_2$ has been frequently noted to be less than 65%. When combined with a serum lactate >2 mmol L^{-1}, further resuscitation is indicated in the early stages. In this study, for the first 6 hours of hospital admission, patients were randomized to receive either "standard care" or fluid and inotropic support to target an $ScvO_2$ value of greater than 70%. The results revealed significantly lower mortality of 31% in this intervention group compared with the control group of 47%. This intervention has now been incorporated into the Surviving Sepsis Campaign "resuscitation bundle."[17]

An observational study of 98 consecutive unplanned admissions to ICU, showed patients with an $ScvO_2$ less than 60% at admission had higher mortality rates.[18] Further work is still required in this patient population to ascertain if $ScvO_2$ can be used to guide treatment.

In non-cardiac surgery, two observational studies have so far shown that reduced $ScvO_2$ may have prognostic significance after major surgery. The first study with 117 patients, carried out in a single center, showed that the lowest measured $ScvO_2$ in the first 8 hours postsurgery was independently associated with postoperative complications.[12] The 8-hour mean $ScvO_2$ value for patients not developing postoperative complications was 75%. In addition, the $ScvO_2$ value was noted to be significantly lower in the first hour postsurgery, despite recording little change in oxygen delivery. This is consistent with results from previous studies in cardiac patients and is attributed to increased oxygen consumption secondary to factors such as cessation of general anesthesia, hypothermia, shivering, and pain.[19]

In another multicenter observational study of 60 patients undergoing either elective or emergency surgery, the mean $ScvO_2$ value at various intervals in the perioperative period was lower in patients developing complications.[20] The mean cut-off value was 73%, with a mean $ScvO_2$ value greater than 74%

Oxygen delivery factors		Oxygen consumption factors	
↑ ScvO₂	↓ ScvO₂	↑ ScvO₂	↓ ScvO₂
Oxygen therapy	Alveolar hypoxia	Analgesia	Pain
Blood transfusion	Anemia	Anesthesia	Agitation
Intravenous fluids	Carboxyhemoglobin	Sedation	Pyrexia
Inotropic agents	Hypovolemia	Warming	Shivering
	Heart failure	Respiratory support	Respiratory failure

Figure 21.2. Summary of common factors that may alter ScvO₂ values.

not developing complications. Again, ScvO₂ values were noted to be significantly lower in the first hour postsurgery.

Limitations

As mentioned earlier, in patients undergoing major surgery, there is significant variation of DO₂ and VO₂ due to a variety of factors both physiological and pathological. Interpretation of the absolute ScvO₂ value therefore requires the observer to consider the causes of deranged values promptly. For example, if ScvO₂ is used as an endpoint to determine inotropic support or administration of intravenous fluids, increasing the inspired oxygen fraction may be erroneously interpreted as adequate hemodynamic resuscitation. VO₂ may fluctuate considerably during the perioperative period. It is therefore imperative that interpretation during the perioperative period takes into account other factors that may also influence the absolute ScvO₂ value. Figure 21.2 gives a summary of common factors to consider and this has been discussed in detail earlier.

Goal directed therapy (GDT) is a term used to describe targeted intravenous fluid administration and inotropic support. The use of GDT in the perioperative period in high-risk surgical patients undergoing non-cardiac surgery has been associated with fewer surgical complications.[21] However, it still remains an under-utilized technique, possibly as a result of debate regarding minimally invasive cardiac output monitoring in the postoperative period. If ScvO₂ is to be successfully incorporated in GDT and as a marker of global tissue perfusion, further studies are required to determine the value or range of ScvO₂ that we should be aiming for.

Overall, central venous saturation monitoring is simple and relatively non-invasive. It reflects circulatory changes and is therefore a useful tool to indicate changes in hypoxia, hemorrhage, and sepsis, thus providing useful information about disease severity and response to treatment. Interpretation of ScvO₂ values requires understanding of venous saturation physiology, and absolute values should be interpreted after considering all the variables that may have altered oxygen delivery and consumption. It is important to remember that it cannot be used interchangeably with SvO₂. Monitoring the trend may be more useful than using absolute values. Further work is required to ascertain the "normal value" range in perioperative patients. Then it may be more routinely used as a hemodynamic monitor and outcome predictor.

References

1. Shepherd S, Pearse R. Role of central and mixed venous oxygen saturation measurement in perioperative care. *Anaesthesiology* 2009;**111**:649–56.

2. Barratt-Boyes B, Wood E. The oxygen saturation of blood in the venae cavae, right-heart chambers and pulmonary vessels of healthy subjects. *J Lab Clin Med* 1957;**50**:93–106.

3. Goldman R, Klughaupt M, Metcalf T, Spivack A, Harrison D. Measurement of central venous oxygen saturation in patients with myocardial infarction. *Circulation* 1968;**38**:941–6.

4. Dueck M, Klimek M, Appenrodt S, Weigand C, Boerner U. Trends but not individual values of central venous oxygen saturation agree with mixed venous oxygen saturation during varying hemodynamic conditions. *Anesthesiology* 2005;**103**: 249–57.

5. Sekkat H, Sohawon S, Noordally S. A comparison of mixed and central venous oxygen saturation in patients during and after cardiac surgery. *J Intens Care Soc* 2009;**10**:99–101.

6. Rivers E, Nguyen B, Havstad S, et al. Early goal directed therapy in the treatment of severe sepsis and

septic shock. *N Eng J Med* 2001;**345**:1368–77.

7. Ho K, Harding R, Chamberlain J, Bulsara M. A comparison of central and mixed venous oxygen saturation in circulatory failure. *J Cardiothor Vasc Anesth* 2010;**24**:434–9.

8. Morgan T, Venkatesh B. Monitoring oxygenation. In Bersten A, Soni N, Oh T, eds. *Intensive Care Manual*, 2003, pp. 95–106.

9. Jenstrup M, Eilersen E, Mogensen T, Secher N. A maximal central venous oxygen saturation (SvO$_2$max) for the surgical patient. *Acta Anaesthesiol Scand Suppl* 1995;**107**:29–32.

10. Madsen P, Iversen H, Secher N. Central venous oxygen saturation during hypovolaemic shock in humans. *Scand J Clin Lab Invest* 1993;**53**:67–72.

11. Ho K, Harding R, Chamberlain J. The impact of arterial oxygen tension on venous oxygen saturation in circulatory failure. *Shock* 2008;**29**:3–6.

12. Pearse R, Dawson D, Fawcett J, et al. Changes in central venous saturation after major surgery and association with outcome. *Crit Care* 2005;**9**:R694–9.

13. Kumba C, Van der Linden P. Effects of sedative drugs on metabolic demand. *Ann Fr Anaesth Reanimation* 2008;**27**:574–80.

14. Ander DS, Jaggi M, Rivers E, et al. Undetected cardiogenic shock in patients with congestive heart failure presenting to the emergency department. *Am J Cardiol* 1998;**82**:888–91.

15. Scalea TM, Hartnett RW, Duncan AO, et al. Central venous oxygen saturation: a useful clinical tool in trauma patients. *J Trauma* 1990;**30**:1539–43.

16. Edwards J, Mayall R. Importance of the sampling site for measurement of mixed venous oxygen saturation in shock. *Crit Care Med* 1998;**26**:1356–60.

17. Dellinger R, Carlet J, Masur H, et al. Surviving sepsis campaign guidelines for management of severe sepsis and septic shock. *Intens Care Med* 2004;**30**(4):536–55.

18. Bracht M, Hänggi M, Jeker B, et al. Incidence of low central venous oxygen saturation during unplanned admissions in a multidisciplinary intensive care unit: an observational study. *Crit Care* 2007;**11**:R2.

19. Polonen P, Hippelainen M, Takala R, Ruokonen E, Takala J. Relationship between intra- and postoperative oxygen transport and prolonged intensive care after cardiac surgery: a prospective study. *Acta Anaesthesiol Scand* 1997;**41**:810–17.

20. Jakob S, Bracht H, Eigenmann V, et al. Multicentre study on peri- and postoperative central venous oxygen saturation in high-risk surgical patients. *Crit Care* 2006;**10**:R158.

21. Pearse R, Dawson D, Fawcett J, et al. Early goal-directed therapy after major surgery reduces complications and duration of hospital stay. A randomised, controlled trial. *Crit Care* 2005;**9**:R687–93.

Chapter

22

Goal directed therapy in the intensive care and emergency settings: what is the evidence?

Joseph Meltzer

Introduction

In 2001, Rivers and colleagues refined the resuscitation of patients with septic shock in a landmark trial of protocolized resuscitation for patients with septic shock in the emergency department.[1] This transformative trial of early goal directed therapy showed profound morbidity and mortality benefit for early and aggressive treatment of the septic patient. These principles have since been applied to many types of "at-risk" patients, and have revolutionized care for patients including those who have undergone major surgery or suffered cardiac arrest, shock, brain injury, or sepsis. This paradigm should be employed for patients manifesting hypotension and/or hyperlactemia.[2] Early aggressive resuscitation of the critically ill patient appears to limit tissue hypoxia, reduce organ failure and improve outcome.[3] There is little controversy that early, target-focused care improves outcome, but controversy does remain in the definition of "early" and which are the appropriate "targets" that the intensivist should be aiming for, and the tools and therapeutics that should be employed to get there.

Intravenous fluid therapy

The cornerstone of treatment for patients with shock is intravenous fluid. This is the initial intervention undertaken by most practitioners when faced with a patient with signs of tissue hypoperfusion in an attempt to reverse their fluid responsive hypodynamic circulation. The saline versus albumin fluid evaluation (SAFE) study reported no difference in the overall risk of death for adults given albumin or saline for intravascular fluid resuscitation in the intensive care unit (ICU).[4] This trial involving nearly 7000 critically ill patients addressed one of the most hotly debated topics in critical care: that of crystalloid versus colloid resuscitation. However, it did not address the outcome benefit of normal saline (NS) versus balanced salt solution resuscitation. The hyperchloremia that is associated with NS resuscitation may increase mortality in perioperative patients.[5,6] The same may be true in the ICU. Yunos and colleagues recently applied this principle of "chloride-restrictive" resuscitation to critically ill patients in the ICU and showed a reduction in acute kidney injury (AKI) and the need for renal replacement therapy (RRT).[7]

Although current guidelines for the treatment of septic shock in adults and children call for initial rapid boluses of large amounts of fluid, some controversy does remain in this arena. The fluid expansion as supportive therapy in critically ill African children (FEAST) trial challenges these guidelines. This trial enrolled eastern African children with a severe febrile illness and evidence of abnormal perfusion.[8] 3141 children without hypotension were randomly assigned to one of three groups: albumin bolus, 0.9% saline bolus or no bolus. The primary endpoint of 48-hour mortality showed a striking difference between the groups. Mortality rates were 10.5%, 10.5%, and 7.3% for the albumin bolus, 0.9% saline bolus and no bolus groups, respectively. The 48-hour mortality in the combined bolus group was increased by 45%. It must be stated that this was a pediatric cohort, with a high rate of malaria without access to ICU monitoring, ventilator support, inotropes, vasopressors, or RRT, but the results are intriguing. At first glance, one might think that these results stand in opposition to early goal directed therapy, but upon closer inspection it can be seen another way. Fluid is a medication thats composition and dose must be titrated appropriately to maximize benefit. The best way to optimize its use

Perioperative Hemodynamic Monitoring and Goal Directed Therapy, ed. Maxime Cannesson and Rupert Pearse.
Published by Cambridge University Press. © Cambridge University Press 2014.

is to avoid a one-size-fits-all approach and use a target-directed management protocol. Resuscitation fluids are the subject of a recent excellent review, but lie outside the scope of this chapter.[9]

Hemodynamic monitoring techniques for the ICU and ED

Three hemodynamic variables lie at the center of River's protocol for early goal directed therapy: central venous pressure (CVP), mean arterial pressure (MAP) and $ScvO_2$.[1] Each of these concepts is addressed in depth in other parts of this textbook. There remains a raging debate as to the ideal hemodynamic monitoring modality to assess fluid responsiveness and adequacy of resuscitation in the hemodynamically unstable patient. The most utilized parameter remains the arterial blood pressure. It is one of the most frequently measured variables in medicine, and is clearly useful in detecting patients in overt shock. A normal blood pressure, however, does not rule out the presence of hypoperfusion, hyperlactemia, and shock.[10] The measurement of the CVP has long been used as a measure of cardiac preload. Unfortunately, there is a paucity of evidence to show that the CVP has any utility for this purpose. Certainly, the CVP is affected by the volume of blood in the central veins; however it is also affected by a multitude of other factors including: venous return, cardiac output, regional vascular tone, right ventricular compliance, tricuspid valve disease, cardiac rhythm, proper leveling of the transducer, and intrathoracic pressure.[11] Because the CVP is affected by so many factors, it is impossible for the intensivist to separate the contribution of cardiac preload from the surrounding "noise." Indeed, the CVP correlates poorly with cardiac index,[12] stroke volume index,[13] or fluid responsiveness.[14,15] The measurement of $ScvO_2$ is simple when a patient has a central venous catheter in place. Critically ill patients often have such catheters for administration of intravenous fluids and potent vasoactive pressor medications. $ScvO_2$ has a demonstrated correlation to SvO_2, and is meant to reflect the balance between oxygen delivery and oxygen consumption.[16,17] $ScvO_2$ is a tool, especially in the early phase of shock to guide fluid management and blood transfusion or inotropic support.[18] Considering such results, it seems that $ScvO_2$, and especially its evolution over time, could be used as an interesting surrogate for SvO_2 monitoring.

Rather than use the above parameters in isolation, several dynamic parameters of fluid responsiveness should be used to guide fluid therapy in mechanically ventilated and spontaneously breathing patients. These are based on pulse contour analysis of the arterial line waveform (PPV, SVV, SPV), aortic blood flow (esophageal Doppler), direct imaging of the heart and inferior vena cava with echocardiography and ultrasound, bioreactance/impedance, or simply performing a passive straight leg raise on a hemodynamically unstable patient. Please refer to other chapters for more detailed description of aforementioned monitoring modalities.

Vasopressors

If fluid resuscitation fails to ameliorate hypoperfusion, vasopressor therapy should be initiated. Adrenergic agonists are the first-line vasopressor in the majority of patients. They are rapid in onset, potent, and have a short half-life. De Backer and colleagues compared dopamine to norepinephrine (NE) in the treatment of shock in almost 1700 patients, over 60% of which were presumed to be septic.[19] There was not a significant difference in the primary endpoint of mortality. There were differences, all favoring NE, in the development of arrhythmias, duration of therapy, and the addition of other pressors. Additionally, in patients with cardiogenic shock, dopamine increased 28-day mortality. The overall improvement in the endpoints of resuscitation make NE the first-line agent over dopamine. De Backer and colleagues have also performed a meta-analysis of pre-existing trial on the use of dopamine versus NE in the treatment of patients with septic shock. I examined their review of five observational and six randomized trials with a total of 2768 patients and found that dopamine was again associated with significant increased risk of mortality.[20]

It has been demonstrated that patients with shock have very low circulating vasopressin levels. The VASST investigators compared NE to vasopressin in a multicenter, randomized, double-blind trial of 778 patients with presumed septic shock.[21] Overall, there was no difference in outcome between the two groups; however, in a prospectively defined stratum of less severely sick patients, the mortality rate was lower in the vasopressin group. They also found that low-dose vasopressin allowed a rapid decrease in the total norepinephrine dose, while maintaining arterial blood pressure. Complication rates in both groups were similar with the possible exception of excess digital ischemia with the use of vasopressin.

Annane et al. compared the effect of combined NE and dobutamine versus epinephrine for the treatment of septic shock.[22] There was no difference in mortality between groups; however, there was less metabolic acidosis in patients who were administered the combination of NE and dobutamine.

The Surviving Sepsis Campaign guidelines recommend norepinephrine as the first-line vasopressor in sepsis.[23] The guidelines go on to recommend epinephrine as the second-line pressor that can be added to NE if additional catecholamine is needed to support a patient's blood pressure. Vasopressin at a dose of 0.01 to 0.03 U/min can be added to further increase the blood pressure or to reduce the NE dose. These guidelines recommend dopamine only for patients with little risk of tachydysrhythmias or overt bradycardia. Phenylephrine is only recommended for salvage cases or when norepinephrine administration results in tachydysrhythmias. It should be stated that vasopressor therapy should always be preceded by volume status assessment and accompanied with fluid administration if required.

Blood transfusion

Anemia is common in the emergency and ICU setting. Approximately two-thirds of patients present to the ICU with a hemoglobin level under 12 g/dL, and 97% become anemic by day 8.[24] The goal of blood transfusion is to improve myocardial and tissue oxygen delivery. One controversial aspect of the study by Rivers and colleagues was the liberal use of RBC transfusion in the group of patients receiving early goal directed therapy.[1] While a strong association exists between anemia and poor outcome, RBC transfusion also comes with significant risk. Adverse effects of allogeneic blood transfusion include reactions, infections, lung injury, circulatory overload, immunomodulation, and death.

The cornerstone of our current knowledge of transfusion thresholds within the ICU is the Transfusion Requirements in Critical Care (TRICC) trial.[25] In this trial, 838 euvolemic and anemic patients without on-going bleeding were randomized to either a restrictive (transfusion at Hb = 7 g/dL and maintained between 7 and 9 g/dL) or liberal (transfusion at Hb = 10 g/dL and maintained between 10–12 g/dL)

transfusion threshold. There was no difference in all-cause mortality between the two groups, but hospital mortality was significantly higher in the liberal strategy group compared with the restrictive strategy group (28.1% vs. 22.2%, $P = 0.05$). In subgroup analysis, young patients (age > 55 years) and less critically ill (APACHE II score > 20) had improved outcome with the restrictive strategy. The TRICC trial is not without flaws. It is underpowered, used non-leukoreduced blood, doesn't have any outcomes related to patient functionality (i.e., ability to mobilize or exercise), had a paucity of patients with coronary disease, and its results are subject to bias due to therapeutic misalignment.[26] Despite these flaws, it has changed practice across specialties in the ICU.

Similar results to the TRICC trial have been shown in patients who have undergone cardiac surgery. The TRACS trial prospectively randomized 502 patients who underwent cardiac surgery with cardiopulmonary bypass.[27] The Hb concentrations were maintained at a mean of 10.5 g/dL in the liberal-strategy group and 9.1 g/dL in the restrictive-strategy group. A total of 198 of 253 patients (78%) in the liberal-strategy group and 118 of 249 (47%) in the restrictive-strategy group received a blood transfusion. Occurrence of the primary endpoint of 30-day all-cause mortality was similar between groups. Independent of transfusion strategy, the number of transfused red blood cell units was an independent risk factor for clinical complications or death at 30 days.

To address the effect of a restrictive approach on functional recovery or risk of myocardial infarction in patients with cardiac disease, as well as get a handle on perioperative transfusion requirements, the Transfusion Trigger Trial for Functional Outcomes in Cardiovascular Patients Undergoing Surgical Hip Fracture Repair (FOCUS) was performed.[28] 2016 patients who were 50 years of age or older (mean age 82) undergoing hip fracture surgery were randomized to either a restrictive (transfusion at Hb = 8 g/dL and maintained between 8 and 10 g/dL) or liberal (transfusion at Hb = 10 g/dL and maintained between 10 and 12 g/dL) transfusion threshold. The primary outcome was death at 30 and 60 days or an inability to walk across a room without human assistance on 60-day follow-up. The liberal transfusion strategy, as compared with a restrictive, did not reduce rates of death or inability to walk independently.

All of these prior trials addressed transfusion requirements for patients that were anemic, euvolemic, and hemostatic. Recently, transfusion requirements in patients with acute upper gastrointestinal (UGI) bleeding have also been investigated, which may have some applicability to patients in the emergency or ICU setting. Villanueva et al. randomized 921 patients with severe acute UGI, 461 of them to a restrictive strategy (transfusion when the Hg level fell below 7g/dL) and 460 to a liberal strategy (transfusion when the Hg fell below 9g/dL).[29] 51% of patients assigned to the restrictive strategy, as compared with 15% assigned to the liberal strategy, did not receive transfusions. The probability of survival at 6 weeks was higher in the restrictive-strategy group than in the liberal-strategy group. Further bleeding occurred in 10% of the patients in the restrictive-strategy group as compared with 16% of the patients in the liberal-strategy group. The probability of survival was slightly higher with the restrictive-strategy than with the liberal-strategy in the subgroup of patients who had bleeding associated with a peptic ulcer, and was significantly higher in the subgroup of patients with cirrhosis and Child–Pugh class A or B disease. While these patients were not suffering from traumatic or surgical hemorrhage, the results may have applicability to unstable patients who are anemic.

Lactate clearance

Hyperlactemia indicates abnormal cellular function and probable tissue hypoxia with increased anaerobic metabolism. Serial lactate measurement and resuscitation directed toward its clearance has been advocated as an endpoint of resuscitation. The data here are conflicting. Jansen and Bakker found that targeting a decrease in serum lactate levels of 20% over 2 hours was associated with decreased in-hospital mortality in propensity-matched patients with undifferentiated shock in the ICU.[30] However, Jones and the Emergency Medicine Shock Research Network Investigators found no benefit to adding lactate clearance to "conventional" early goal directed therapy with a target of $ScvO_2 > 70\%$ in septic patients in the emergency department.[31] In this trial 300 patients were randomized to one of two protocols. The $ScvO_2$ group was resuscitated to normalize central venous pressure, mean arterial pressure, and $ScvO_2$ of at least 70%; and the lactate clearance group was resuscitated to normalize central venous pressure, mean arterial pressure, and lactate clearance of at least 10%. Both protocols were continued until all goals were achieved or for up to 6 hours. In-hospital mortality was reduced in the lactate-clearance cohort but the results did not reach statistical significance.

Broad spectrum antibiotic administration

Shock has multiple etiologies, and goal directed approaches should be implemented in all patients. However, if severe sepsis is suspected, then the algorithm must employ antibiotics directed to treat the infection. All too often, this life-saving therapy is delayed. In sepsis, the duration of hypotension without the administration of antibiotics is associated with mortality.[32] Early administration of appropriate antibiotics reduces mortality in patients with gram-positive and gram-negative bacteremia.[33] Appropriate antimicrobials should be administered within the first hour of recognition of septic shock. When antibiotic administration is paired with early goal directed therapy in the emergency department, it decreases time to antibiotic administration and improves patient outcome.[34] The most common causes of infection in severe sepsis are pneumonia and intra-abdominal infections. In patients with ventilator-acquired pneumonia, those who receive antibiotics later have greater ICU and in-hospital mortality.[35] The choice of antibiotics should be guided by local antibiograms and the patient's clinical presentation. Full loading doses of each antimicrobial should be given, and only later adjusted for changing renal or hepatic function. The availability of pre-mixed formulations of antimicrobials should be available for the physicians in the emergency department, ICU and rapid response team.

Tight glycemic control

Evidence suggests that there is no benefit and probable harm to glycemic control below 140–180mg/dL. The largest trial of tight glycemic control performed by the NICE-SUGAR investigators clearly demonstrated that target blood glucose levels of 81–108mg/dL were associated with a significantly higher mortality rate than with a target of less than 180mg/dL.[36] Additionally, in follow-up analysis of the same data set, any moderate (41–70mg/dL) or severe hypoglycemic (<41md/dL) episodes were associated with a higher mortality rate and were more common in the 81–108 mg/dL group.[37]

Sedation in the ICU

Just as we have goal directed targets for hemodynamic parameters, we must apply the same focus to our patients' physical and psychological comfort. Significant advances in our understanding of pain, agitation, and delirium in the ICU have recently been made.[38] We now know that delirium is associated with increased hospital mortality, prolonged length of stay, and the development of long-term cognitive impairment.[39] The implementation of protocols with target-directed titration of sedatives, analgesics, and anxiolytics leads to improved clinical outcomes in terms of delirium reduction, early mobilization,[40] and decreased times of mechanical ventilation.[41]

Conclusion

Early goal directed therapy is a hemodynamic resuscitation technique used to correct tissue hypoxia before organ failure develops. Comprehensive protocols and pathways for patients with hypotension, hypoperfusion and/or shock presenting to the ICU or emergency department are required to maximize patient survival.

References

1. Rivers E, Nguyen B, Havstad S, et al. Early goal-directed therapy in the treatment of severe sepsis and septic shock. *N Engl J Med* 2001;**345**:1368–77.

2. Rhodes A, Bennett D. Early goal-directed therapy: an evidence-based review. *Crit Care Med* 2004;**32**(Suppl):S448–50.

3. Levy M, Macias W, Russell J, et al. Failure to improve during the first day of therapy is predictive of 28-day mortality in severe sepsis. *Chest* 2004;**124** (Suppl):120S.

4. The SAFE Study Investigators. A comparison of albumin and saline for fluid resuscitation in the intensive care unit. *N Engl J Med* 2004;**350**:2247–56.

5. McCluskey S, Karkouti K, Wijeysundera D, et al. Hyperchloremia after noncardiac surgery is independently associated with increased morbidity and mortality: a propensity-match cohort study. *Anesth Analg* 2013;**117**:412–21.

6. Shaw A, Bagshaw S, Goldstein S, et al. Major complications, mortality, and resource utilization after open abdominal surgery: 0.9% saline compared to Plasma-Lyte. *Ann Surg* 2012;**255**:821–9.

7. Yunos N, Bellomo R, Hegarty C, et al. Association between a chloride-liberal vs. chloride-restrictive intravenous fluid administration strategy and kidney injury in critically ill adults. *JAMA* 2012;**308**:1566–72.

8. Maitland K, Kiguli S, Opoka R, et al. Mortality after fluid bolus in African children with severe infection. *N Engl J Med* 2011;**364**:2483–95.

9. Myburgh J, Mythen M. Resuscitation Fluids. *N Engl J Med* 2013;**369**:1243–51.

10. Bennett D. Arterial pressure: a personal View. In Pinsky M, Payen D, Vincent JL, eds. *Update in Intensive Care Medicine: Functional Hemodynamic Monitoring.* Berlin: Springer, 2005.

11. Smith T, Grounds R, Rhodes A. Central venous pressure: uses and limitations. In Pinsky M, Payen D, Vincent JL, eds. *Update in Intensive Care Medicine: Functional Hemodynamic Monitoring.* Berlin, Springer, 2005.

12. Ishihara H, Suzuki A, Okawa H, et al. The initial distribution volume of glucose rather than indocyanine green derived plasma volume is correlated with cardiac output following major surgery. *Intens Care Med* 2000;**26**:1441–8.

13. Michard F, Ayala S, Zarka V, et al. Global end diastolic function as an indicator of cardiac preload in patients with septic shock. *Chest* 2003;**124**;1900–8.

14. Marik P, Baram M, Vahid B. Does central venous pressure predict fluid responsiveness? A systematic review of the literature and the tale of seven mares. *Chest* 2008;**134**:172–8.

15. Marik P, Cavallazzi R. Does central venous pressure predict fluid responsiveness? An updated meta-analysis and a plea for some common sense. *Crit Care Med* 2013;**41**:1774–81.

16. Reinhart K, Kuhn H, Hartog C, Bredle D. Continuous central venous and pulmonary artery oxygen saturation monitoring in the critically ill. *Intens Care Med* 2004;**30**;1572–8.

17. Martin C, Auffray J, Badetti C, et al. Monitoring of central venous oxygen saturation versus mixed venous oxygen saturation in critically ill patients. *Inten Care Med* 1992;**18**:101–4.

18. Nebout S, Pirracchio R. Should we monitor ScvO$_2$ in critically ill patients? *Cardiol Res Pract* 2012; Article ID 370697, 7 pages.

19. De Backer D, Biston P, Deviendt J, et al. Comparison of dopamine and norepinephrine in treatment of shock. *N Engl J Med* 2010;**362**:779–89.

20. De Backer D, Aldecoa C, Njimi H, Vincent JL. Dopamine versus norepinephrine in the treatment of septic shock. *Crit Care Med* 2012;**40**:725–30.

21. Russell J, Walley K, Singer J, et al. Vasopressin versus norepinephrine infusion in patients with septic shock. *N Engl J Med* 2008;**358**:877–87.

22. Annane D, Vignon P, Renault A, et al. Norepinephrine plus dobutamine versus epinephrine alone for the management of septic shock: a randomized trial. *Lancet* 2007;**370**:676–84.

23. Dellinger R, Levy M, Rhodes A, et al. Surviving sepsis campaign: international guidelines for management of severe sepsis and septic shock: 2012. *Crit Care Med* 2013;**41**:580–637.

24. Hayden S, Albert T, Watkins T, Swenson E. Anemia in critical illness: insights into etiology, consequences, and management. *Am J Respir Crit Care Med* 2012;**185**:1049–57.

25. Hebert P, Wells G, Blajchman M, et al. A multicenter, randomized, controlled clinical trial of transfusion requirements in critical care. *N Engl J Med* 1999;**340**:409–17.

26. Dean K, Minneci P, Danner R, Eichacker P, Natanson C. Practice misalignments in randomized controlled trials: identification, impact, and potential solutions. *Anesth Analg* 2010;**111**:444–50.

27. Hajjar L, Vincent JL, Auler J, et al. Transfusion requirements after cardiac surgery. *JAMA* 2010;**304**:1559–67.

28. Carson J, Terrin M, Noveck H, et al. Liberal or restrictive transfusion in high-risk patients after hip surgery. *N Engl J Med* 2011;**365**:2453–62.

29. Villanueva C, Colomo A, Guarner C, et al. Transfusion strategies for acute upper gastrointestinal bleeding. *N Engl J Med* 2013;**368**:11–21.

30. Jansen T, van Bommel J, Schoonderbeek F, et al. Early lactate-guided therapy in intensive care unit patients: a multicenter, open-label, randomized controlled trial. *Am J Respir Crit Care Med* 2010;**182**:752–61.

31. Jones A, Shapiro N, Kline J, et al. Lactate clearance vs. central venous oxygen saturation as goals of early sepsis therapy: a randomized clinical trial. *JAMA* 2010;**303**:739–46.

32. Kumar A, Roberts D, Wood K, et al. Duration of hypotension prior to initiation of effective antimicrobial therapy is the critical determinant of survival in human septic shock. *Crit Care Med* 2006;**34**:1589–96.

33. Ibrahim E, Sherman G, Ward S, et al. The influence of inadequate antimicrobial treatment of bloodstream infections on patient outcomes in the ICU setting. *Chest* 2000;**118**:146–55.

34. Gaieski D, Pines J, Band R, Goyal M. Impact of time to antibiotics on survival in patients with severe sepsis or septic shock in whom early goal-directed therapy was initiated in the emergency department. *Crit Care Med* 2010;**38**:1–9.

35. Clec'h C, Timsit J, De Lassence A. Efficacy of adequate early antibiotic therapy in ventilator-associated pneumonia: influence of disease severity. *Int Care Med* 2004;**30**:1327–33.

36. Finfer S, Chittock D, Su S, et al. Intensive versus conventional glucose control in critically ill patients. *N Engl J Med* 2009;**360**:1283–97.

37. Finfer S, Liu B, Chittock D, et al. Hypoglycemia and risk of death in critically ill patients. *N Engl J Med* 2012;**367**:1108–18.

38. Barr J, Fraser G, Jaeschke R, et al. Clinical practice guidelines for the management of pain, agitation, and delirium in adult patients in the intensive care unit. *Crit Care Med* 2013;**13**:263–306.

39. Pandharipande P, Girard T, Ely E, et al. Long-term cognitive impairment after critical illness. *N Engl J Med* 2013;**369**:1306–16.

40. Needham D, Korupolu R, Zanni J, et al. Early physical medicine and rehabilitation for patients with acute respiratory failure: a quality improvement project. *Arch Phys Med Rehabil* 2010;**91**:53.

41. Girard T, Kress J, Fuchs B, et al. Efficacy and safety of a paired sedation and ventilator weaning protocol for mechanically ventilated patients in the intensive care (Awakening and Breathing Controlled trial): a randomized controlled trial. *Lancet* 2008;**371**:126–34.

Goal directed therapy in the perioperative setting: what is the evidence?

Eric Edison and Andrew Rhodes

Introduction

Goal directed therapy involves the perioperative optimization of cardiac output (CO) and total oxygen body delivery (DO_2) to improve postoperative outcomes. This philosophy was originally based on the observations that CO and DO_2 were much better predictors of mortality than conventionally measured parameters such as heart rate, blood pressure, and central venous pressure,[1,2] and that artificially improving these variables to predetermined limits seemed to help patients survive following surgery.[3]

In order to optimize CO and DO_2, there are multiple options available for the type of monitoring (pulmonary artery catheter, Doppler velocimetry, lithium dilution, pressure waveform analysis), therapy (fluids, with or without inotropes), specific therapeutic goals (such as CO, DO_2, maximum stroke volume), and resuscitation targets (normal vs. "supranormal"). The technique was initially developed in high-risk patients, for example, patients with multiple co-morbidities undergoing major surgery. Based on the concept of an "oxygen debt," GDT is initiated either during or soon after surgery, but as a preventative rather than as a curative measure for postoperative complications.

The evidence for GDT is subject to methodological limitations that are inherent to research in critical care, such as difficulty in double-blinding complex interventions. The myriad variants, changes in practice over time, and heterogeneity between studies provide challenges to meta-analysis. Despite these limitations, there is convincing evidence that GDT reduces the rate of complications and hospital stay, and thus potentially reduces long-term mortality and cost.

The benefit to short-term or in-hospital mortality is less clear-cut but may be limited to the highest-risk patients. Further work is needed to characterize which patients are high risk and what versions of GDT specifically have an impact on mortality.

The evidence for benefit of GDT
Complications and length of hospital stay

A number of different meta-analyses have convincingly demonstrated a reduction in morbidity with goal directed therapy.

A recent Cochrane analysis[4] calculated that, for every 100 patients given GDT, 13 would avoid complications following surgery. This meta-analysis further attempted to elucidate specifically which complications were avoided, finding significant reductions in renal failure, respiratory failure, and wound infection but not in other types of infections, cardiovascular complications, or veno-thromboembolism. However, caution should be taken with the more specific characterization of complications, as no significant difference was seen when a sensitivity analysis was performed, which removed studies where the intervention groups were less well controlled, i.e., control groups not matched to intervention. There remained a significant difference in the total number of complications in this sensitivity analysis.

Another recent meta-analysis of GDT in moderate and high-risk non-cardiac surgical patients has confirmed a reduction in overall complication rate, with an odds ratio of 0.43 ([0.34–0.53]; $P < 0.0001$) in GDT group compared to control.[5] Similarly, a meta-analysis comparing GDT between patients in different risk-groups found an overall odds ratio of 0.45 ([0.34–0.60]; $P < 0.00001$). Furthermore, the benefit appeared more pronounced in higher-risk patients. Note, however, that the difference in odds ratio between risk groups was not reported as significant

Perioperative Hemodynamic Monitoring and Goal Directed Therapy, ed. Maxime Cannesson and Rupert Pearse.
Published by Cambridge University Press. © Cambridge University Press 2014.

despite the trend seen.[6] Subgroup analyses in both studies demonstrate that reductions in complications are seen, regardless of the type of monitoring, therapy and therapeutic goals used. These findings have been replicated in cardiac surgery[7] It would follow a priori that a reduction in complication rates would lead to a reduction in length of hospital stay, and this has been demonstrated empirically. For non-cardiac surgery patients stay 1 day less on average,[4] while cardiac patients stay 2.4 days less.[7] Of note, Hamilton et al. demonstrated that the complication rate has remained consistent over the last 30 years, despite mortality roughly halving every decade.[5] This suggests that progress in medical practice has reduced short-term mortality but not the rate of complications, and has perhaps delayed mortality. Goal directed therapy might provide a genuine opportunity to reduce these complication rates.

In summary, there is convincing evidence for a reduction in the rate of complications with GDT, which may be more so with higher-risk patients. More work is needed to elucidate specifically which complications are reduced.

Difficulties in reporting and collating complications

Across meta-analyses, the reduction in the rate of complications is convincing. However, further work is needed because it has been difficult to identify exactly which complications are reduced because of two main issues: heterogeneous definitions and unit of analysis issues.

There is no consistency in how complications are defined or measured across papers. The Cochrane report points out that no two studies used the same criteria, in most cases no specific criteria were listed for morbidities, and no two studies used the same list of morbidities. There are standardized methods to report morbidity such as the postoperative morbidity survey.[8] Future studies should use such standardized methods to facilitate future meta-analysis.

It is difficult to collate complications sometimes as some studies report number of complications, but others report number of patients with complications. These numbers cannot be combined. The Cochrane report was only able to pool the overall complication rate from 17 of the 31 eligible studies due to such unit of analysis issues, and there were similar problems with each of the individual complications investigated.

Short-term mortality in unselective patient cohorts

Unlike complications, reductions in short-term mortality may be limited to high-risk patients and specific types of goal directed therapy. The recent Cochrane report is equivocal with regards to the effect of GDT on short-term mortality. Its primary outcome, longest available mortality, did not demonstrate a statistically significant difference in their primary analysis. However, it was significant when alternative statistical models were used. The difference also became significant when a sensitivity analysis was performed to remove studies with obvious confounding factors between intervention and control groups (RR = 0.65; 95% [0.48–0.89] $P = 0.007$)). Similarly, 28-day mortality tended toward significance (RR 0.81; [0.65–1.00] $P = 0.06$) and again became significant with other statistical models.

Short-term mortality in high-risk patients

The Cochrane report does not stratify patients according to risk. Other meta-analyses demonstrate that there is an overall short-term mortality benefit in the higher-risk patients. Hamilton et al. calculated the odds ratio for overall mortality in moderate to high-risk patients as 0.48([0.33–0.78]; $P = 0.0002$)).[5] Similarly, Cecconi et al. found an overall odds ratio of 0.52 ([0.36 to 0.74] $P = 0.003$). This latter study stratified patients according to risk, and further demonstrated that the benefit may be greatest with higher-risk patients.[6] Only studies with extremely high-risk patients had a significant mortality benefit (OR 0.20[0.09 to 0.41] $P < 0.0001$)), while there was a trend toward mortality benefit in the high-risk group (OR 0.65 [0.39 to 1.07] $P = 0.09$) and there was no mortality benefit in the lowest-risk patients. There is a growing body of evidence that high-risk and critically ill patients benefit from pre-emptive optimization before organ dysfunction sets in after major physiological insults other than surgery, such as trauma and septic shock.[9]

Despite these findings, further work is needed to explore potential mortality benefit in high-risk patients. First, subgroup analyses by Hamilton et al. demonstrated that high-quality RCTs did not demonstrate a significant mortality benefit.[5] A time-dependent analysis demonstrated that no mortality benefit was seen if studies were only used that were published after 2000. The nature of the meta-analyses did not separate and stratify individual patients from studies, but used the aggregate findings. This means that significant confounding factors cannot be ruled out; the factors that contributed to higher mortality in certain papers may have also contributed to the increased efficacy of GDT, such as treatment in more specialist centers. In fact, baseline mortality more than 20% is unusual in current practice and neither of the studies with extremely high-risk patients in the last decade demonstrated a significant mortality benefit. It is important to note that the morbidity benefit in all these studies is not affected by time- or quality-dependent analyses.

Selecting who the high-risk patients are is one of the major challenges of modern perioperative care. It has been estimated that, in the UK, 12% of all patients undergoing surgery account for almost 80% of all surgery and deaths.[10] These studies demonstrate that there may be a survival benefit if therapy can be targeted to these patients. However, there is a lack of consensus over what exactly defines high risk. Cecconi et al. stratified risk according to the mortality of the control group: intermediate (<5%), high (5%–20%) and extremely high (>20%). On the other hand, Hamilton et al. defined high-risk patients according to a set of predetermined inclusion criteria including co-morbidities, underlying pathology, type of surgery and acute complications, described previously.[11]

Subgroup analyses: the effects of type of monitoring, therapy, therapeutic goals, and resuscitation targets on mortality

As a complex intervention, GDT has a number of variable factors that may contribute to the survival benefit, including type of monitoring, therapy, therapeutic goals, and resuscitation targets. Subgroup analysis in those meta-analyses that demonstrated a survival benefit were consistent in the factors identified.[5,6] A survival benefit was seen in studies where inotropes were part of the protocol; no benefit was seen when fluids were used alone. Studies defining therapeutic goals by cardiac index or oxygen delivery saw a survival benefit. Studies using other goals did not confer a benefit; these goals included oxygen extraction ratio, pulse pressure variation, $S_V O_2$, lactate, plethysmographic variability index, pulmonary artery occlusion pressure, and intrathoracic blood volume. Studies using supranormal resuscitation targets (oxygen delivery index of >600 mL/min/m^2) saw a survival benefit,

whereas those using normal resuscitation targets did not. Only studies using pulmonary artery catheters for monitoring had a survival benefit. The meta-analysis of optimization in cardiac surgery did not have enough studies to perform rigorous subgroup analyses for mortality, but it is interesting to note that no studies used supra-normal resuscitation targets, as there is no evidence for benefit in cardiac patients.

Note that subgroup analyses can be difficult to interpret. First, they must be recognized as hypothesis-generating analyses and not definitive evidence. Second, in such complex interventions, it is difficult to avoid confounding between these factors. For example, in the meta-analysis by Cecconi et al., all eight studies using the esophageal Doppler used fluids alone, reflected by the lack of mortality benefit with the use of FTc or SV as a target.[6] Similarly, the authors state that the survival benefit associated with the use of PACs is unlikely to be due to the use of the PACs *per se*, but to other factors such as the ability to measure and therefore achieve supranormal DO2, and the use of inotropes in addition to fluids in all studies using a PAC. It is interesting to note that the morbidity benefit is seen across all subgroups.

Long-term mortality

It may be the case that reducing short-term complications reduces long-term mortality. The occurrence of short term postoperative complications is, in fact, a more important predictor of long term survival than preoperative patient risk.[12] This suggests that interventions that reduce complications may impact on long-term mortality even if not on short-term mortality. A 15-year follow-up of an RCT demonstrated a significant survival benefit for the GDT group (1107 days $P = 0.005$). Long-term survival was associated with avoidance of postoperative cardiac complications suggesting that GDT may reduce long-term mortality in part due to its ability to reduce postoperative complications.[13]

Cost

It would be expected that reduced complications and length of hospital stay would lead to a reduced overall cost. The Cochrane report found five cost analyses of RCTs.[4] These give a mixed picture, but studies that do not find a difference in cost have a number of limitations. Two have results at odds with the meta-analysis overall, i.e., either do not find a difference in morbidity or mortality[14] or find no difference in length of hospital stay.[15] These both also have a small sample size and only follow-up during hospital stay, not accounting for medium to long-term benefits. One of these papers was published in 1991 and the reduced cost from complications was offset by expensive monitoring, which is less invasive and cheaper now.[15] Similarly, one of the oldest RCTs has an equivocal cost analysis due to invasive monitoring techniques.[3]

Those studies that have findings consistent with that of the meta-analyses overall do demonstrate a reduced cost. One such cost analysis in sterling found that there was a mean saving of over £1000 in the GDT group, much of which was attributable to the reduced cost of treating postoperative complications (saving almost £500 per patient). The cost of obtaining a survivor was 31% lower in the protocol group.[16] The cost analysis with the longest follow-up, of 2 years, found a saving of £5000 per patient.[17] Importantly, this RCT had findings consistent with the meta-analyses: no significant difference in short-term mortality, but significant improvements in morbidity and length of hospital stay.

Comments on the evidence and its quality

There are over 30 RCTs describing the efficacy of perioperative goal directed therapy. As a complex multifaceted intervention carried out in a critical care environment, there are a number of limitations that are important to appreciate. In the context of these limitations, the effect of GDT on short-term mortality is equivocal. The effect on morbidity, however, remains convincing despite limitations including quality, time dependency, and heterogeneity between studies.

Quality of RCTs

The Jadad score is a useful tool to quantify the quality of RCTs. It is scored from 0 to 5 on appropriate randomization, blinding, and handling of withdrawals.[18] Cecconi et al. calculated the average Jadad score as 3 for non-cardiac papers,[6] whilst no cardiac studies scored above 3.[7] It is well recognized that low-quality RCTs overestimate potential treatment effects. This was demonstrated by Hamilton et al., where higher-quality papers (Jadad $\geq$ 3) did not demonstrate a significant reduction in mortality, whereas lower quality papers did.[5] It is interesting to note that both subgroups

showed reductions in morbidity. Aya et al. had similar findings with cardiac surgical trials; all trials being Jadad 3 or less. None of those scoring 2 or 3 found a reduction in mortality. However, again there was a reduction in morbidity regardless of Jadad.[7]

Part of the reason for low Jadad scores are inherently unavoidable problems. It is difficult to blind care providers and patients when control and intervention groups involve different therapies and therapy targets. A Cochrane study found that the blinding of participants was adequate in only 12/31 (39%) studies and blinding of outcome assessments was adequate in 8/31 (26%) studies. Furthermore, the majority of studies are single-center and underpowered; but most are small (<100).[4]

The limitations in not providing adequate blinding are inherent to the intervention being studied, but almost certainly open the studies up to bias. However, a significant minority of studies demonstrated improper randomization, which is avoidable and is, perhaps, even worse. Adequate randomization was only seen in 17/31 (55%), while robust allocation concealment was adequate in only 20/31 (65%). In addition, selection bias cannot be ruled out in the significant minority of studies where exclusion happened after randomization. RCTs constructed in the future must have more robust protocols for randomization in place.

The largest study[19] included in the recent Cochrane report[4] (1994/5292 patients) has a number of systematic biases, which limits its conclusions. The intervention group was not well controlled and the protocol failed to achieve the hemodynamic goals in 80% at the preoperative and 20% at the postoperative time periods. Furthermore, a large number of participants were lost to follow-up, meaning significant attrition bias cannot be excluded. Although this study dominated the meta-analysis, a sensitivity analysis performed that excluded this study, or assumed that all the excluded died, demonstrated no difference in mortality (long-term or 28 days), reassuring that the conclusions are valid.

Heterogeneity and changes in practice over time

As a complex intervention, there are a number of factors that vary between studies. It can be difficult to reliably collate results from studies that use different parameters. For example, each meta-analysis uses different parameters to define the perioperative period in which GDT must be started. Cecconi and colleagues define it as from immediately before to immediately after the operation, the Cochrane study as 24 hours before up to 6 hours after, and Aya et al. 24 hours before to 24 hours after. Note that, despite differences, there is consensus that GDT is a pre-emptive strategy and is not beneficial after complications develop.[20]

Another aspect of heterogeneity generally not reported in the meta-analyses is the proportion of patients that actually achieved therapy targets. This may confound conclusions of individual studies and meta-analyses. Aya et al. found that one study, where only around half of the patients achieved treatment goals, caused significant heterogeneity in the calculated effect of GDT on hospital stay (using the I2 method).

Suggestions for future work

Current studies are limited by quality, sample size, and heterogeneity. Future work should be focused on high quality, multicenter trials to elaborate on which factors may contribute to short-term mortality, if at all. Complications are not often reported as the primary outcome in randomized controlled trials, partly due to the issues of heterogeneous definitions and unit of analysis described above. In-hospital mortality is often used as primary endpoint as it is easily defined and reliable across studies. As the major benefit of GDT appears to be a reduction in complications, future studies should consider using standardized definitions to investigate reduction in complication rates with GDT. Finally, despite the best evidence of benefit being in high-risk patients, there is surprisingly little work in emergency surgery.

References

1. Shoemaker WC, Czer LS. Evaluation of the biologic importance of various hemodynamic and oxygen transport variables: which variables should be monitored in postoperative shock? *Crit Care Med* 1979;**7**(9):424–31.

2. Shoemaker WC, Appel PL, Kram HB. Hemodynamic and oxygen transport responses in survivors and nonsurvivors of high-risk surgery. *Crit Care Med* 1993;**21**(7):977–90.

3. Shoemaker WC, Appel PL, Kram HB, Waxman K, Lee TS. Prospective trial of supranormal values of survivors as therapeutic goals in high-risk surgical patients. *Chest* 1988;**94**(6):1176–86.

4. Grocott MP, Dushianthan A, Hamilton MA, et al. Perioperative increase in global blood flow to explicit defined goals and outcomes after surgery: a Cochrane Systematic Review. *Br J Anaesth* 2013;**111**(4):535–48.

5. Hamilton MA, Cecconi M, Rhodes A. A systematic review and meta-analysis on the use of preemptive hemodynamic

intervention to improve postoperative outcomes in moderate and high-risk surgical patients. *Anesth Analg* 2011;**112**(6):1392–402.

6. Cecconi M, Corredor C, Arulkumaran N, et al. Clinical review: goal-directed therapy-what is the evidence in surgical patients? The effect on different risk groups. *Crit Care (Lond, UK).* 2013;**17**(2):209.

7. Aya HD, Cecconi M, Hamilton M, Rhodes A. Goal-directed therapy in cardiac surgery: a systematic review and meta-analysis. *Br J Anaesth* 2013;**110**(4):510–17.

8. Grocott MP, Browne JP, Van der Meulen J, et al. The Postoperative Morbidity Survey was validated and used to describe morbidity after major surgery. *J Clin Epidemiol* 2007;**60**(9):919–28.

9. Kern JW, Shoemaker WC. Meta-analysis of hemodynamic optimization in high-risk patients. *Crit Care Med* 2002;**30**(8):1686–92.

10. Pearse RM, Harrison DA, James P, et al. Identification and characterisation of the high-risk surgical population in the United Kingdom. *Crit Care (Lond, UK).* 2006;**10**(3):R81.

11. Pearse R, Dawson D, Fawcett J, et al. Early goal-directed therapy after major surgery reduces complications and duration of hospital stay. A randomised, controlled trial [ISRCTN38797445]. *Crit Care (Lond, UK).* 2005;**9**(6):R687–93.

12. Khuri SF, Henderson WG, DePalma RG, et al. Determinants of long-term survival after major surgery and the adverse effect of postoperative complications. *Ann Surg* 2005;**242**(3):326–41; discussion 41–3.

13. Rhodes A, Cecconi M, Hamilton M, et al. Goal-directed therapy in high-risk surgical patients: a 15-year follow-up study. *Intens Care Med* 2010;**36**(8):1327–32.

14. Bender JS, Smith-Meek MA, Jones CE. Routine pulmonary artery catheterization does not reduce morbidity and mortality of elective vascular surgery: results of a prospective, randomized trial. *Ann Surg* 1997;**226**(3):229–36; discussion 36–7.

15. Berlauk JF, Abrams JH, Gilmour IJ, et al. Preoperative optimization of cardiovascular hemodynamics improves outcome in peripheral vascular surgery. A prospective,

randomized clinical trial. *Ann Surg* 1991;**214(3)**:289–97; discussion 98–9.

16. Guest JF, Boyd O, Hart WM, Grounds RM, Bennett ED. A cost analysis of a treatment policy of a deliberate perioperative increase in oxygen delivery in high risk surgical patients. *Intens Care Med.* 1997;**23(1)**:85–90.

17. Fenwick E, Wilson J, Sculpher M, Claxton K. Pre-operative optimisation employing dopexamine or adrenaline for patients undergoing major elective surgery: a cost-effectiveness analysis. *Intens Care Med* 2002;**28(5)**: 599–608.

18. Jadad AR, Moore RA, Carroll D, et al. Assessing the quality of reports of randomized clinical trials: is blinding necessary? *Contr Clini Trials* 1996;**17(1)**:1–12.

19. Sandham JD, Hull RD, Brant RF, et al. A randomized, controlled trial of the use of pulmonary-artery catheters in high-risk surgical patients. *N Engl J Med* 2003;**348(1)**:5–14.

20. Gattinoni L, Brazzi L, Pelosi P, et al. A trial of goal-oriented hemodynamic therapy in critically ill patients. SvO_2 Collaborative Group. *N Engl J Med* 1995;**333 (16)**:1025–32.

Chapter

24

Endpoints of goal directed therapy in the OR and in the ICU

Nathan H. Waldron, Timothy E. Miller, and Tong J. Gan

Goals of goal directed therapy

Ultimately, the aim of goal directed therapy (GDT) is to improve patient outcomes by optimizing tissue perfusion and end-organ function. Adverse outcomes are associated with both under- and over-resuscitation.[1] Inadequate intraoperative resuscitation can lead to decreased circulating volume and resultant hypoperfusion of end-organs,[2] which may predispose patients to adverse perioperative outcomes.[1] On the other hand, excessive intraoperative fluid volumes can result in increased intra- as well as extravascular volumes, which may lead to peripheral and/or pulmonary edema. Of particular importance in gastrointestinal surgery, excessive crystalloid infusion has been associated with bowel wall edema,[3] which may delay gastrointestinal function.[1] Multiple studies have shown that GDT is associated with improved outcomes following moderate to major surgery, with shorter hospital stays, fewer ICU admissions, earlier return of bowel function, and less postoperative nausea and vomiting.[1,4–9] There are emerging data that demonstrate a long-term survival benefit (up to 15 years postoperatively) in ICU patients who underwent GDT postoperatively after high-risk surgery.[10] This survival benefit may be due to the ability of GDT to reduce the initial number of postoperative complications.

Optimal perfusion may be dependent upon disease process, with various types of shock as well as sepsis being times of high metabolic demand. Shoemaker et al. demonstrated that patients surviving shock states had higher oxygen delivery than non-surviving patients. This realization led to the concept of super-optimization, or using vasopressors and/or inotropic agents to increase oxygen delivery to supranormal values.[11] Outcomes associated with "super-optimization" have been

mixed. Some investigators have found that the use of epinephrine and/or dopexamine to increase oxygen delivery (DO_2) during surgery decreased perioperative morbidity and mortality.[12,13] Similar attempts to super-optimize oxygen delivery in septic ICU patients[14] as well as a mixed group of critically ill patients[15] have not shown to significantly impact mortality. It is notable, however, that these patients generally had their resuscitation started approximately 12 hours after presentation. Follow-up studies in which optimization began immediately upon arrival to the ICU showed a decreased hospital length of stay (LOS) for patients undergoing cardiothoracic surgery[16] as well as high-risk patients undergoing major general surgery.[17]

Ideal endpoint for GDT

There is still no consensus on optimal endpoint for GDT. Ideally, the perfect endpoint would be accurate, reproducible, easily measured in either the OR as well as the ICU, continuous or at least rapidly available, and reflective of end-organ perfusion. Perhaps the most widely embraced endpoints for GDT are those set out by the Surviving Sepsis Campaign, which suggest targeting: central venous pressure (CVP) 8–12 mmHg, mean arterial pressure (MAP) > 65 mmHg, urine output (UOP) $\geq$ 0.5 mL/kg/hr, superior vena cava oxygenation saturation ($ScvO_2$) or mixed venous oxygen saturation (SvO_2) 70% or 65%, respectively, and normalizing lactate if elevated.[18,19] However, some of these goals were obtained from single center studies and have been questioned as being optimal endpoints for resuscitation of sepsis.[20] Furthermore, as will be discussed below, many of these endpoints do not necessarily reflect the adequacy of tissue perfusion.

Perioperative Hemodynamic Monitoring and Goal Directed Therapy, ed. Maxime Cannesson and Rupert Pearse. Published by Cambridge University Press. © Cambridge University Press 2014.

Available endpoints for GDT (Table 24.1)

Traditional and pressure-based parameters

Traditional parameters by which GDT has been accomplished include heart rate (HR), blood pressure (typically measured as MAP), urine output (UOP), CVP, and pulmonary artery occlusion pressure (PAOP or "wedge pressure"). In general, these endpoints are either routinely measured (HR, MAP, UOP) or readily available (CVP, PAOP) in both the OR and ICU settings. In the ICU, HR, MAP, and UOP are monitored frequently as part of every patient's routine assessment, where they often function as a kind of rough indicator of patient status that can trigger further investigation.[21] Heart rate is continuously monitored in the OR as well as in the ICU. Traditional teaching says that increasing heart rate may represent hypovolemia or hemorrhage, among other things, though this has been called into question. In a study where healthy subjects lost 15%–20% blood volume, there were no changes in conventional hemodynamic parameters, including HR, and it appeared that blood was preferentially lost from the splanchnic circulation rather than from the central blood volume.[22] In another study where healthy volunteers were phlebotomized to approximately 75% of their baseline blood volume, neither HR nor blood pressure changed appreciably after blood loss, though gastric tonometry decreased reliably.[23] In short, HR cannot be reliably used to measure changes in central blood volume or as an indicator of hypovolemia.[24]

Mean arterial pressure is monitored on a minute-by-minute basis in the OR, where providers generally aim for relatively tight (intraoperative MAP within 20% of baseline MAP) control, though this may vary. MAP is also monitored frequently in the ICU, where the goals fluctuate, based on patient condition. As mentioned above, Surviving Sepsis guidelines call for MAP > 65 mmHg, though true MAP goals vary based on patient co-morbidities and baseline blood pressure.[18] Follow-up studies have examined the effects of super-optimization of MAP in septic shock, namely targeting a MAP > 85 mmHg, and found that there were no benefits in terms of improved tissue oxygenation, splanchnic perfusion,[25] or indices of renal function.[26] Similar to HR, MAP is not a reliable indicator of central blood volume or hypovolemia,[24] though profound hypotension can certainly contribute to decreased tissue perfusion. In a 2013 review, researchers observed that targeting normotension was likely inferior to GDT designed to optimize preload or stroke volume.[27]

Urine output is monitored as a crude marker of renal function. In the perioperative period, oliguria (defined as UOP <0.5 mL/kg/hr) is extremely common and often occurs as a neurohormonal response to surgical stress, rendering it an unreliable marker of acute kidney injury.[28] In the ICU, oliguria and acute kidney injury (AKI) are both quite common, but despite standardized definitions that require oliguria (i.e., RIFLE or AKIN criteria), decreased urine output has not been fully embraced as representative of kidney injury.[29] In the resuscitation of sepsis, urine output is probably best used as part of a combination of variables (i.e., MAP, mental status, skin perfusion) rather than in isolation.[30]

There are multiple reasons to perform central venous cannulation, but monitoring of CVP and/or PAOP is performed relatively frequently by anesthesiologists and intensivists.[28] "Normal" values for CVP as well as PAOP are standard fodder during introduction physiology classes and beyond. Indeed, CVP has been integrated into the Surviving Sepsis algorithm, where it is advised that fluid resuscitation be targeted toward a CVP 8–12mmHg.[18] However, there are data showing that CVP as well as PAOP[31] are not accurate measures of volume status or predictors of fluid responsiveness in both critically ill patients[32] or healthy volunteers.[33] A 2002 meta-analysis including 12 studies and 334 patients did not find indicators of ventricular preload, such as CVP or PAOP, to be valuable as a predictor of fluid responsiveness in critically ill patients.[34] In resuscitation of shock, it is not recommended that preload measures are used as the sole predictors of fluid responsiveness.[35] Moreover, there are data that there are no differences in outcomes between ICU patients whose management was guided by pulmonary artery catheter (PAC) versus central venous catheter (CVC)[36] or PAC versus usual care,[37] and also that PACs have a higher risk of arrhythmia.[36] Similarly, PAC-guided GDT provided no mortality or morbidity benefit in elderly high-risk patients having major surgery, though patients in the PAC group did have a higher incidence of pulmonary embolism.[38]

Optimization of flow-based parameters with cardiac output (CO) monitors

Flow-based measures by which GDT has been accomplished include stroke volume (SV) and cardiac output (CO). At present, there are multiple monitors capable of measuring SV and CO. The "gold standard" for measuring cardiac output as well as filling pressures is a PAC,

Table 24.1. Advantages, disadvantages and clinical utility of hemodynamic and tissue variable endpoints

Hemodynamic and tissue variables	Pros	Cons	Utility for GDT
Traditional/pressure-based parameters			
Heart rate (HR)	Easily obtained	Unreliable, altered by pharmacotherapy	–
Mean arterial pressure (MAP)	Easily obtained	Unreliable, not indicative of flow	–
Urine output (UOP)	Easily obtained	Unreliable, particularly in the perioperative setting	–
Central venous pressure (CVP)	CVC is multi-functional	Invasive, a suboptimal measure of preload	– / +
Pulmonary artery occlusion pressure (PAOP)	PAC is multi-functional	Invasive, a suboptimal measure of preload	– / +
Flow-based parameters			
Pulse contour techniques (LiDCO, Vigileo, PiCCO)	Accurate, minimally invasive	Requires an arterial line	++
Esophageal Doppler monitor	Accurate, minimally invasive, well validated in GDT	Need focusing to obtain optimal signal	++
Transthoracic bioreactivity (NICOM)	Accurate, non-invasive	Body habitus may make monitoring difficult	++
Finger cuff plethysmographic techniques (Nexfin)	Accurate, non-invasive	Not well studied for GDT	+
Dynamic parameters			
Stroke volume variation (SVV)	Accurate	Requires constant R–R interval and tidal volumes	++
Pulse pressure variation (PPV)	Accurate	Requires constant R–R interval and tidal volumes	++
Pleth variability index (PVI)	Accurate, non-invasive	Requires constant R–R interval and tidal volumes	++
Passive leg raise (PLR)	Can be performed awake	Not easy to perform during surgery	++
Markers of tissue well-being			
Lactate	Can reveal dysoxia	Non-specific, time lag	+ / ++
Base deficit	Can reveal acidosis	Non-specific, time lag	+ / ++
Mixed venous oxygen saturation (SvO_2)	Superior marker of dysoxia	Invasive	++
Central venous oxygen saturation ($SCvO_2$)	Can reveal dysoxia	Invasive	++
Gastric tonometry	Representative of splanchnic perfusion	Time-consuming, time lag	+

(– Not useful as an endpoint for GDT; + Potentially useful as an endpoint for GDT in some circumstances; ++ Likely useful as an endpoint for GDT). Accurate is interpreted as clinically acceptable.

but they are invasive and can be associated with complications.[39] As such, investigators have sought out less invasive measures, such as pulse contour techniques (e.g., LiDCO, Vigileo, and PiCCO), esophageal Doppler techniques, bioimpedance, and bioreactance techniques (e.g., NICOM), and finger cuff and plethysmographic technologies. A 2011 meta-analysis including nearly 5000 patients found that pre-emptive hemodynamic optimization using flow-based techniques or a PAC resulted in decreased morbidity and mortality in moderate- to high-risk patients compared to standard perioperative care.[40]

Most pulse contour techniques (e.g., LiDCO, Vigileo, PiCCO) require an arterial line and use the arterial waveform to calculate SV, CO, as well as dynamic measures of preload responsiveness, such as pulse pressure variation (PPV) and stroke volume variation (SVV). They have shown moderate accuracy in determining cardiac output in cardiothoracic surgery patients when compared to a PAC.[41] Goal directed intraoperative hemodynamic optimization using the PiCCO (a pulse contour technique that also utilizes transpulmonary thermodilution) has been shown to decrease requirement for inotropes/vasopressors and shorten mechanical ventilation time in patients undergoing routine cardiac surgery.[42] GDT using the Vigileo has also been shown to decrease duration of mechanical ventilation, ICU LOS, and hospital LOS in patients undergoing cardiac surgery.[43] Similarly, GDT using the LiDCO is associated with a decrease in hospital LOS and postoperative complications in patients having major general surgery.[17]

The esophageal Doppler is a thin, flexible probe inserted into a patient's mid-esophagus, where it measures blood flow velocity in the descending thoracic aorta. It uses a nomogram to calculate aortic cross-sectional area based on the patient's height, weight, and age.[44] The EDM is a valid measure of cardiac output when compared with a pulmonary artery catheter,[45] and is also appropriate for measuring hemodynamic response to fluid boluses in GDT.[5,46] Multiple studies have compared GDT using the EDM to usual care and found favorable results in terms of reduced morbidity and decreased LOS or earlier fitness for discharge.[5,7,8] However, experience is required to become skilled in using this device, and an optimal signal may be difficult to obtain. In addition, there is some concern that the device only measures flow through the descending aorta and that some of the mathematical assumptions may make it somewhat inaccurate.[47]

Transthoracic bioimpedance technology is used to measure changes in amplitude of high frequency waves transmitted across the thorax. It has been available as a measure of cardiac output for approximately 20 years, but it has not been widely used due to problems with electrical interference and because the algorithm relies on hemodynamic stability and the absence of cardiac dysrhythmias.[47] Newer monitors, such as the non-invasive cardiac output monitor (NICOM), use an improved algorithm based on bioreactance, which measures phase shifts in high-frequency waves transmitted across the thorax, with a nearly 100-fold improvement in the signal-to-noise ratio.[48] The device consists of four pads placed across the thorax that simultaneously emit and detect high-frequency low-amplitude electrical currents, and are connected to the monitor via a single cable. The NICOM has been validated for clinically acceptable precision and accuracy when compared to the PAC in critically ill postoperative cardiothoracic surgery patients.[48,49] In addition, it is a sensitive and specific method for assessing fluid responsiveness[48,50] as well as hemodynamic response to passive leg raise (PLR).[51,52] The NICOM has been found to perform similarly to the EDM in monitoring hemodynamic response as part of an intraoperative GDT protocol.[53]

A new development in non-invasive monitoring is the Nexfin, a completely non-invasive monitor that utilizes finger-cuff arterial pressure monitoring and pulse contour analysis to calculate cardiac output, stroke volume, and blood pressure. This monitor has been validated against a PAC for measuring arterial pressure and CO in postoperative cardiac surgery patients with favorable results,[54] and has also been shown to have suitable agreement with intraoperative esophageal Doppler measurements of CO.[55] However, the Nexfin has had mixed results for measuring fluid responsiveness, with some studies supporting its use,[56] while others suggesting that it is not reliable to measure fluid responsiveness in postoperative cardiac surgical patients[57] or critically ill ICU patients.[58]

Echocardiography is another possibility for measuring response to GDT in the ICU. Echocardiography (both transthoracic and transesophageal) offer a plethora of information in critically ill patients.[59] In addition, the use of transesophageal echocardiography (TEE) has been shown to impact the care of patients in surgical ICUs.[60]

Dynamic parameters

Dynamic parameters by which GDT has been accomplished include SVV, PPV, plethysmography variability index (PVI), and PLR. SVV and PPV both rely on the principle that in mechanically ventilated patients with no spontaneous respiratory effort, inspiration causes an increase in intrathoracic pressure that causes an increase in right atrial pressure and, in volume depleted patients, a concomitant decrease in right ventricular (and thus left-ventricular) filling. This is reflected in a cyclical variation of left ventricular stroke volume and thus arterial pulse pressure.[21] These technologies are limited in the fact that they require a constant R–R interval (i.e., normal sinus rhythm) as well as constant tidal volumes (> 6 mL/kg). PLR is performed by raising a patient's legs above their chest and holding them for 1 minute, which causes autotransfusion from the lower extremities that simulates a fluid bolus, and increases RV preload. PLR has the advantage that it can be performed in spontaneously breathing patients.[61]

Stroke volume variation is calculated as $(SV_{max}-SV_{min})/SV_{mean}$ over multiple breaths or a defined time period.[62] With a tidal volume of 6mL/kg, a SVV $>10\%$ predicts a 15% increase in CO after a 500 mL fluid bolus.[21] Intra- and postoperative GDT using SVV as an endpoint in cardiac surgery patients has been shown to result in shorter ICU LOS as well as fewer postoperative complications.[63] In addition, intraoperative GDT with the aim of minimizing SVV improved GI function in low-to-moderate risk patients undergoing major abdominal surgery[64] and decreased wound complications in high-risk surgical patients.[65]

Pulse pressure variation is calculated as $(PP_{max}-PP_{min})/PP_{mean}$ over multiple breaths or a defined time period.[62] With a tidal volume of 6 mL/kg, a PPV $>13\%$ predicts a 15% increase in CO after a 500 mL fluid bolus.[21] Use of PPV has been found to be useful in predicting fluid responsiveness after cardiothoracic surgery.[66] Intraoperative GDT using PPV as an endpoint in patients undergoing high-risk surgery has been shown to decrease ICU and hospital LOS, duration of mechanical ventilation, as well as postoperative complications.[67]

Pleth variability index and pulse oximetry plethysmographic waveform amplitude (ΔPOP) are non-invasive measures obtained from pulse oximeters that, similar to SVV, take advantage of changes in preload during mechanical ventilation. It has previously been shown that ΔPOP is closely related to PPV, which predicts fluid responsiveness.[68] Furthermore, a 2012 meta-analysis of ten studies investigating PVI and ΔPOP found that, in mechanically ventilated adult patients in normal sinus rhythm, both indices were predictive of hemodynamic response to a 500 mL fluid bolus.[69] PVI has successfully been used to predict fluid responsiveness in colorectal surgery patients.[70] Intraoperative GDT using PVI has been associated with lower intra- and postoperative lactate levels in patients undergoing major abdominal surgery.[71] PVI and ΔPOP have the distinct advantage of not requiring invasive monitoring, namely an arterial line.

Hemodynamic changes during passive leg raise (PLR) can be monitored in multiple different ways depending on patient and provider preference, but a proper PLR does require continuous hemodynamic monitoring as changes are transient and reversible. An increase in aortic blood flow $>10\%$ with PLR, as measured by esophageal Doppler monitoring, predicted fluid response with 97% sensitivity, and 94% specificity.[72] More recently, it was found that an increase in pulse pressure $>9\%$ was predictive of volume responsiveness in critically ill ICU patients.[73] Unfortunately, PLR may be difficult to perform intraoperatively, where necessary position changes may prove prohibitive to surgical progress.

Markers of tissue well-being

Markers of tissue well-being that have been used for GDT include lactate, base deficit, mixed venous oxygen saturation (SvO_2), central venous oxygen saturation ($ScvO_2$), and gastric tonometry. These endpoints have the advantage of providing a more refined look at tissue perfusion than simple hemodynamic measures. Lactate is thought to generally represent the tissue oxygen debt or an imbalance between tissue oxygen requirements and delivery. In sepsis, lactate is associated with tissue dysoxia.[74] Moreover, elevated lactate as well as a failure of lactate to normalize during resuscitation is associated with poorer outcomes.[35,75,76] A 2010 study of septic patients in the ED whose resuscitation was guided by either lactate clearance or $ScvO_2$ found no difference in mortality between the two approaches.[20] Similar to lactate, an increased base deficit often heralds tissue dysoxia, and normalization may be helpful as a marker for adequate resuscitation.[35] In trauma, worsened base deficit is an independent predictor of mortality, perhaps because it reflects severity and duration of hypoperfusion.[77] Unfortunately, elevated lactate and base deficit are sensitive but not specific, i.e., lactate may be elevated because of other conditions, e.g., hepatic dysfunction, glycogen storage diseases, malignancy, or drugs (biguanides or nucleoside reverse transcriptase inhibitors), rather than tissue dysoxia.[78] Similarly, renal dysfunction may also cause metabolic acidosis and elevated base deficit, as can drugs (cocaine) and bicarbonate wasting. Finally, the turn-around time for laboratory variables such as lactate and base deficit may be longer than some hemodynamic measurements, which are obtained almost instantaneously.

Mixed venous oxygen saturation, taken from a pulmonary artery catheter, can give an estimate of oxygen consumption and can also be used to calculate CO.[79]

A study of cardiac surgery patients found that GDT aimed at normalizing SvO_2 and lactate in the first 8 hours after surgery decreased LOS and perioperative organ dysfunction.[80] SvO_2 has the disadvantage of requiring a PAC, which comes with its own inherent risks.[39] Central venous oxygen saturation ($ScvO_2$), taken from a catheter in the internal jugular or subclavian vein, has also been shown to parallel SvO_2.[81,82] Moreover, intra- and immediately postoperative GDT utilizing $ScvO_2$ (specifically calculating oxygen extraction using $SaO_2 - ScvO_2 / SaO_2$) reduced hospital LOS and postoperative organ failure compared with standard care in patients undergoing abdominal surgery.[83] In terms of measuring $ScvO_2$, it should be noted that there are significant differences between $ScvO_2$ measurements obtained from a femoral catheter ($SfvO_2$) and those obtained via an internal jugular or subclavian catheter ($ScvO_2$).[84]

Gastric tonometry is performed by inserting a specialized nasogastric tube with a silicon balloon at the end that allows for measurement of gastric pCO_2 and resultant calculation of mucosal pH or measurement of the pCO_2 gap,[85] both of which are thought to reflect the adequacy of splanchnic perfusion and are predictors of morbidity and mortality in critically ill patients.[86] A 1995 study of cardiac surgical patients showed that pre- and intraoperative colloid volume expansion with the goal of optimizing SV and CVP resulted in less gastric mucosal hypoperfusion as well as shorter ICU LOS and fewer adverse events.[2] One study investigating cardiac index-based versus gastric mucosal pH-based resuscitation in ICU patients with septic shock found no survival advantage of the tonometry-guided resuscitation approach, but did note that patients who reach or maintain a normal mucosal pH have a higher probability of survival.[87] In addition to gastric tonometry, there are a number of other techniques for monitoring microvascular perfusion, including regional (sublingual) capnometry as well as near-infrared spectroscopy, though these techniques are not well studied as endpoints for GDT.[78]

Recommendations

At present, there are no ideal endpoints for goal directed therapy. Clinicians are advised to consider patient factors, location (i.e., OR versus ICU), and nature of the physiological insult (i.e., surgery versus shock state) to design the optimal schema for GDT. Despite their relative lack of sensitivity and specificity for changes in central blood volume, routine monitoring of HR and MAP in the OR and ICU setting is appropriate. Changes in these parameters may prompt further investigation for hypovolemia and/or hypoperfusion with more advanced techniques, and therefore impact GDT. Urine output is not a helpful indicator of hypovolemia in the OR, but may prove useful as a rough indicator of tissue perfusion in the ICU. At present, there is scant evidence to support routine use of CVP or PAOP as an endpoint for GDT. Flow-based minimally or non-invasive measures are promising endpoints for GDT. In patients who have an arterial line, pulse-contour analysis techniques are appropriate for titrating GDT. In unconscious patients, optimizing SV, CO, or corrected flow time (FTc) via esophageal Doppler techniques are appropriate endpoints for GDT. Completely non-invasive modalities, including bioreactance techniques (NICOM) and finger cuff pressures (Nexfin) are potentially promising endpoints for awake patients who have not been instrumented with an arterial line. Dynamic techniques such as SVV, PPV, PVI, and response to PLR will likely be increasingly utilized in the coming years. PVI has the advantage of being non-invasive, compared with the other dynamic techniques, which require continuous flow monitoring. Measuring hemodynamic response to PLR would be challenging for intraoperative GDT, but may prove to be a useful tool for postoperative GDT or for assessing degree of hypovolemia preoperatively. Lactate clearance and correction of base deficit may prove useful as an additional endpoint in both intraoperative and ICU-based GDT. Similarly, SvO_2 and $ScvO_2$ may be useful as an additional endpoint reflective of tissue perfusion, but placement of a PAC or central venous line strictly for this purpose should likely be avoided. Gastric tonometry represents an innovative way of measuring perfusion in an at-risk vascular bed (splanchnic), but is limited as an endpoint for GDT due to prolonged delay in its response.

There is some suggestion that closed-loop fluid administration systems may help to more effectively administer GDT, but this concept deserves further exploration.[88] Further issues with education and familiarity abound. In a multinational survey of anesthesiologists, hesitancy to adapt GDT was more commonly due to lack of appropriate monitors or lack of experience with these monitors than to a belief that GDT was ineffective.[89] At present, we advise readers to create institutionally adopted GDT algorithms utilizing literature-supported endpoints with the aim of improving patient outcomes.

References

1. Grocott MP, Mythen MG, Gan TJ. Perioperative fluid management and clinical outcomes in adults. *Anesth Analg* 2005;**100**:1093–106.

2. Mythen MG, Webb AR. Perioperative plasma volume expansion reduces the incidence of gut mucosal hypoperfusion during cardiac surgery. *Arch Surg* 1995;**130**:423–9.

3. Prien T, Backhaus N, Pelster F, et al. Effect of intraoperative fluid administration and colloid osmotic pressure on the formation of intestinal edema during gastrointestinal surgery. *J Clin Anesth* 1990;**2**:317–23.

4. Abbas SM, Hill AG. Systematic review of the literature for the use of oesophageal Doppler monitor for fluid replacement in major abdominal surgery. *Anaesthesia* 2008;**63**:44–51.

5. Gan TJ, Soppitt A, Maroof M, et al. Goal-directed intraoperative fluid administration reduces length of hospital stay after major surgery. *Anesthesiology* 2002;**97**:820–6.

6. Mythen MG, Webb AR. Intra-operative gut mucosal hypoperfusion is associated with increased post-operative complications and cost. *Intens Care Med* 1994;**20**:99–104.

7. Sinclair S, James S, Singer M. Intraoperative intravascular volume optimisation and length of hospital stay after repair of proximal femoral fracture: randomised controlled trial. *BMJ* 1997;**315**:909–12.

8. Venn R, Steele A, Richardson P, et al. Randomized controlled trial to investigate influence of the fluid challenge on duration of hospital stay and perioperative morbidity in patients with hip fractures. *Br J Anaesth* 2002;**88**:65–71.

9. Giglio MT, Marucci M, Testini M, Brienza N. Goal-directed haemodynamic therapy and gastrointestinal complications in major surgery: a meta-analysis of randomized controlled trials. *Br J Anaesth* 2009;**103**:637–46.

10. Rhodes A, Cecconi M, Hamilton M, et al. Goal-directed therapy in high-risk surgical patients: a 15-year follow-up study. *Intens Care Med* 2010;**36**:1327–32.

11. Shoemaker WC, Montgomery ES, Kaplan E, Elwyn DH. Physiologic patterns in surviving and nonsurviving shock patients. Use of sequential cardiorespiratory variables in defining criteria for therapeutic goals and early warning of death. *Arch Surg* 1973;**106**:630–6.

12. Boyd O, Grounds RM, Bennett ED. A randomized clinical trial of the effect of deliberate perioperative increase of oxygen delivery on mortality in high-risk surgical patients. *JAMA* 1993;**270**:2699–707.

13. Wilson J, Woods I, Fawcett J, et al. Reducing the risk of major elective surgery: randomised controlled trial of preoperative optimisation of oxygen delivery. *BMJ* 1999;**318**:1099–103.

14. Tuchschmidt J, Fried J, Astiz M, Rackow E. Elevation of cardiac output and oxygen delivery improves outcome in septic shock. *Chest* 1992;**102**:216–20.

15. Gattinoni L, Brazzi L, Pelosi P, et al. A trial of goal-oriented hemodynamic therapy in critically ill patients. SvO₂ Collaborative Group. *N Engl J Med* 1995;**333**:1025–32.

16. McKendry M, McGloin H, Saberi D, et al. Randomised controlled trial assessing the impact of a nurse delivered, flow monitored protocol for optimisation of circulatory status after cardiac surgery. *BMJ* 2004;**329**:258.

17. Pearse R, Dawson D, Fawcett J, et al. Early goal-directed therapy after major surgery reduces complications and duration of hospital stay. A randomised, controlled trial [ISRCTN38797445]. *Crit Care* 2005;**9**:R687–93.

18. Dellinger RP, Levy MM, Rhodes A, et al. Surviving sepsis campaign: international guidelines for management of severe sepsis and septic shock: 2012. *Crit Care Med* 2013;**41**:580–637.

19. Rivers E, Nguyen B, Havstad S, et al. Early goal-directed therapy in the treatment of severe sepsis and septic shock. *N Engl J Med* 2001;**345**:1368–77.

20. Jones AE, Shapiro NI, Trzeciak S, et al. Lactate clearance vs central venous oxygen saturation as goals of early sepsis therapy: a randomized clinical trial. *JAMA* 2010;**303**:739–46.

21. Pinsky MR. Hemodynamic evaluation and monitoring in the ICU. *Chest* 2007;**132**:2020–9.

22. Price HL, Deutsch S, Marshall BE, et al. Hemodynamic and metabolic effects of hemorrhage in man, with particular reference to the splanchnic circulation. *Circ Res* 1966;**18**:469–74.

23. Hamilton-Davies C, Mythen MG, Salmon JB, et al. Comparison of commonly used clinical indicators of hypovolaemia with gastrointestinal tonometry. *Intens Care Med* 1997;**23**:276–81.

24. Bundgaard-Nielsen M, Holte K, Secher NH, Kehlet H. Monitoring of peri-operative fluid administration by individualized goal-directed therapy. *Acta Anaesth Scand* 2007;**51**:331–40.

25. LeDoux D, Astiz ME, Carpati CM, Rackow EC. Effects of perfusion pressure on tissue perfusion in septic shock. *Crit Care Med* 2000;**28**:2729–32.

26. Bourgoin A, Leone M, Delmas A, et al. Increasing mean arterial pressure in patients with septic shock: effects on oxygen variables and renal function. *Crit Care Med* 2005;**33**:780–6.

27. Bartels K, Thiele RH, Gan TJ. Rational fluid management in today's ICU practice. *Crit Care* 2013;**17 Suppl 1**:S6.

28. Miller RD. *Miller's Anesthesia*. Philadelphia, PA: Churchill Livingstone/Elsevier, 2010:1 online resource (2 v. (xxii, 3084, I-89 p.)).

29. Cruz DN, Ricci Z, Ronco C. Clinical review: RIFLE and AKIN – time for reappraisal. *Crit Care* 2009;**13**:211.

30. Vincent JL, Gerlach H. Fluid resuscitation in severe sepsis and septic shock: an evidence-based review. *Crit Care Med* 2004;**32**: S451–4.

31. Osman D, Ridel C, Ray P, et al. Cardiac filling pressures are not appropriate to predict hemodynamic response to volume challenge. *Crit Care Med* 2007;**35**:64–8.

32. Marik PE, Baram M, Vahid B. Does central venous pressure predict fluid responsiveness? A systematic review of the literature and the tale of seven mares. *Chest* 2008;**134**:172–8.

33. Kumar A, Anel R, Bunnell E, et al. Pulmonary artery occlusion pressure and central venous pressure fail to predict ventricular filling volume, cardiac performance, or the response to volume infusion in normal subjects. *Crit Care Med* 2004;**32**:691–9.

34. Michard F, Teboul JL. Predicting fluid responsiveness in ICU patients: a critical analysis of the evidence. *Chest* 2002;**121**:2000–8.

35. Antonelli M, Levy M, Andrews PJ, et al. Hemodynamic monitoring in shock and implications for management. International Consensus Conference, Paris, France, 27–28 April 2006. *Intens Care Med* 2007;**33**:575–90.

36. Wheeler AP, Bernard GR, Thompson BT, et al. Pulmonary-artery versus central venous catheter to guide treatment of acute lung injury. *N Engl J Med* 2006;**354**:2213–24.

37. Harvey S, Harrison DA, Singer M, et al. Assessment of the clinical effectiveness of pulmonary artery catheters in management of patients in intensive care (PAC-Man): a randomised controlled trial. *Lancet* 2005;**366**:472–7.

38. Sandham JD, Hull RD, Brant RF, et al. A randomized, controlled trial of the use of pulmonary-artery catheters in high-risk surgical patients. *N Engl J Med* 2003;**348**:5–14.

39. Bowdle TA. Complications of invasive monitoring. *Anesthesiol Clin North Am* 2002;**20**:571–88.

40. Hamilton MA, Cecconi M, Rhodes A. A systematic review and meta-analysis on the use of preemptive hemodynamic intervention to improve postoperative outcomes in moderate and high-risk surgical patients. *Anesth Analg* 2011;**112**:1392–402.

41. Zimmermann A, Kufner C, Hofbauer S, et al. The accuracy of the Vigileo/FloTrac continuous cardiac output monitor. *J Cardiothoracic Vasc Anesth* 2008;**22**:388–93.

42. Goepfert MS, Reuter DA, Akyol D, et al. Goal-directed fluid management reduces vasopressor and catecholamine use in cardiac surgery patients. *Intens Care Med* 2007;**33**:96–103.

43. Kapoor PM, Kakani M, Chowdhury U, et al. Early goal-directed therapy in moderate to high-risk cardiac surgery patients. *Ann Cardiac Anaesth* 2008;**11**:27–34.

44. Singer M. Esophageal Doppler monitoring of aortic blood flow: beat-by-beat cardiac output monitoring. *Internat Anesth Clin* 1993;**31**:99–125.

45. Dark PM, Singer M. The validity of trans-esophageal Doppler ultrasonography as a measure of cardiac output in critically ill adults. *Intens Care Med* 2004;**30**:2060–6.

46. Roche AM, Miller TE, Gan TJ. Goal-directed fluid management with trans-oesophageal Doppler. *Best Pract Res Clin Anaesth* 2009;**23**:327–34.

47. Funk DJ, Moretti EW, Gan TJ. Minimally invasive cardiac output monitoring in the perioperative setting. *Anesth Analg* 2009;**108**:887–97.

48. Squara P, Denjean D, Estagnasie P, et al. Noninvasive cardiac output monitoring (NICOM): a clinical validation. *Intens Care Med* 2007;**33**:1191–4.

49. Marque S, Cariou A, Chiche JD, Squara P. Comparison between Flotrac-Vigileo and Bioreactance, a totally noninvasive method for cardiac output monitoring. *Crit Care* 2009;**13**:R73.

50. Raval NY, Squara P, Cleman M, et al. Multicenter evaluation of noninvasive cardiac output measurement by bioreactance technique. *J Clin Monit Comput* 2008;**22**:113–19.

51. Benomar B, Ouattara A, Estagnasie P, Brusset A, Squara P. Fluid responsiveness predicted by noninvasive bioreactance-based passive leg raise test. *Intens Care Med* 2010;**36**:1875–81.

52. Marik PE, Levitov A, Young A, Andrews L. The use of bioreactance and carotid Doppler to determine volume responsiveness and blood flow redistribution following passive leg raising in hemodynamically unstable patients. *Chest* 2013;**143**: 364–70.

53. Waldron NH, Miller TE, Nardiello J, Manchester AK, Gan TJ. NICOM versus EDM guided goal directed fluid therapy in the perioperative period. *Anesthesiology* 2011.

54. Bogert LW, Wesseling KH, Schraa O, et al. Pulse contour cardiac output derived from non-invasive arterial pressure in cardiovascular disease. *Anaesthesia* 2010;**65**:1119–25.

55. Chen G, Meng L, Alexander B, et al. Comparison of noninvasive cardiac output measurements using the Nexfin monitoring device and the esophageal Doppler. *J Clin Anesth* 2012;**24**:275–83.

56. Bubenek-Turconi SI, Craciun M, Miclea I, Perel A. Noninvasive continuous cardiac output by the nexfin before and after preload-modifying maneuvers: a comparison with intermittent thermodilution cardiac output. *Anesth Analg* 2013;**117**:366–72.

57. Fischer MO, Coucoravas J, Truong J, et al. Assessment of changes in cardiac index and fluid responsiveness: a comparison of Nexfin and transpulmonary thermodilution. *Acta Anaesth Scand* 2013;**57**:704–12.

58. Monnet X, Picard F, Lidzborski E, et al. The estimation of cardiac output by the Nexfin device is of poor reliability for tracking the effects of a fluid challenge. *Crit Care* 2012;**16**:R212.

59. Romero-Bermejo FJ, Ruiz-Bailen M, Guerrero-De-Mier M, Lopez-Alvaro J. Echocardiographic hemodynamic monitoring in the critically ill patient. *Curr Cardiol Rev* 2011;**7**:146–56.

60. Bruch C, Comber M, Schmermund A, et al. Diagnostic usefulness and impact on management of transesophageal echocardiography in surgical intensive care units. *Am J Cardiol* 2003;**91**:510–13.

61. Teboul JL, Monnet X. Prediction of volume responsiveness in critically ill patients with spontaneous breathing activity. *Curr Opin Crit Care* 2008;**14**:334–9.

62. Hofer CK, Cannesson M. Monitoring fluid responsiveness. *Acta Anaesth Taiwan* 2011;**49**:59–65.

63. Goepfert MS, Richter HP, Eulenburg CZ, et al. Individually optimized hemodynamic therapy reduces complications and length of stay in the intensive care unit: a prospective, randomized controlled trial. *Anesthesiology* 2013;**119**(4):824–36.

64. Ramsingh DS, Sanghvi C, Gamboa J, Cannesson M, Applegate RL, 2nd. Outcome impact of goal directed fluid therapy during high risk abdominal surgery in low to moderate risk patients: a randomized controlled trial. *J Clin Monit Comput* 2013;**27**:249–57.

65. Scheeren TW, Wiesenack C, Gerlach H, Marx G. Goal-directed intraoperative fluid therapy guided by stroke volume and its variation in high-risk surgical patients: a prospective randomized multicentre study. *J Clin Monit Comput* 2013;**27**:225–33.

66. Auler JO, Jr., Galas F, Hajjar L, et al. Online monitoring of pulse pressure variation to guide fluid therapy after cardiac surgery. *Anesth Analg* 2008;**106**:1201–6.

67. Lopes MR, Oliveira MA, Pereira VO, Lemos IP, Auler JO, Jr., Michard F. Goal-directed fluid management based on pulse pressure variation monitoring during high-risk surgery: a pilot randomized controlled trial. *Crit Care* 2007;**11**:R100.

68. Cannesson M, Besnard C, Durand PG, Bohe J, Jacques D. Relation between respiratory variations in pulse oximetry plethysmographic waveform amplitude and arterial pulse pressure in ventilated patients. *Crit Care* 2005;**9**: R562–8.

69. Sandroni C, Cavallaro F, Marano C, et al. Accuracy of plethysmographic indices as predictors of fluid responsiveness in mechanically ventilated adults: a systematic review and meta-analysis. *Intens Care Med* 2012;**38**:1429–37.

70. Hood JA, Wilson RJ. Pleth variability index to predict fluid responsiveness in colorectal surgery. *Anesth Analg* 2011;**113**:1058–63.

71. Forget P, Lois F, de Kock M. Goal-directed fluid management based on the pulse oximeter-derived pleth variability index reduces lactate levels and improves fluid management. *Anesth Analg* 2010;**111**:910–14.

72. Monnet X, Rienzo M, Osman D, et al. Passive leg raising predicts fluid responsiveness in the critically ill. *Crit Care Med* 2006;**34**:1402–7.

73. Preau S, Saulnier F, Dewavrin F, Durocher A, Chagnon JL. Passive leg raising is predictive of fluid responsiveness in spontaneously breathing patients with severe sepsis or acute pancreatitis. *Crit Care Med* 2010;**38**:819–25.

74. da Silva Ramos FJ, Azevedo LC. Hemodynamic and perfusion end points for volemic resuscitation in sepsis. *Shock* 2010;**34 Suppl 1**:34–9.

75. Nguyen HB, Kuan WS, Batech M, et al. Outcome effectiveness of the severe sepsis resuscitation bundle with addition of lactate clearance as a bundle item: a multi-national evaluation. *Crit Care* 2011;**15**: R229.

76. Nguyen HB, Rivers EP, Knoblich BP, et al. Early lactate clearance is associated with improved outcome in severe sepsis and septic shock. *Crit Care Med* 2004;**32**:1637–42.

77. Rutherford EJ, Morris JA, Jr., Reed GW, Hall KS. Base deficit stratifies mortality and determines therapy. *J Trauma* 1992;**33**:417–23.

78. Holley A, Lukin W, Paratz J, et al. Review article: Part two: Goal-directed resuscitation – which goals? Perfusion targets. *Emerg Med Aust* 2012;**24**:127–35.

79. Longnecker DE. *Anesthesiology*. New York: McGraw-Hill Medical, 2008.

80. Polonen P, Ruokonen E, Hippelainen M, Poyhonen M, Takala J. A prospective, randomized study of goal-oriented hemodynamic therapy in cardiac surgical patients. *Anesth Analg* 2000;**90**:1052–9.

81. Dueck MH, Klimek M, Appenrodt S, Weigand C, Boerner U. Trends but not individual values of central venous oxygen saturation agree with mixed venous oxygen saturation during varying hemodynamic conditions. *Anesthesiology* 2005;**103**:249–57.

82. Reinhart K, Kuhn HJ, Hartog C, Bredle DL. Continuous central venous and pulmonary artery oxygen saturation monitoring in the critically ill. *Intens Care Med* 2004;**30**:1572–8.

83. Donati A, Loggi S, Preiser JC, et al. Goal-directed intraoperative therapy reduces morbidity and length of hospital stay in high-risk surgical patients. *Chest* 2007;**132**:1817–24.

84. Davison DL, Chawla LS, Selassie L, et al. Femoral-based central venous oxygen saturation is not a reliable substitute for subclavian/internal jugular-based central venous oxygen saturation in patients who are critically ill. *Chest* 2010;**138**:76–83.

85. Marik PE. Sublingual capnography: a clinical validation study. *Chest* 2001;**120**:923–7.

86. Marik PE. Regional carbon dioxide monitoring to assess the adequacy of tissue perfusion. *Curr Opin Crit Care* 2005;**11**: 245–51.

87. Palizas F, Dubin A, Regueira T, et al. Gastric tonometry versus cardiac index as resuscitation goals in septic shock: a multicenter, randomized, controlled trial. *Crit Care* 2009;**13**: R44.

88. Rinehart J, Liu N, Alexander B, Cannesson M. Review article: closed-loop systems in anesthesia: is there a potential for closed-loop fluid management and hemodynamic optimization? *Anesth Analg* 2012;**114**:130–43.

89. Srinivasa S, Kahokehr A, Soop M, Taylor M, Hill AG. Goal-directed fluid therapy-a survey of anaesthetists in the UK, USA, Australia and New Zealand. *BMC Anesth* 2013;**13**:5.

Chapter

25

What is a fluid challenge and how to perform it?

Maurizio Cecconi and Hollman D. Aya

Introduction

Hemodynamic instability is a common cause for intensive care unit admission. This instability is often described as an inadequate arterial blood pressure, or as unspecific signs of inadequate perfusion of organs and tissues such as metabolic acidosis, hyperlactemia, decreased urine output, and prolonged capillary repletion time. Sustained in time, hemodynamic instability will result in inadequate oxygen delivery and activation of cellular apoptosis and organ failure, so that hemodynamic stabilization represents a life-saving intervention.

The causes of cardiovascular dysfunction can be grouped into three categories:

1. Hypovolemia
2. Cardiac dysfunction
3. Obstructive pathology.

Hypovolemia can also be divided into two groups:

- Absolute hypovolemia: secondary to
  - External fluid losses (hemorrhage or losses from gastrointestinal or urinary tracts or skin surface) or
  - Internal fluid losses (exudation or transudation of body fluids into a third space).
- Relative hypovolemia secondary to an increase in venous capacitance due to side effects of medications or due to release of endogenous vasodilators as in septic states.[1]

Excluding cases of cardiac failure, administration of intravascular fluids represents the first-line treatment for most hemodynamic instability conditions. Not surprisingly, fluid repletion is also the first therapeutic intervention in the context of goal directed therapy.[2-7] However, intravascular fluids, as any other medication, must be administered in the right dose in order to avoid adverse effects. Actually, it has been increasingly recognized that fluid overload increases the incidence of acute lung injury, tissue healing complications, intra-abdominal hypertension, and mortality in critically ill patients.[8-14] Hence, a method for guiding fluid administration comes to be of great importance. In this chapter, we will present the "fluid challenge" concept, its historic evolution, and physiological rationale, and finally some of the issues that are still uncertain about this diagnostic test for fluid responsiveness.

What is a fluid challenge?

A fluid challenge is the administration of a small quantity of fluid, over a short period of time for the purpose of testing the cardiovascular response to an increase in intravascular volume. This test is still considered the "gold standard" for assessing fluid responsiveness.

Historic review

The term "fluid challenge" was first coined by Max H. Weil and Robert J. Henning.[15] They suggested the administration of 200, 100, or 50 mL of fluid (if central venous pressure [CVP] was less than 8 mm H_2O, between 8 and 14, or greater than 14 cm H_2O, respectively) over 10 minutes through a peripheral venous cannula. For assessing the response they also conceived the "5–2" rule: if, after the infusion, the CVP rose no more than 2 cm H_2O, the fluid challenge was repeated; if the CVP rose between 2 and 5 cm H_2O and remained at that level for more than 10 minutes, no more fluid challenges were necessary; if at any point during the fluid infusion the CVP increased by more than 5 cm H_2O, the infusion had

Perioperative Hemodynamic Monitoring and Goal Directed Therapy, ed. Maxime Cannesson and Rupert Pearse.
Published by Cambridge University Press. © Cambridge University Press 2014.

to be stopped. In a similar way, they proposed the use of the "3–7" rule for the pulmonary artery occlusion pressure (PAOP).

Since then, the "fluid challenge" term has been widely used in connection with the administration of intravenous fluids in order to test preload dependence, and similar terms – such as "volume expansion," "volume loading," or "volume-loading step" – have been used interchangeably in the literature.[16–53]

Table 25.1 shows how the fluid challenge technique was reported in the studies included in the meta-analysis recently performed by Marik et al.:[54] 95% of the fluid challenges reported were performed with colloids (6% hydroxyethyl starch mainly); the range of volume given was from 100 mL to 3 liters, although the most frequent volumes were 500 mL (36%), 7 mL/kg (17%), 250 mL (10%), 20 mL/kg (7%), or 10 mL/kg (7%). The rate of infusion is similarly variable, from 1 minute of infusion to 1000 mL/hour. The most frequent rate reported was 30 minutes of infusion. For assessment of fluid responsiveness, an increase in cardiac index (CI) equal to or greater than 15% is the most frequently used (28%), followed by an increase in stroke volume index (SVI) equal to or greater than 15%. Other authors used cardiac output (CO) or stroke volume (SV) with different cutoffs, and only one study defined the target as an absolute increase in CI of 300 mL/min/m.[23,24] 52 % of authors assessed the effect of the fluid challenge immediately after the fluid infusion, 21% did it between 1 and 10 minutes, while the rest of the authors reported the assessment time at 12, 30, or even 47 minutes after the fluid infusion. The most common method used to evaluate the response was the pulmonary artery catheter, although in recent studies other devices such as PiCCO, LiDCO, Vigileo FloTrac, or echocardiographic techniques have also been reported. Only three studies reported a parameter as a safety limit for the fluid infusion: RAP, PAP, PAOP, or ELWI.[25,32,50]

Not surprisingly, far from being a homogeneous intervention, this review reveals an important variability in performance of what seems to be a simple technique. The protocol initially proposed by Weil et al.[15] was reviewed in 2006 and, although the same principle was maintained, several modifications were proposed.[55] First, the rate of infusion was reduced to 500 mL of colloids over 30 minutes. Second, the clinical target is not clearly stated, but mean arterial pressure (MAP), heart rate, urine output, or even parameters of tissue perfusion such as toe temperature

and sublingual CO_2 are mentioned. Third, as a safety limit, the authors advocated for CVP, although then as a single value rather than as a relative increase from baseline value.

In light of all this heterogeneity, it seems important to gain a better understanding of the physiological concepts behind this technique in order to perform the technique correctly.

History of physiological rationale

Carl Ludwig was the first to describe the relationship between diastolic volume and cardiac performance.[56] Later, S. W. Patterson and E. H. Starling[57] studied the relationships between venous inflow, venous pressure, and ventricular output, and they concluded "…*with increasing* (venous) *inflow,* (venous pressure) *rises at first only slightly, so long as the amount of blood flowing in is not more than sufficient to exert a minimal distension of the relaxing ventricles.*" They continued, "*As soon as the inflow exceeds the rate at which it can keep pace with the relaxation of the ventricle muscle, the pressure at the auricular orifice of the great veins must begin to rise, and this pressure will exert an active distending influence on the ventricular walls, so still further quickening the rate of filling of their cavities and increasing the output from the ventricles.*" Interestingly, the curve known as the "cardiac function curve" or the "Frank–Starling curve" was first drawn with the cardiac output variable on the *x*-axis and the venous pressure on the *y*-axis (Figure 25.1). However, in this curve the controlled variable is actually the venous inflow. Patterson et al.[57] pointed out that the *optimum* venous pressure is the amount necessary to produce "maximal" dilatation of the heart during diastole, which is determined by its muscular anatomy. Thus, if we can increase "venous inflow," for example, with a fluid challenge, we could expect to increase CVP and CO, and importantly, we would expect a greater increase in CVP once the ventricle has achieved its maximal dilatation. That *optimum* amount of pressure is intrinsically related to the characteristics of each ventricle, so that no absolute value of CVP can be identified as "optimum" for a group of patients. As demonstrated by Marik et al.,[54,58] CVP cannot be used to assess intravascular volume state or to predict fluid responsiveness. However, as pointed out by Patterson,[57] CVP can still play a role in assessing the response of a fluid challenge, particularly on the venous side of the circulation.

Table 25.1. Fluid challenges reported in the literature

Study	Year	FCh / patients	Fluid	Volume	Rate	Target / assessment	Time of assessment	Method of assessment	Safety
Calvin et al.[21]	1981	28/28	5% albumin	250 mL	30 min	Increase SV	N/A	PAC	N/A
Reuse et al.[45]	1990	24/24	4.5% albumin	300 mL	30 min	Increase CI	N/A	PAC	N/A
Wagner et al.[50]	1998	25/25	NS 5% albumin	938 mL ± 480 584 ± 187	N/A	SV > 10%	47 min	PAC	3 mmHg PPAO
Michard et al.[36]	2000	40/40	6% HES	500 mL	N/A	CI > 15%	30 min	PAC	N/A
Reuter et al.[46]	2002	20/20	3.5% oxypolygelatine	20 mL x BMI	N/A	SVI > 15%	N/A	PiCCO	N/A
Barbier et al.[17]	2004	20/20	4% gelatine	7 mL/kg	30 min	CI >15%	Immediately after	TTE	N/A
Kramer et al.[30]	2004	21/21	Blood	500 mL	10 – 15 min	CO > 12%	Immediately after	PAC	N/A
Marx et al.[35]	2004	10/10	10% HES	500 mL	30 min	Not defined	Immediately after	PiCCO / PAC	N/A
Perel et al.[43]	2005	14/14	Colloid	7mL/kg	30 min	CI ≥15%	N/A	PAC	N/A
De Backer et al.[25]	2005	60/60	HES or crystalloid	500 or 1000 mL	30 min	CI > 15%	Immediately after	PAC	PAP or RAP increase above individual value or > 3 mmHg.
Osman et al.[42]	2007	96/96	6% HES	500 mL	20 min	CI ≥15%	N/A	PAC	N/A
Magder et al.[34]	2007	135/83	N/A	368 mL	10 – 30 min	CI 300 mL/ min/m²	30 min	PAC	N/A
Wyffels et al.[52]	2007	32/32	6% HES	500 mL	20 min	CI ≥15%	Immediately after	PAC	N/A
Auler et al.[16]	2008	59/59	Ringer's lactate	20 mL/kg	20 min	CI ≥15%	Immediately after	PAC	N/A
Muller et al.[40]	2008	35/35	6% HES	250 – 500 mL	999 mL/h	CI ≥15%	0–10 min	PiCCO	Clinical
Huang et al.[29]	2008	22/22	10% pentastarch	500 mL	10 mL/ kg/h	CI ≥15%	Immediately after	PAC / PiCCO	N/A

Table 25.1. (cont.)

Study	Year	FCh / patients	Fluid	Volume	Rate	Target / assessment	Time of assessment	Method of assessment	Safety
Monge Garcia et al.[37]	2009	38/38	6% HES	500 mL	30 min	SVI ≥ 15%	Immediately after	Vigileo	N/A
Thiel et al.[49]	2009	102/89	NS, HAR, hetastarch	500 mL or more	N/A	SV ≥ 15%	Immediately after	USCOM (transthoracic Doppler)	N/A
Monge Garcia et al.[38]	2009	30/30	6% HES	500 mL	30 min	SVI ≥ 15%	Immediately after	Vigileo	N/A
Moretti et al.[39]	2010	31/31	6% HES	7 mL/kg	N/A	CI ≥15%	Immediately after	PiCCO	N/A
Muller et al.[41]	2011	39/39	6% HES	100 mL 400 mL	1 min 14 min	VTI ≥15%	Immediately after	TTE	N/A
Lakhal et al.[32]	2011	65/65	Colloid	300 mL 200 mL	18 min 12 min	CO > 10%	Immediately after	PiCCO / PAC	ELWI > 22 mL/Kg PPAO > 18 mmHg
Berkenstatd et al.[19]	2001	140/15	6% HES	100 mL	2 min	SV > 5%	1 min after	PiCCO	N/A
Preisman et al.[44]	2005	70/18	3.5% gelatine	250 mL	5 – 7 min	SVI > 15%	3 min after	PiCCO	N/A
Hofer et al.[28]	2005	35/35	6% HES	10 mL/kg Ideal BW	20 min	SVI > 25%	Immediately after	PAC / PiCCO	N/A
Wiesenack et al.[51]	2005	20/20	6% HES	7 mL/kg	1 mL/kg/min	SVI > 20%	Immediately after	PiCCO	N/A
Solus-Biguenet et al.[48]	2006	54/8	4% gelatine	250 mL	10 – 15 min	SVI ≥ 10%	2 – 3 min after	PAC	N/A
Lee et al.[33]	2007	20/20	6% HES	7 mL/kg	1 mL/kg/min	SVI ≥ 10%	12 min after	TOE	N/A
Cannesson et al.[22]	2007	25/25	6% HES	500 mL	10 min	CI ≥ 15%	0–3 min after	PAC	N/A

Study	Year	N	Fluid	Volume	Rate	Threshold	Timing	Monitor	
Belloni et al.[18]	2008	20/20	6% HES	7 mL/kg	5 min	CI > 15%	Immediately after	PAC / LiDCO	N/A
Biais et al.[20]	2008	35/35	4% albumin	20 mL /BMI	20 min	CO ≥ 15%	Immediately after	TTE	N/A
De Waal et al.[26]	2009	36/18	6% HES	10 mL/kg	10 min	SVI ≥ 12%	Immediately after	PiCCO	N/A
Cannesson et al.[24]	2009	25/25	6% HES	500 mL	10 min	CI ≥ 15%	0 – 3 min	PAC	N/A
Zimmermann et al.[53]	2010	20/20	6% HES	7 mL/kg	1mL/kg/min	SVI ≥ 15%	Immediately after	FloTrac Vigileo	N/A
Desgranges et al.[27]	2011	28/28	6% HES	500 mL	10 min	CI ≥ 15%	5 min after	PAC	N/A
Shin et al.[47]	2011	35/35	6% HES	10 mL/kg	5 min	CI ≥ 15%	12 min after	PAC / Vigileo	N/A
Cannesson et al.[23]	2011	413/413	6% HES modified gelatine	500 mL	10 – 20 min	CO ≥ 15%	2 – 5 min after	PAC / PiCCO / esophageal Doppler	N/A
Kumar et al.[31]	2004	44/44	Normal saline	3 L	1 L / hour	N/A	Immediately after	PAC, TTE	N/A

HES hydroxyethyl starch; CI cardiac index; CO cardiac output; SV stroke volume; SVI stroke volume index; VTI velocity time integral; PAC pulmonary artery catheter; TTE transthoracic echocardiography; TOE transesophageal echocardiography; PPAO pulmonary artery occluded pressure; PAP pulmonary artery pressure; RAP right atrial pressure; ELWI extra-lung water index.

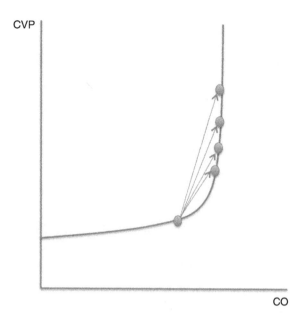

Figure 25.1. Cardiac function curve, as it was initially published by Patterson and Starling in 1914.[57] A fluid challenge can induce an increase in CO, achieving many different levels of CVP, depending on the ventricle compliance.

In 1955 Guyton[59,60] proposed that the venous return (VR) is directly proportional to the pressure gradient of venous return and inversely proportional to the resistance to venous return (RVR). The pressure gradient of the venous return is the difference between the mean systemic filling pressure (Pmsf) and the right atrial pressure (RAP). This can also be mathematically represented as follows:

$$VR = \frac{Pmsf - RAR}{RVR}$$

The Pmsf is the pressure in the cardiovascular system when there is no blood motion and it is directly proportional to the *stressed* blood volume (Vs) and conversely proportional to the compliance (C) of the cardiovascular system.

$$Pmsf = \frac{Vs}{C}$$

The stressed volume is the volume that distends the blood vessel walls, generating an increase of intravascular pressure. It constitutes the volume hemodynamically effective and normally represents 30% – 40% of the total blood volume. The unstressed volume is inactive hemodynamically, since it is the volume that fills up the intravascular space without any increase of intravascular pressure.

It constitutes a blood reserve that can be used by changes in vascular compliance.

Thus, in order to increase cardiac output or venous return, a fluid challenge, which is an increase in blood volume, must increase the stress blood volume, increase the Pmsf and increase the pressure gradient of venous return, given that the ventricle wall distends and the stroke volume in the next systole increases. If the heart ventricle is no longer preload dependent, the ventricle will not accommodate that volume and the CVP will increase avoiding any increase of pressure gradient of venous return. This has recently been studied by our group[61] with 101 fluid challenges where the Pmsf analog increased similarly among responders and non-responders, whereas the gradient of venous return increased only among responders.

The fluid challenge technique: new perspectives

The ideal fluid challenge would have to take into account the following considerations:

- Type of fluid
- Volume
- Rate of infusion
- Assessment of response
- Safety limits.

Type of fluid

After a long debate, it seems now largely accepted that colloids do not offer a clear advantage with respect to crystalloids for fluid resuscitation. There is also evidence that in septic patients their administration is associated with a higher incidence of acute kidney injury.[62]

Among crystalloids, normal saline (sodium chloride 0.9%) can cause more metabolic acidosis compared with balanced solutions (normal strong ion difference) such as Hartmann's or Plasmalyte.[63] Therefore, we would suggest the use of balanced crystalloid solutions for a fluid challenge technique.

Volume and rate of infusion: validity of a fluid challenge

It is important to differentiate a fluid challenge from "volume load" or "volume expansion." The main objective of the fluid challenge is to test the cardiovascular response, and should be performed in a relatively controlled environment in order to obtain a trustable interpretation. This is not the case in an emergency resuscitation. The volume must be small in order to avoid fluid overload in the case of a negative response. However, the volume must be big enough to be able to increase Pmsf and perform a "valid" test of the hemodynamic response. The Pmsf can be calculated using the methods described by Maas et al.,[64] Anderson and colleagues,[65] or it can also be estimated using a non-invasive software as described by Parkin et al.[66] Magder et al.,[34] proposed using the CVP to assess the validity of the fluid challenge, although there is limited evidence about the utility of CVP to assess the validity of the test. A fluid challenge can generate an increase of cardiac output without any change in CVP because the heart is increasing its efficiency and keeping CVP at the same level. In that case, CVP would not reflect the changes on intravascular volume at all and would not be a reliable variable for assessing the validity of the technique. However, in the absence of an increase of CO (non-responders), the change in CVP basically reflects the changes in Pmsf. Our group[61] recently demonstrated that the Pmsf analog (Pmsa) increases similarly in responders and non-responders, but in non-responders the changes in CVP are similar to the change in Pmsa after a fluid challenge of 250 mL performed in less than 5 minutes. Given that the "validity" question mainly rises in the case of lack of response, an increase of CVP in the absence of an increase of CO could be considered as evidence of "validity" of the test. From unpublished data of that study,[61] a fluid challenge of 250 mL administered in less than 5 min increased Pmsa in 95% of 101 events in postsurgical patients. It remains unclear, however, how much the Pmsf or CVP should increase to consider a fluid challenge as valid.

Assessment of response: target and time

The response to a fluid challenge is frequently assessed by an increase in flow-related variables, such as CO or SV. This is physiologically reasonable, as the objective of the fluid therapy is increasing the oxygen delivery by increasing the blood flow. Vincent et al.[55] suggested the use of mean arterial pressure (MAP), but this parameter poorly correlates with changes in CI or pulse pressure (PP) after a fluid challenge,[67] particularly in young patients,[68] where the

compliance of the arterial wall can compensate for the changes in stroke volume.

Positive response has been defined by an increase of 15%, according to a literature review based on 14 studies reported by Stetz et al.[69] in 1982, where they revealed that there must be a minimal difference of 12% to 15% (average, 13%) between determinations of cardiac output (three measurements per determination) with thermodilution devices (PAC at that point) to suggest a real clinical difference. Later, Ostergaard et al.[70] performed a study on 25 patients in atrial fibrillation (AF) and 25 in sinus rhythm (SR) using PAC and concluded that two measurements must differ by 15% in AF patients and 9% in SR patients before one can be 95% confident that a real change has taken place.

The choice of CO or SV as a target allows the clinician the performance of a "maximization" of SV with fluids, rather than a proper optimization. Ideally, we should be able to detect not only the changes in CO or SV, but also changes in CVP, as both parameters are affected by the fluid challenge. The slope of the cardiac function curve might be more informative in order to avoid unnecessary elevated pressures on the venous side of the circulation.

With regard to the time of assessment, more than half of the studies included in our review reported the assessment immediately after the fluid challenge. This approach has the advantage of avoiding the stress–relaxation effect that the infusion of fluid may produce on the vascular wall[71] and the Anrep effect on myocardial muscle.[72,73] However, the "average" time that every device uses to measure the CO must be taken into consideration.

Safety

The main concern in the administration of fluid is the generation of fluid overload. Ideally, even the administration of a small amount of fluid, such as in a fluid challenge, should be accompanied by a parameter that allows the clinician to detect the harmful impact of the volume on the circulation.

Patterson and Starling[57] had already pointed out that CVP can increase not only in response to an increase of blood volume which effectively increase cardiac output, but also as a consequence of cardiac failure. From the guytonian point of view, the RAP (or the CVP as its surrogate) was considered to be a reverse force to venous return when it increased under isovolumetric conditions. As the variation of CVP increases as we are approaching the flat part of cardiac function curve, CVP could be used to detect an alarming increase of pressure in the absence of an increase of flow. The variation of CVP in response to a fluid challenge was originally proposed by Weil et al.[15] Limited evidence is available for this approach, but it has been used in a clinical trial of goal directed therapy on orthopedic surgery[74] and, interestingly, similar results were observed compared with the group guided by SV obtained by esophageal Doppler ultrasound. It remains unclear how much CVP must increase to stop the fluid infusion, but a single value of CVP is poorly informative and not applicable to every patient.[54]

Practical conclusions

- Use balanced crystalloids in small quantity for fluid challenge

- To minimize the amount of fluid, the volume must be given quickly, for example, 250 mL over 5 minutes.
- To assess the validity of the test (for research purposes), a change in Pmsf should be observed.
- To assess the response, CO or SV must be observed immediately, for as long as CVP. The threshold to identify a positive response depends on every device.
- The change in CVP should be observed during a fluid challenge. An increase in CVP in the absence of increase in CO confirms a negative response and a valid test. The magnitude of this increase remains unclear and probably depends on the amount of fluid given and the compliance of the cardiovascular system. No single value of CVP should be used to predict fluid responsiveness or to stop fluid infusion.

References

1. Grisham MB, Jourd'Heuil D, Wink DA. Nitric oxide. I. Physiological chemistry of nitric oxide and its metabolites: implications in inflammation. *Am J Physiol* 1999;**276(2 Pt 1)**: G315–21.

2. Cecconi M, Fasano N, Langiano N, et al. Goal-directed haemodynamic therapy during elective total hip arthroplasty under regional anaesthesia. *Crit Care* 2011;**15(3)**:R132.

3. Donati A, Loggi S, Preiser JC, et al. Goal-directed intraoperative therapy reduces morbidity and length of hospital stay in high-risk surgical patients. *Chest* 2007; **132(6)**:1817–24.

4. Gan TJ, Soppitt A, Maroof M, et al. Goal-directed intraoperative fluid administration reduces length of hospital stay after major surgery. *Anesthesiology* 2002; **97(4)**:820–6.

5. McKendry M, McGloin H, Saberi D, et al. Randomised controlled trial assessing the impact of a nurse delivered, flow monitored protocol for optimisation of circulatory status after cardiac surgery. *BMJ* 2004; **329(7460)**:258.

6. Pearse R, Dawson D, Fawcett J, et al. Early goal-directed therapy after major surgery reduces complications and duration of hospital stay. A randomised, controlled trial [ISRCTN38797445]. *Crit Care* 2005;**9(6)**:R687–93.

7. Sinclair S, James S, Singer M. Intraoperative intravascular volume optimisation and length of hospital stay after repair of proximal femoral fracture: randomised controlled trial. *BMJ* 1997;**315(7113)**:909–12.

8. Payen D, de Pont AC, Sakr Y, et al. A positive fluid balance is associated with a worse outcome in patients with acute renal failure. *Crit Care* 2008;**12(3)**:R74.

9. Hughes CG, Weavind L, Banerjee A, et al. Intraoperative risk factors for acute respiratory distress syndrome in critically ill patients. *Anesth Analg* 2010; **111(2)**:464–7.

10. Jia X, Malhotra A, Saeed M, Mark RG, Talmor D. Risk factors for ARDS in patients receiving mechanical ventilation for > 48 h. *Chest* 2008;**133(4)**:853–61.

11. Holte K, Jensen P, Kehlet H. Physiologic effects of intravenous fluid administration in healthy volunteers. *Anesth Analg* 2003; **96(5)**:1504–9.

12. Vincent JL, Sakr Y, Sprung CL, et al. Sepsis in European intensive care units: results of the SOAP study. *Crit Care Med* 2006; **34(2)**:344–53.

13. Brandstrup B, Tonnesen H, Beier-Holgersen R, et al. Effects of intravenous fluid restriction on postoperative complications: comparison of two perioperative fluid regimens: a randomized assessor-blinded multicenter trial. *Annals Surg* 2003; **238(5)**:641–8.

14. Malbrain ML, Chiumello D, Pelosi P, et al. Incidence and prognosis of intraabdominal hypertension in a mixed population of critically ill patients: a multiple-center epidemiological

study. *Crit Care Med* 2005; **33**(2):315–22.

15. Weil MH, Henning RJ. New concepts in the diagnosis and fluid treatment of circulatory shock. Thirteenth annual Becton, Dickinson and Company Oscar Schwidetsky Memorial Lecture. *Anesth Analg* 1979;**58**(2):124–32.

16. Auler JO, Jr., Galas F, Hajjar L, Santos L, Carvalho T, Michard F. Online monitoring of pulse pressure variation to guide fluid therapy after cardiac surgery. *Anesth Analg* 2008;**106**(4):1201–6.

17. Barbier C, Loubieres Y, Schmit C, et al. Respiratory changes in inferior vena cava diameter are helpful in predicting fluid responsiveness in ventilated septic patients. *Intens Care Med* 2004;**30**(9):1740–6.

18. Belloni L, Pisano A, Natale A, et al. Assessment of fluid-responsiveness parameters for off-pump coronary artery bypass surgery: a comparison among LiDCO, transesophageal echochardiography, and pulmonary artery catheter. *J Cardiothorac Vasc Anesth* 2008;**22**(2):243–8.

19. Berkenstadt H, Margalit N, Hadani M, et al. Stroke volume variation as a predictor of fluid responsiveness in patients undergoing brain surgery. *Anesth Analg* 2001;**92**(4):984–9.

20. Biais M, Nouette-Gaulain K, Cottenceau V, Revel P, Sztark F. Uncalibrated pulse contour-derived stroke volume variation predicts fluid responsiveness in mechanically ventilated patients undergoing liver transplantation. *Br J Anaesth* 2008;**101**(6):761–8.

21. Calvin JE, Driedger AA, Sibbald WJ. The hemodynamic effect of rapid fluid infusion in critically ill patients. *Surgery* 1981; **90**(1):61–76.

22. Cannesson M, Attof Y, Rosamel P, et al. Respiratory variations in pulse oximetry plethysmographic waveform amplitude to predict fluid responsiveness in the operating room. *Anesthesiology* 2007;**106**(6):1105–11.

23. Cannesson M, Le Manach Y, Hofer CK, et al. Assessing the diagnostic accuracy of pulse pressure variations for the prediction of fluid responsiveness: a "gray zone" approach. *Anesthesiology* 2011; **115**(2):231–41.

24. Cannesson M, Musard H, Desebbe O, et al. The ability of stroke volume variations obtained with Vigileo/FloTrac system to monitor fluid responsiveness in mechanically ventilated patients. *Anesth Analg* 2009;**108**(2):513–17.

25. De Backer D, Heenen S, Piagnerelli M, Koch M, Vincent JL. Pulse pressure variations to predict fluid responsiveness: influence of tidal volume. *Intens Care Med* 2005;**31**(4):517–23.

26. de Waal EE, Rex S, Kruitwagen CL, Kalkman CJ, Buhre WF. Dynamic preload indicators fail to predict fluid responsiveness in open-chest conditions. *Crit Care Med* 2009;**37**(2):510–15.

27. Desgranges FP, Desebbe O, Ghazouani A, et al. Influence of the site of measurement on the ability of plethysmographic variability index to predict fluid responsiveness. *Br J Anaesth* 2011;**107**(3):329–35.

28. Hofer CK, Muller SM, Furrer L, et al. Stroke volume and pulse pressure variation for prediction of fluid responsiveness in patients undergoing off-pump coronary artery bypass grafting. *Chest* 2005;**128**(2):848–54.

29. Huang CC, Fu JY, Hu HC, et al. Prediction of fluid responsiveness in acute respiratory distress syndrome patients ventilated with low tidal volume and high positive end-expiratory pressure. *Crit Care Med* 2008;**36**(10):2810–16.

30. Kramer A, Zygun D, Hawes H, Easton P, Ferland A. Pulse pressure variation predicts fluid responsiveness following coronary artery bypass surgery. *Chest* 2004;**126**(5):1563–8. Epub 2004/ 11/13.

31. Kumar A, Anel R, Bunnell E, et al. Pulmonary artery occlusion pressure and central venous pressure fail to predict ventricular filling volume, cardiac performance, or the response to volume infusion in normal subjects. *Crit Care Med* 2004; **32**(3):691–9.

32. Lakhal K, Ehrmann S, Benzekri-Lefevre D, et al. Respiratory pulse pressure variation fails to predict fluid responsiveness in acute respiratory distress syndrome. *Crit Care* 2011;**15**(2):R85.

33. Lee JH, Kim JT, Yoon SZ, et al. Evaluation of corrected flow time in oesophageal Doppler as a predictor of fluid responsiveness. *Br J Anaesth* 2007;**99**(3):343–8.

34. Magder S, Bafaqeeh F. The clinical role of central venous pressure measurements. *J Intens Care Med* 2007;**22**(1):44–51.

35. Marx G, Cope T, McCrossan L, et al. Assessing fluid responsiveness by stroke volume variation in mechanically ventilated patients with severe sepsis. *Eur J Anaesthesiol* 2004;**21** (2):132–8.

36. Michard F, Boussat S, Chemla D, et al. Relation between respiratory changes in arterial pulse pressure and fluid responsiveness in septic patients with acute circulatory failure. *Am J Resp Crit Care Med* 2000;**162**(1):134–8.

37. Monge Garcia MI, Gil Cano A, Diaz Monrove JC. Brachial artery peak velocity variation to predict fluid responsiveness in mechanically ventilated patients. *Crit Care* 2009;**13**(5):R142.

38. Monge Garcia MI, Gil Cano A, Diaz Monrove JC. Arterial pressure changes during the Valsalva maneuver to predict fluid responsiveness in spontaneously

breathing patients. *Intens Care Med* 2009;**35**(1):77–84.

39. Moretti R, Pizzi B. Inferior vena cava distensibility as a predictor of fluid responsiveness in patients with subarachnoid hemorrhage. *Neurocrit Care* 2010;**13**(1):3–9.

40. Muller L, Louart G, Bengler C, et al. The intrathoracic blood volume index as an indicator of fluid responsiveness in critically ill patients with acute circulatory failure: a comparison with central venous pressure. *Anesth Analg* 2008;**107**(2):607–13.

41. Muller L, Toumi M, Bousquet PJ, et al. An increase in aortic blood flow after an infusion of 100 ml colloid over 1 minute can predict fluid responsiveness: the mini-fluid challenge study. *Anesthesiology* 2011;**115**(3):541–7.

42. Osman D, Ridel C, Ray P, et al. Cardiac filling pressures are not appropriate to predict hemodynamic response to volume challenge. *Crit Care Med* 2007;**35**(1):64–8.

43. Perel A, Minkovich L, Preisman S, et al. Assessing fluid-responsiveness by a standardized ventilatory maneuver: the respiratory systolic variation test. *Anesth Analg* 2005;**100**(4):942–5.

44. Preisman S, Kogan S, Berkenstadt H, Perel A. Predicting fluid responsiveness in patients undergoing cardiac surgery: functional haemodynamic parameters including the Respiratory Systolic Variation Test and static preload indicators. *Br J Anaesth* 2005;**95**(6):746–55.

45. Reuse C, Vincent JL, Pinsky MR. Measurements of right ventricular volumes during fluid challenge. *Chest* 1990;**98**(6):1450–4.

46. Reuter DA, Felbinger TW, Kilger E, et al. Optimizing fluid therapy in mechanically ventilated patients after cardiac surgery by on-line monitoring of left ventricular stroke volume variations. Comparison with aortic systolic

pressure variations. *Br J Anaesth* 2002;**88**(1):124–6.

47. Shin YH, Ko JS, Gwak MS, et al. Utility of uncalibrated femoral stroke volume variation as a predictor of fluid responsiveness during the anhepatic phase of liver transplantation. *Liver Transpl* 2011;**17**(1):53–9.

48. Solus-Biguenet H, Fleyfel M, Tavernier B, et al. Non-invasive prediction of fluid responsiveness during major hepatic surgery. *Br J Anaesth* 2006;**97**(6):808–16.

49. Thiel SW, Kollef MH, Isakow W. Non-invasive stroke volume measurement and passive leg raising predict volume responsiveness in medical ICU patients: an observational cohort study. *Crit Care* 2009;**13**(4):R111.

50. Wagner JG, Leatherman JW. Right ventricular end-diastolic volume as a predictor of the hemodynamic response to a fluid challenge. *Chest* 1998;**113**(4):1048–54.

51. Wiesenack C, Fiegl C, Keyser A, Prasser C, Keyl C. Assessment of fluid responsiveness in mechanically ventilated cardiac surgical patients. *Eur J Anaesthesiol* 2005;**22**(9):658–65.

52. Wyffels PA, Durnez PJ, Helderweirt J, Stockman WM, De Kegel D. Ventilation-induced plethysmographic variations predict fluid responsiveness in ventilated postoperative cardiac surgery patients. *Anesth Analg* 2007;**105**(2):448–52.

53. Zimmermann M, Feibicke T, Keyl C, et al. Accuracy of stroke volume variation compared with pleth variability index to predict fluid responsiveness in mechanically ventilated patients undergoing major surgery. *Eur J Anaesthesiol* 2010; **27**(6):555–61.

54. Marik PE, Cavallazzi R. Does the central venous pressure predict fluid responsiveness? An updated meta-analysis and a plea for some

common sense. *Crit Care Med* 2013;**41**(7):1774–81.

55. Vincent JL, Weil MH. Fluid challenge revisited. *Crit Care Med* 2006;**34**(5):1333–7.

56. Ludwig CFW. *Lehrbuch der Physiologie des Menschen.* Leipzig: Heidelberg, C.F. Winter, 1858.

57. Patterson SW, Starling EH. On the mechanical factors which determine the output of the ventricles. *J Physiol* 1914; **48**(5):357–79.

58. Marik PE, Baram M, Vahid B. Does central venous pressure predict fluid responsiveness? A systematic review of the literature and the tale of seven mares. *Chest* 2008;**134**(1):172–8.

59. Guyton AC. Determination of cardiac output by equating venous return curves with cardiac response curves. *Physiol Rev* 1955;**35**(1):123–9.

60. Guyton AC, Lindsey AW, Kaufmann BN. Effect of mean circulatory filling pressure and other peripheral circulatory factors on cardiac output. *Am J Physiol* 1955;**180**(3):463–8.

61. Cecconi M, Aya HD, Geisen M, et al. Changes in the mean systemic filling pressure during a fluid challenge in postsurgical intensive care patients. *Intens Care Med* 2013;**39**(7):1299–305.

62. Myburgh JA, Finfer S, Bellomo R, et al. Hydroxyethyl starch or saline for fluid resuscitation in intensive care. *N Engl J Med* 2012;**367**(20):1901–11.

63. Hasman H, Cinar O, Uzun A, et al. A randomized clinical trial comparing the effect of rapidly infused crystalloids on acid-base status in dehydrated patients in the emergency department. *Int J Med Sci* 2012;**9**(1):59–64.

64. Maas JJ, Geerts BF, van den Berg PC, Pinsky MR, Jansen JR. Assessment of venous return curve and mean systemic filling pressure in postoperative cardiac

surgery patients. *Crit Care Med* 2009;**37**(3):912–18.

65. Anderson RM. *The Gross Physiology of the Cardiovascular System*. Tucson, AZ: Racquet Press, 1993.

66. Parkin WG, Leaning MS. Therapeutic control of the circulation. *J Clin Monit Comput* 2008;**22**(6):391–400.

67. Pierrakos C, Velissaris D, Scolletta S, et al. Can changes in arterial pressure be used to detect changes in cardiac index during fluid challenge in patients with septic shock? *Intens Care Med* 2012; **38**(3):422–8.

68. Monnet X, Letierce A, Hamzaoui O, et al. Arterial pressure allows monitoring the changes in cardiac output induced by volume expansion but not by norepinephrine. *Crit Care Med* 2011;**39**(6):1394–9.

69. Stetz CW, Miller RG, Kelly GE, Raffin TA. Reliability of the thermodilution method in the determination of cardiac output in clinical practice. *Am Rev Resp Dis* 1982;**126**(6):1001–4.

70. Ostergaard M, Nilsson LB, Nilsson JC, Rasmussen JP, Berthelsen PG. Precision of bolus thermodilution cardiac output measurements in patients with atrial fibrillation. *Acta Anaesth Scand* 2005;**49**(3):366–72.

71. Prather JW, Taylor AE, Guyton AC. Effect of blood volume, mean circulatory pressure, and stress relaxation on cardiac output. *Am J Physiol* 1969;**216**(3):467–72.

72. Alvarez BV, Perez NG, Ennis IL, Camilion de Hurtado MC, Cingolani HE. Mechanisms underlying the increase in force and Ca(2+) transient that follow stretch of cardiac muscle: a possible explanation of the Anrep effect. *Circ Res* 1999; **85**(8):716–22.

73. Cingolani HE, Perez NG, Cingolani OH, Ennis IL. The Anrep effect: 100 years later. *Am J Physiol Heart Circ Physiol* 2013;**304**(2):H175–82.

74. Venn R, Steele A, Richardson P, et al. Randomized controlled trial to investigate influence of the fluid challenge on duration of hospital stay and perioperative morbidity in patients with hip fractures. *Br J Anaesth* 2002;**88**(1):65–71.

Chapter

26

The relationships between anesthesia, hemodynamics and outcome

Tom Abbott and Gareth L. Ackland

Introduction

The impact of anesthetic depth on hemodynamics has always been suspected to be a potentially pivotal factor in determining perioperative outcome, albeit with little systematically garnered evidence to support that assertion. Several studies have emerged in the last 5 years providing important hypothesis generating data that highlight the possible relationships between depth of anesthesia, hypotension, and 30-day mortality – coined the "triple low" hypothesis.[1] Here, we review the evidence that may support these relationships and re-examine the data on the basis of basic scientific and clinical research, which suggests a plausible deleterious interaction between hemodynamic alterations and depth of anesthesia.

Impact of anesthetic depth on neuro-cardiovascular control

Before considering patient-centered data, it is worth revisiting the role of anesthesia and the perioperative period (Figure 26.1) in modulating central and peripheral neuro-cardiovascular control. Several studies – that can only be conducted in laboratory models – have confirmed the impact of anesthesia on central neural control of cardiovascular function by assessing how anesthesia affects physiologic function in decerebrate preparations.[2] These experiments reveal several important neurophysiologic features of anesthesia of direct relevance to the interpretation of linking depth of clinical anesthesia to hemodynamic changes. First, anesthetic agents unequivocally reduce blood pressure and heart rate in decerebrate preparations. However, the same anesthetic agents tested profoundly alter various baro- and chemoreflex responses,[3–7] at much lower anesthetic dose. Thus,

the hemodynamic effects observed under general anesthesia may not be solely due to central depressant effects of anesthesia. There is a wealth of evidence that even low levels of various anesthetic agents impair peripheral neural function, including the detection of hypoxia and hypercapnia by the peripheral chemo-receptors.[8,9] These physiologic changes impact profoundly on a range of hemodynamic responses, as explored extensively in both human and animal laboratory models.[10] A range of physiologic responses may therefore be altered under anesthesia, that occur independently of excessive anesthetic depth and/or central integration of neural afferent information. Second, peripheral neural function may be altered via anesthetic and non-anesthetic mechanisms. For example, neuromuscular blockade may affect the measurement of depth of anesthesia.[11] Similarly, higher levels of spinal blockade are positively correlated with bispectral index values in elderly patients.[12] While high spinal anesthesia predictably decreases systolic blood pressure, bispectral index values also decrease, despite concomitantly preserved cardiac output.[12] Thus, several confounding perioperative factors can impact on both depth of anesthesia and hemodynamics, either alone or in combination (Figure 26.1). With these important potential caveats and confounders in mind, we next consider each element of the "triple low" hypothesis.

Intraoperative hypotension

Although it is widely held that low blood pressure can lead to inadequate tissue perfusion, the clinical threshold at which this happens in a patient-specific manner remains unclear. Important experimental medicine studies in unanesthetized volunteers have added critical physiologic insights and help clarify

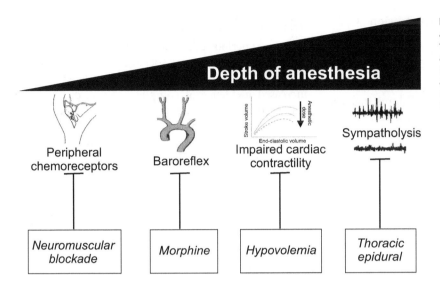

Figure 26.1. In addition to increasing anesthetic dose, other perioperative factors influence both the depth of anesthesia and its interaction with hemodynamic parameters. Ablation, or attenuation, of central pressor control mechanisms can cause hypotension, independently of anesthetic depth.

the importance of the relationship between arterial blood pressure and end-organ perfusion. These studies have demonstrated clear disconnects between blood pressure, end-organ injury, and global hemodynamic variables. A landmark human experimental study demonstrated that there was no consistent change in blood pressure even after removal of ~25% blood volume over a period of 1h.[13] In other words, the intuitive assumption that intraoperative hypotension is likely to be associated with adverse perioperative and postoperative outcomes will remain merely an association until future studies document measures of flow – including cardiac output – but also focus in the same studies on measures of end-organ perfusion and biomarkers of organ dysfunction. Certainly, current clinical and experimental data demonstrate that significant abnormalities in tissue oxygenation/function can occur at arterial blood pressures apparently maintained within normal range despite detrimental falls in perfusion.[14]

Defining intraoperative hypotension (IOH)

Various thresholds and limits with regard to both the degree and duration of hypotension have been used; consequently, the incidence of IOH is unknown. A systematic review examined 130 journal articles providing 140 different definitions! None of these studies documented measurements of cardiac output. Only 50% of papers using a definition of IOH

by comparing intraoperative values to baseline actually defined that baseline value. When the authors applied the published definitions of IOH to a cohort of 15 509 patients undergoing non-cardiac surgery, they found the incidence of IOH to be between 5% and 99% depending on which definition was used.[15] Thus, it is clear that a wide variety of definitions have been used, and variations between research studies will influence the incidence of associated complications.

IOH and mortality

Several retrospective observational studies have linked IOH to perioperative mortality. A survey of anesthesia-related mortality used the French national mortality database, and sent questionnaires to both the anesthetist and the doctor completing the death certificate. The incidence of death at least partially attributable to anesthesia was 4.7/100 000 (3.1 – 6.3/100 000). The most commonly cited factors contributing to death were aspiration of gastric contents, arbitrarily defined IOH, cardiac complications, and anemia.[16] The POISE multicenter, randomized controlled trial ($n = 8351$) examining the role of beta-blockade in non-cardiac surgery identified "clinically significant hypotension" as an independent intraoperative and postoperative predictor of death (OR 4.97; 95% CI 3.62 – 6.81) or stroke (OR 2.14; 95% CI 1.15 – 3.96) at 30 days postoperatively.[17] Cohort studies have also identified both systolic hypotension (<80 mmHg) and a 20% reduction in baseline BP and mean arterial pressure as risk factors for post-operative death.[18–20] However, whether these are independent of factors such as occult hypovolemia and/or blood loss remains unclear. Interestingly, a study that considered a priori 48 different definitions of IOH, by taking into account absolute and relative hypotension and their respective durations, failed to find an increased risk of death within a year of surgery.[21]

Perioperative myocardial and cerebrovascular events

Estimates of subclinical perioperative myocardial injury are as high as 22% using highly sensitive troponin assays[22] and there is growing evidence to suggest that the peak troponin level in the immediate postoperative period is an important marker of the risk of postoperative mortality.[23] The most robust dataset exploring the potential role of intraoperative blood pressure on cardiac morbidity used electronically recorded data acquired minute-by-minute in 15 000 patients, and every 2–5 min in a further ~18 000 patients.[24] The authors of this study report that "MAP<55 mmHg was associated with the development of myocardial injury and cardiac complications" and that "any amount of time at a MAP<55 mmHg was associated with adverse outcomes." In addition, they suggest that, although these data cannot exclude "residual confounding," including the effect of antihypertensive medication, their results mirror other work in this area. Multivariate logistic regression analysis of a multicenter, prospective dataset of 3387 patients undergoing non-cardiac surgery that identified 146 (4.3%) cases of major adverse cardiac events also identified IOH as a risk factor (OR 2.3; 95% CI 1.5 – 3.7).[25] However, these data also showed that six other variables were linked to major adverse cardiac events (history of coronary artery disease, congestive cardiac failure, cerebrovascular disease, chronic kidney disease, abnormal preoperative ECG, and red cell transfusion), suggesting that IOH may merely represent the underlying cardiovascular substrate associated with the complex, established multi-organ dysfunction of medical co-morbidities.[25]

IOH and other perioperative complications

Prolonged periods of hypotension, lasting longer than 10 minutes, have been associated with an increased length of hospital stay,[26] perhaps related to an increased incidence of complications. A prospective cohort study of 504 patients undergoing gastric bypass surgery found an association between IOH (one reading of MAP <60 mmHg) and postoperative Acute Kidney Injury (AKI) (P = 0.01), defined as "a 50% increase in serum creatinine relative to baseline during the first 3 postoperative days or requirement of dialysis."[27] As for myocardial ischemia, a mean arterial pressure <55 mmHg was also associated with the development of acute kidney injury, although whether the co-development of renal and cardiac postoperative complications is linked remains unclear.

Depth of anesthesia and intraoperative electroencephalography

The most widely used measure of anesthetic depth exploiting intraoperative electroencephalography (EEG) to measure brain activity is the Bispectral Index (BIS) (BIS Covidien, Boulder, Colorado, USA). However, recent evidence from studies comparing BIS-guided anesthesia with conventional methods of gauging the depth of anesthesia, including end-tidal anesthetic concentration (ETAC) guided approaches, remains equivocal.[28,29] The rationale for the use of BIS-guided anesthesia is based on the premise that anesthesia produces a consistent and reproducible effect on the EEG waveform in a concentration dependent manner. However, a recent study of 1100 patients with a high risk of intraoperative awareness challenged this assumption. By comparing intraoperative BIS values with ETACs using a generalized estimating equation, the authors found that, while there was a correlation between BIS and ETAC at a population level, "BIS frequently correlates poorly with ETAC" at an individual level and was "often insensitive to clinically significant changes in ETAC."[30] These findings serve to highlight the lack of real understanding of how anesthetic agents exert their hypnotic action on the brain.[28] In fact, unexpectedly low BIS at low end-tidal concentrations of volatile anesthetic could suggest sensitivity to the anesthetic agent. The same could be true of the relationship between ETAC and intraoperative blood pressure.[1]

The monitor represents a measurement of EEG activity as a number on a scale of 0 to 100, where

100 equates to normal, wakeful brain activity and 0 represents an absence of brain activity. The manufacturer suggested BIS normal range during anesthesia is between 40 and 60,[28] with a reading of 45 or less indicating a deep hypnotic state.[1] Initial studies into the use of BIS monitoring focused on the incidence of awareness and recall after anesthesia. A Cochrane review suggested that BIS may enhance recovery from deep anesthesia.[31] A more recent review suggests that, while early studies supported the use of BIS monitoring to reduce the incidence of awareness with recall, contemporary studies have shown no difference between BIS and conventional techniques.[28] There certainly is doubt as to how BIS equates to the suppression of neural activity involved in cardiovascular control.

Bispectral index and mortality

Conflicting data exist over whether depth of anesthesia is associated with postoperative morbidity and mortality,[18,32-35] reviewed in detail by Monk et al.[28] Three analyses support the association of low BIS and postoperative mortality. One prospective study of 1064 patients undergoing non-cardiac surgery identified cumulative time with BIS <45 as an independent predictor of 1-year postoperative mortality (RR = 1.24/hour, 95% CI: 1.06 – 1.44) using multivariate analysis. In addition, IOH defined as systolic BP < 80mmHg (RR 1.04/min, 95% CI: 1.01 – 1.07) and Charlson Comorbidity Score (RR = 16.2, 95% CI: 10.1– 33.7) were also identified.[18] A smaller retrospective analysis of 460 cardiac surgery patients identified cumulative time with BIS <45 as an independent predictor of 3-year postoperative mortality using multivariate regression analysis (hazard ratio 1.29/hour; 95% CI 1.1 – 1.5).[28,32] Leslie et al. performed a retrospective analysis on data collected as part of a RCT, including 1230 patients that were randomized to receive intraoperative BIS monitoring. The authors report that, while there was no difference in mortality between BIS and non-BIS groups, BIS <40 for longer than 5 minutes duration was associated with postoperative death by propensity score analysis, comparing BIS <40 with BIS >40 (hazard ratio 1.41; 95%CI: 1.02 – 1.95) with a mean length of follow-up of 4.1 years.[34] In contrast, two studies do not support low BIS as a predictor of postoperative mortality. Lindholm et al. performed a retrospective analysis of data from a prospective study of 4087 patients undergoing non-cardiac surgery. Initial findings associated low intraoperative BIS with postoperative mortality. After controlling for concurrent malignant disease using multivariable analysis, the association between BIS and mortality ceased to be significant.[35] A similar study in 1500 non-cardiac surgery patients also failed to find a relationship between the duration of low BIS (<45) and 1-year mortality.[33]

Bispectral index and postoperative recovery

In addition to mortality, the use of intraoperative BIS monitoring in predicting length of hospital stay has also been explored. A randomized controlled trial of 2949 patients at high risk of intraoperative awareness compared BIS with ETAC monitoring as the mechanism for judging the depth of anesthesia. The authors failed to demonstrate a benefit of BIS monitoring compared to ETAC with respect to five endpoints: time to discharge from the postanesthesia care unit; time to postoperative recovery; length of ICU stay; incidence of postoperative nausea or vomiting; or incidence of postoperative pain.[36]

The intraoperative "triple low"

Intraoperative hypotension, reduced electroencephalogram activity (quantified by Bispectral index), and low end-tidal volatile anesthetic concentration (mean alveolar concentration [MAC]), have been postulated to be a triad of intraoperative factors associated with a poor postoperative outcome.[1] As illustrated throughout this review, a complex relationship exists among these three factors – each of which is difficult to separate from intraoperative management strategies that are heavily influenced by underlying patient characteristics. A landmark study consisting of a retrospective analysis of 24 120 patients undergoing non-cardiac surgery at a single center in the USA raised the issue of potentially deleterious intraoperative anesthetic practice causing adverse outcomes.[1] Using both "case-based" and "time-based" analyses, no association between either intraoperative hypotension or low BIS was found, consistent with the findings from other recent studies.[21,33,35] However, the population-derived definition of IOH used as part of the "case-based" analysis was substantially greater than definitions used in other studies (MAP<87mmHg). "Case-based" analysis identified associations between all three pairs of low values, for example, low MAP and low BIS, and 30-day mortality. A "double-low" was associated with an increased risk of mortality after surgery.[37] The addition of a third low value further increased the likelihood of postoperative death such that "triple low" carried a four-fold increase in mortality compared to controls. "Time-based" analysis demonstrated that the total duration of "triple-low" needed to be longer than 31 minutes in order to see a significant increase in 30-day mortality. The authors also identified increased lengths of hospital stay for patients with "triple low" durations longer than 30 minutes.[1] As this study was observational, it is clearly not possible to infer causation from the results.

Plausible hypotheses to explain the intraoperative "triple low" relationship

Various hypotheses have been put forward in an attempt to explain the associations between the intraoperative "triple low" state and postoperative mortality. The authors of the "triple low" study suggest that patients with sensitivity to volatile anesthetic agents might exhibit low BIS values at low concentrations of anesthetic, where the decrease in BIS was unexpected or uncharacteristic for the low level of anesthetic. An alternative cause of low BIS values is cerebral hypoperfusion, which might occur during periods of intraoperative hypotension. Furthermore, the degree of anesthesia or hypoperfusion induced by low BIS is likely to be more severe if the patient is particularly sensitive to the anesthetic agent, through pharmacologic interactions or genetic predisposition. Thus the "triple low" carries a greater likelihood of postoperative death when compared with pairs of low intraoperative values.[1] Alternatively, the triad of low intraoperative blood pressure, BIS, and anesthetic concentration could merely "reflect the underlying disease" state;[37] thus, existing morbidity predisposes these patients to postoperative death rather than the "triple low" itself.[37,38] For example, impaired cerebral perfusion or cerebral hypoxia may be more likely to be associated with postoperative outcome than with low BIS. The same argument is made for IOH in respect of the reason for low blood pressure; for example, the hypotension may be cardiogenic in origin or due to hypovolemia, and therefore associated with postoperative mortality.[38] If low BIS values are causally linked to postoperative mortality, a clearer mechanistic link between intraoperative BIS and postoperative outcome needs to emerge.

Summary

The impact of depth of anesthesia on perioperative outcome remains unclear. In the absence of physiologically rational measures of oxygen delivery and cellular utilization, the relevance of arbitrarily defined hypotension remains questionable. While the associations between the triad of intraoperative hypotension, reduced EEG activity quantified by bispectral index, and low concentrations of end-tidal volatile anesthetic have been linked with an increased risk of 30-day postoperative mortality and increased length of hospital stay, mechanisms responsible for these observational findings currently evade compelling pathophysiologic explanations. Adoption of cardiac output measurement (and hence oxygen delivery), and the robust determination of tissue-specific bioenergetic status, are required to help establish plausible pathophysiologic mechanism(s). In the absence of such data, further prospective exploration and validation of current clinical research findings are required to provide compelling data that result in evidence-based or empiric changes in intraoperative management.[37]

References

1. Sessler DI, Sigl JC, Kelley SD, et al. Hospital stay and mortality are increased in patients having a "triple low" of low blood pressure, low bispectral index, and low minimum alveolar concentration of volatile anesthesia. *Anesthesiology* 2012;**116**:1195–203.

2. Rampil IJ, Mason P, Singh H. Anesthetic potency (MAC) is independent of forebrain structures in the rat. *Anesthesiology* 1993;**78**:707–12.

3. Skovsted P, Price ML, Price HL. The effects of short-acting barbiturates on arterial pressure, preganglionic sympathetic activity and barostatic reflexes. *Anesthesiology* 1970;**33**:10–18.

4. Fukunaga AF, Epstein RM. Sympathetic excitation during nitrous-oxide-halothane anesthesia in the cat. *Anesthesiology* 1973;**39**:23–36.

5. Katzin DB, Rubinstein EH. Reversal of hypoxic bradycardia by halothane or midcollicular

decerebration. *Am J Physiol* 1976;**231**:179–84.

6. Blake DW, Korner PI. Effects of ketamine and Althesin Anesthesia on baroreceptor—heart rate reflex and hemodynamics of intact and pontine rabbits. *J Auton Nerv Syst* 1982;**5**:145–54.

7. Faber JE, Harris PD, Wiegman DL. Anesthetic depression of microcirculation, central hemodynamics, and respiration in decerebrate rats. *Am J Physiol* 1982;**243**:H837–43.

8. Davies RO, Edwards MW, Jr., Lahiri S. Halothane depresses the response of carotid body chemoreceptors to hypoxia and hypercapnia in the cat. *Anesthesiology* 1982;**57**:153–9.

9. Pandit JJ. The variable effect of low-dose volatile anaesthetics on the acute ventilatory response to hypoxia in humans: a quantitative review. *Anaesthesia* 2002;**57**:632–43.

10. Taylor EW, Jordan D, Coote JH. Central control of the cardiovascular and respiratory systems and their interactions in vertebrates. *Physiol Rev* 1999;**79**:855–916.

11. Messner M, Beese U, Romstock J, Dinkel M, Tschaikowsky K. The bispectral index declines during neuromuscular block in fully awake persons. *Anesth Analg* 2003;**97**:488–91.

12. Nishikawa K, Hagiwara R, Nakamura K, et al. The effects of the extent of spinal block on the BIS score and regional cerebral oxygen saturation in elderly patients: a prospective, randomized, and double-blinded study. *J Clin Monit Comput* 2007;**21**:109–14.

13. Hamilton-Davies C, Mythen MG, Salmon JB, et al. Comparison of commonly used clinical indicators of hypovolaemia with gastrointestinal tonometry. *Intens Care Med* 1997;**23**:276–81.

14. Pearse RM, Ackland GL. Perioperative fluid therapy. *BMJ* 2012;**344**:e2865.

15. Bijker JB, van Klei WA, Kappen TH, et al. Incidence of intraoperative hypotension as a function of the chosen definition: literature definitions applied to a retrospective cohort using automated data collection. *Anesthesiology* 2007;**107**:213–20.

16. Lienhart A, Auroy Y, Pequignot F, et al. Survey of anesthesia-related mortality in France. *Anesthesiology* 2006 **105**:1087–97.

17. POISE study group, Devereaux PJ, Yang H, et al. Effects of extended-release metoprolol succinate in patients undergoing non-cardiac surgery (POISE trial): a randomised controlled trial. *Lancet* 2008;**371**:1839–47.

18. Monk TG, Saini V, Weldon BC, Sigl JC. Anesthetic management and one-year mortality after noncardiac surgery. *Anesth Analg* 2005;**100**:4–10.

19. Younes RN, Rogatko A, Brennan MF. The influence of intraoperative hypotension and perioperative blood transfusion on disease-free survival in patients with complete resection of colorectal liver metastases. *Ann Surg* 1991;**214**:107–13.

20. Ziser A, Plevak DJ, Wiesner RH, et al. Morbidity and mortality in cirrhotic patients undergoing anesthesia and surgery. *Anesthesiology* 1999;**90**:42–53.

21. Bijker JB, van Klei WA, Vergouwe Y, et al. Intraoperative hypotension and 1-year mortality after noncardiac surgery. *Anesthesiology* 2009;**111**:1217–26.

22. Alcock RF, Kouzios D, Naoum C, Hillis GS, Brieger DB. Perioperative myocardial necrosis in patients at high cardiovascular risk undergoing elective non-cardiac surgery. *Heart* 2012;**98**:792–8.

23. Vascular Events In Noncardiac Surgery Patients Cohort Evaluation (VISION) Study, Devereaux PJ, Chan MT, et al. Association between postoperative troponin levels and 30-day mortality among patients undergoing noncardiac surgery. *JAMA* 2012;**307**:2295–304.

24. Walsh M, Devereaux PJ, Garg AX, et al. Relationship between intraoperative mean arterial pressure and clinical outcomes after noncardiac surgery: toward an empirical definition of hypotension. *Anesthesiology* 2013; **119**(3): 507–15.

25. Sabate S, Mases A, Guilera N, et al. Incidence and predictors of major perioperative adverse cardiac and cerebrovascular events in non-cardiac surgery. *Br J Anaesth* 2011;**107**:879–90.

26. Tassoudis V, Vretzakis G, Petsiti A, et al. Impact of intraoperative hypotension on hospital stay in major abdominal surgery. *J Anesth* 2011;**25**:492–9.

27. Thakar CV, Kharat V, Blanck S, Leonard AC. Acute kidney injury after gastric bypass surgery. *Clin J Am Soc Nephrol* 2007;**2**:426–30.

28. Monk TG, Weldon BC. Does depth of anesthesia monitoring improve postoperative outcomes? *Curr Opin Anaesthesiol* 2011;**24**:665–9.

29. Avidan MS, Jacobsohn E, Glick D, et al. Prevention of intraoperative awareness in a high-risk surgical population. *N Engl J Med* 2011;**365**:591–600.

30. Whitlock EL, Villafranca AJ, Lin N, et al. Relationship between bispectral index values and volatile anesthetic concentrations during the maintenance phase of anesthesia in the B-Unaware trial. *Anesthesiology* 2011;**115**:1209–18.

31. Punjasawadwong Y, Boonjeungmonkol N, Phongchiewboon A. Bispectral index for improving anaesthetic delivery and postoperative

recovery. *Cochrane Database Syst Rev* 2007;**CD003843**.

32. Kertai MD, Pal N, Palanca BJ, et al. Association of perioperative risk factors and cumulative duration of low bispectral index with intermediate-term mortality after cardiac surgery in the B-Unaware Trial. *Anesthesiology* 2010;**112**:1116–27.

33. Kertai MD, Palanca BJ, Pal N, et al. Bispectral index monitoring, duration of bispectral index below 45, patient risk factors, and intermediate-term mortality after noncardiac surgery

34. Leslie K, Myles PS, Forbes A, Chan MT. The effect of bispectral index monitoring on long-term survival in the B-aware trial. *Anesth Analg* 2010;**110**:816–22.

35. Lindholm ML, Traff S, Granath F, et al. Mortality within 2 years after surgery in relation to low intraoperative bispectral index values and preexisting malignant disease. *Anesth Analg* 2009;**108**:508–12.

36. Fritz BA, Rao P, Mashour GA, et al. Postoperative recovery with

in the B-Unaware Trial. *Anesthesiology* 2011 **114**:545–56.

bispectral index versus anesthetic concentration-guided protocols. *Anesthesiology* 2013;**118**:1113–22.

37. Kheterpal S, Avidan MS. "Triple low": murderer, mediator, or mirror. *Anesthesiology* 2012;**116**:1176–8.

38. Yu H, Liu B. Is "triple low" of low blood pressure, low bispectral index, and low minimum alveolar concentration of volatile anesthesia an independent predictor for postoperative mortality? *Anesthesiology* 2013;**118**:225–6.

Chapter

27

Goal directed fluid and hemodynamic therapy in cardiac surgical patients

Byron D. Fergerson and Gerard R. Manecke Jr.

Goal directed therapy (GDT) is the practice of using parameters such as stroke volume (SV), cardiac output (CO), stroke volume variation, and pulse pressure variation to optimize tissue blood flow and oxygen delivery in critically ill and high-risk surgical patients. Optimization of oxygen delivery in the perioperative period was first explored by Shoemaker, who, in the 1980s, examined the hemodynamic parameters of shock survivors, finding that they had a significantly higher cardiac index (CI), oxygen delivery (DO_2), and oxygen consumption (VO_2) than non-survivors.[1] He then hypothesized that achieving supranormal hemodynamic values in high-risk surgical patients would compensate for increased perioperative metabolic requirements, thus decreasing morbidity and mortality. His landmark paper in 1988[2] showed a significant reduction in mortality and hospital length of stay (LOS) in high-risk surgical patients managed with GDT. Other investigators have had similar results, although the "supranormal" approach to GDT is still debated.

Anesthetic management using targets and goals is standard practice. Anesthesiologists use conventional parameters such as mean arterial pressure (MAP), heart rate (HR), urine output (UOP), and more invasive ones such as central venous pressure (CVP) and pulmonary capillary wedge pressure (PCWP) as surrogates of cardiac output, preload, and oxygen delivery. They then manipulate these variables with volume administration, vasopressors, and inotropes to achieve and maintain goal values. For low- to moderate-risk patients and surgeries, normalization of these markers is probably sufficient for maintaining tissue perfusion. However, tissue hypoxia may manifest in high-risk surgical patients, despite normal conventional parameters. It is now generally accepted

that markers such as PCWP,[3] CVP,[4] UOP,[5] HR,[6] and BP[7] often do not reflect end-organ perfusion. Tissue hypoxia is a key component in activating systemic inflammatory response in postsurgical patients and may not manifest clinically for days. The objective of GDT is to use flow-directed hemodynamic parameters to guide fluid and inotropic administration to maintain adequate circulating volume and oxygen delivery. Normal tissue perfusion helps prevent systemic inflammation and end-organ dysfunction and thus reduces perioperative morbidity and mortality.[8] GDT has been evaluated in numerous randomized controlled trials, with the vast majority showing improvement in outcomes in high-risk patients undergoing non-cardiac surgery.[9] The obvious next step is to evaluate the effectiveness of GDT in the cardiothoracic surgical population. These patients represent a high-risk group that should benefit from hemodynamic optimization using "alternative" parameters.

At the time of this writing there are five studies that specifically examine the effectiveness of GDT in cardiac surgery. The first is a prospective, randomized trial by Mythen et al.[10] studying the effect of perioperative volume expansion on gut mucosal pH during cardiac surgery. Low gut mucosal pH had been previously shown to be a sensitive predictor of poor outcome in cardiac surgery.[11] Mythen studied 60 American Society of Anesthesiologists (ASA) class 3 patients presenting for elective cardiac surgery with ejection fraction (EF) of >50%, randomly allocating them to control and protocol groups. The anesthetic management of the control group was based on management using HR, MAP, UOP, and CVP. In addition to the standard practice, patients in the protocol group received 200 mL boluses of 6% hydroxyethyl starch solution based on CVP and SV measurements using esophageal Doppler. Colloid boluses were repeatedly administered throughout the pre- and postbypass period if there was evidence of an increase in SV without a significant increase in CVP. Gut mucosal perfusion was assessed by gastric tonometry. Mythen found that the incidence of gut mucosal hypoperfusion was significantly less in the protocol group (7% vs. 56%). In addition, the protocol group had fewer major complications (0 vs. 6), had shorter hospital LOS (6.4 vs. 10.1), and spent fewer days in the intensive care unit (1 vs. 1.7). The protocol group received significantly more colloid than the control group. Mythen suggested that volume expansion based on SV and CVP can reduce gut hypoperfusion and thus perioperative complications in cardiac surgery. Of note, despite significant differences in SV and gastric pH at the end of surgery, the blood pressures and heart rates were similar between groups. Moreover, the CVP was lower in the protocol group, even with the increase in fluid administration. This confirms that BP, HR, and CVP are not, in themselves, effective measures of oxygen delivery and preload.

Polonen et al.[12] studied mixed venous oxygen saturation (SvO_2) and serum lactate as parameters for GDT in the 8 hours following surgery. Four hundred and three elective cardiac surgical patients presenting for revascularization were randomly assigned to control and protocol groups. The control group was treated based on the standard institutional practice including maintenance of CI >2.5 L/min/m^2, PCWP between 12 and 18 mmHg, and MAP between 60 and 90 mmHg. The goals of the protocol group were to maintain the SvO_2 greater than 70% and serum lactate concentration below 2.0 mmol/L using fluids, adding dobutamine if fluid administration alone was ineffective. Although discharge time from the ICU was similar in both groups, the patients in the protocol group had a shorter mean hospital LOS (6 vs. 7 days) with less morbidity at the time of discharge (1.1% vs. 6.1%). Mortality between the groups was statistically similar, but showed a trend toward a reduction in the protocol patients at 28 days (2 deaths in the protocol group vs. 6 in the control group), 6 months (3 vs. 7), and 12 months (4 vs. 9). One problem with this study is that both groups were managed in a "goal directed" manner. The outcome differences between the groups thus reflect the effectiveness of the chosen goals and not GDT itself.

Another issue with this study is the similarity in outcome between the control and protocol groups when hemodynamic targets were met. Only about half the protocol patients achieved the predetermined goals. In addition, a significant portion of the control group also achieved these goals despite a lack of directed therapy. Patients who achieved these goals in both groups tended to be younger, have a better ejection fraction (EF), and were less likely to have diabetes. All patients who achieved these targets had better outcomes. Therefore, it may be that the therapy itself is not the cause of the improved outcome, but rather that the ability to achieve these hemodynamic goals is a marker for healthier patients (who will thus have better outcome).

McKendry et al.[13] studied how GDT in the postoperative period affects outcome. He randomly allocated 174 postcardiac surgery patients to either conventional hemodynamic management using BP, HR, CVP, UOP, and arterial base deficit, or protocol driven management using a stroke volume index (SVI) > 35 mL/m^2 as the goal. The protocol was nurse-directed in the ICU using esophageal Doppler. Two hundred mL colloid boluses were the primary method of optimizing the SVI, although, if unsuccessful, vasodilator or inotropic therapy was used. With this protocol McKendry showed a reduction in the hospital LOS (11.4 vs. 13.9 days). There was also a trend toward a reduction in ICU LOS and a reduction in major complications (17% vs. 26%), including atrial fibrillation and acute renal failure. The protocol group had significantly higher CO, SV, and colloid administration. Although not statistically significant, there were fewer deaths in the control group (2 vs. 4). It is important to note that only 61% of the protocol patients achieved a target SVI > 35 mL/m^2, attesting to the fact that achieving the goals in GDT can be difficult. Also of note is that 44% of the control group achieved an SVI > 35 mL/m^2.

Kapoor et al.[14] studied 27 patients with a Euro-SCORE $\geq$ 3 undergoing on-pump coronary artery bypass surgery. They randomly allocated patients to control and GDT groups. Both groups were monitored and treated throughout the intraoperative period and for up to 8 hours postoperatively. As with the earlier studies, the control group had therapy guided by BP, HR, CVP, and UOP. In addition to these parameters, the GDT group received FloTrac™ and PreSep™ monitoring to maintain the CI 2.5–4.2 L/min/m^2, SVI 30–65 mL/beat/m^2, systemic vascular resistance index (SVRI) 1500–2500 dynes/s/cm^5/m^2, oxygen delivery index (DO$_2$I) 450–600 mL/min/m^2, ScO$_2$ > 70%, and stroke volume variation (SVV) < 10% through administration of fluids, blood (if the hematocrit was < 30%), and inotropic and vasodilator agents. The GDT group received more fluids and more adjustments to their inotropic agents. The patients in the GDT group had a shorter average duration of mechanical ventilation (13.8 vs. 20.7 hours), fewer days of use of inotropic agents (1.6 vs. 3.8), shorter ICU LOS (2.6 vs 4.9 days), and shorter hospital LOS (5.6 vs. 8.9 days). Morbidity was low in both groups and there were no deaths. The authors stated the data in their study was inconclusive with regard to the benefit of GDT in cardiac surgery patients, although the study size was so small as to make any conclusions difficult. Of note, although the inotropic agents were adjusted more frequently in the GDT group, the overall duration of inotropic use was less, indicating that diligence with regards to endpoints when using cardiovascular drugs may limit the duration of their use.

Smetkin et al.[15] studied 40 patients presenting for off-pump coronary artery bypass grafting and randomized them to a control group where therapy was guided by CVP (6–14 mmHg), MAP (60–100 mmHg), and HR (< 90 beats per minute), and a GDT group guided by MAP, HR, ScO$_2$ (>60%), and intrathoracic blood volume index (850–1000 mL/m^2) assessed by transpulmonary thermodilution. Intrathoracic blood volume index (ITBVI) is an estimate of preload, SV, SVV, and extravascular pulmonary fluid.[16] Measurements were performed pre-, intra-, and 2, 4, and 6 hours postoperatively. The parameters in the GDT group were optimized by volume administration (hydroxyethylstarch) and dobutamine. The GDT group received more colloid and dobutamine with resultant increases in ScO$_2$, CI, and DO$_2$. ICU and hospital LOS were decreased by 15% and 25%, respectively in the GDT group, although these differences were not statistically significant. There were no deaths in either group. This paper, like Kapoor's, suggests that GTD may be beneficial in cardiac surgery patients and indicates that larger trials are in order.

Aya et al.[17] performed a systematic review and meta-analysis on GDT in cardiac surgery using these five articles. Taken together, these studies evaluated 699 patients and revealed a reduction in postoperative complication rate (21 patients in the GDT group vs. 51 in the control) and hospital length of stay (2.21 fewer days). As mentioned above, two of the trials had no reported deaths leaving 632 patients to evaluate mortality. The overall effect on mortality was not statistically significant. In a similar meta-analysis, Giglio et al.[18] came to the same conclusion revealing that these trials showed a reduction in postoperative complications using GDT, but no reduction in mortality.

Aya cites several limitations of the data pooled from these trials. None of these trials was considered to have a high methodological quality because of difficulty in properly double blinding. All the studies were single centered and thus subject to the effects of the patient population, operative team experience, and complexity of the surgeries performed. The overall sample size in each was small which, in the setting of a low baseline operative mortality, may explain why there was no effect on mortality, despite the fact that GDT used in high-risk non-cardiac surgery has been reported to reduce mortality.[9] The effect of the small sample size might have been reduced with pooling of the data had there not been significant heterogeneity among the five trials. Nevertheless, these trials taken as a whole suggest that GDT in cardiac surgery can reduce postoperative complication rate and thus ICU and hospital LOS.

Given that the data on the effects of GDT in improving outcome in non-cardiac surgery is so robust, where do the comparatively modest results of GDT in cardiac surgery leave us? The first thing to consider is whether we even need an alternative to the current management model. Mortality is relatively low in cardiac surgery, despite the high-risk nature of the procedures and the severity of illness in the patients. Welsby et al.[19] found a mortality rate of approximately 3.6% in cardiac patients who undergo a procedure using cardiopulmonary bypass. Shoemaker suggests that GDT is best applied to high-risk surgical patients with a predicted mortality of upwards of 20%. If mortality is the primary reason to use GDT, the low mortality rate in cardiac surgery would not warrant its use.

The rate of complications in cardiac surgery, however, remains high. Approximately 36.5% of the patients studied in Welsby's article had complications and 15.7% had an adverse outcome. In the cardiac surgery GDT trials noted above, even those with no mortality had relatively high rates of non-cardiac organ dysfunction. Welsby also showed that patients who suffered non-cardiac complications had more than twice the mortality rate of those with cardiac complications alone, and nearly seven times that of patients without complications. Looking at causes of prolonged ICU LOS after coronary artery bypass grafting (CABG), Michalopoulos et al.[20] suggested that low cardiac output syndrome, as evidenced by the need for multiple inotropes, was the primary cause of postoperative complications and thus prolonged ICU LOS. Goepfert et al.[21] showed that GDT in cardiac surgery reduces the need for vasopressor and inotropic support. It appears from these articles that tissue hypoperfusion secondary to low cardiac output and the organ dysfunction that ensues is the primary cause of complications, prolonged ICU stays, and, likely, postoperative mortality. It follows that GDT, with its primary goal being to improve cardiac output, reduces the prevalence of low cardiac output syndrome and thus non-cardiac complications and hospital LOS. Given this, it is reasonable to suspect that larger trials would show a reduction in overall mortality.

Even if GDT does not prove to reduce postoperative mortality in cardiac patients, the data currently available is enough to warrant its consideration simply from an economic standpoint. Depending on a hospital's caseload, a 1-day reduction in a cardiac surgery patient's hospital LOS can amount to hundreds of thousands to several million dollars saved annually. In addition, reduced ICU and bed usage would allow for more cases and thus more reimbursement. Probably most importantly, a reduction in complications significantly reduces the costs associated with those complications. Respiratory failure requires mechanical ventilation; renal failure requires dialysis; and neurocognitive dysfunction requires rehabilitation, just to name a few of the more expensive interventions. A reduction in complications such as these can result in enormous cost savings to the hospital.

The data for GDT in cardiac surgery argues for larger trials to determine its effectiveness. The next thing to consider is whether the additional fluid load often (although not always) associated with GDT is dangerous for cardiac surgical patients with compromised physiology. The Frank–Starling mechanism is the concept often used to describe how cardiac output varies in relation to preload. The heart is thought to increase its force of contraction in response to changes in preload up to a point. After this point, the Starling curve levels off and additional fluid does not enhance SV. Heart failure is associated with a "stretching" of the myocardium that leads to a reduction in overlapping actin and myosin units. This flattens the Starling curve, causing the point of diminishing returns and potential complications to be reached at a lower preload. For this reason, as well as the fact that cardiopulmonary bypass (CPB) machines are "primed" with fluid, fluids are often restricted in cardiac surgical patients.

There are, however, several problems with this model. The first is that the contractile response of the heart to preload is not solely based on stretching of the sarcomere. It is multifactorial and includes calcium homeostasis, neurohormonal responses, and alterations in genetic expression.[22] There is no single curve on which a ventricle operates. The contractile state of the heart can vary from day to day, even minute to minute. The second issue is that, although the Starling curve in heart failure is flatter, it is still a curve. Even the compromised myocardium can have an improved contractile response to volume.[23] Lastly, hypo- or hypervolemia is nearly impossible to predict from conventional parameters and cannot be assumed based on preoperative fasting, theoretical "third-spacing," or estimated blood loss.[24] Cardiac surgical patients can be hypovolemic and the extra fluid associated with CPB may not optimize the myocardial response. Using a flow-based parameter to aid in determining the volume and hemodynamic status in cardiac surgical patients therefore makes physiologic sense.

The use of GDT does not imply pre-existing hypovolemia. Instead, it offers additional parameters to help determine what level of venous return an individual heart requires. GDT follows the CO or other end-organ perfusion measures to determine the result of fluid administration. Moreover, fluid restriction is not at odds with the concept of GDT. One can fluid restrict by significantly limiting the background fluid administration and guide volume resuscitation solely by flow-related parameters. The key point in GDT is individualization of volume administration, not high volume resuscitation. In fact, the concept "goal directed fluid restriction" is rapidly gaining acceptance.

Cardiothoracic anesthesiologists already use (relatively invasive) flow and cardiac volume related parameters, and use goals in applying them.

Management based on CO, intracardiac volume, and ejection fraction as measured by pulmonary artery catheters and echocardiography is ubiquitous in cardiac surgery. A significant portion of the control groups in the above articles met the CO goals set for the protocol groups. In McKendry's study, 44% of the control patients met SV index goal value of > 35 mL/m^2 at 4 hours postoperatively. In Polonen's work, 42% of the control patients reached the hemodynamic goals as compared to 57% of the protocol patients. These data show two things:[1] the current standard of practice is geared toward optimizing SV and CO, and[2] depending upon the targets of GTD, optimizing flow is difficult. The question may not be whether GDT is safe and beneficial in cardiac surgery, but instead which parameters should be used to guide management.

Conclusion

Goal directed therapy is a method of managing fluid administration based on parameters that trend flow, preload responsiveness, and/or oxygen delivery. Its utility in reducing morbidity, mortality, and hospital length of stays has been conclusively shown in noncardiac surgical patients. The data for its use in cardiac patients suggest benefit as well, but are limited. Larger studies will be necessary to determine the future role of goal directed therapy in cardiac surgery patients.

References

1. Shoemaker WC, Montgomery ES, Kaplan E, Elwyn DH. Physiologic patterns in surviving and nonsurviving shock patients. Use of sequential cardiorespiratory variables in defining criteria for therapeutic goals and early warning of death. *Arch Surg* (Chicago, Il: 1960) 1973;**106**(5):630–6.

2. Shoemaker WC. Prospective trial of supranormal values of survivors as therapeutic goals in high-risk surgical patients. *Chest* 1988;**94**(6):1176.

3. Kumar A, Anel R, Bunnell E, et al. Pulmonary artery occlusion pressure and central venous pressure fail to predict ventricular filling volume, cardiac performance, or the response to volume infusion in normal subjects. *Crit Care Med* 2004;**32**(3):691–9.

4. Marik PE, Baram M, Vahid B. Does central venous pressure predict fluid responsiveness? A systematic review of the literature and the tale of seven mares. *Chest* 2008;**134**(1):172–8.

5. Alpert RA, Roizen MF, Hamilton WK, Stoney RJ. Intraoperative urinary output does not predict postoperative renal function in patients undergoing abdominal aortic revascularization. *Surgery* 1987;**15**(2):153–6.

6. Victorino GP, Battistella FD, Wisner DH. Does tachycardia correlate with hypotension after trauma? *J Am Coll Surg* 2003;**196**(5):679–84.

7. Wo CC, Shoemaker WC, Appel PL, et al. Unreliability of blood pressure and heart rate to evaluate cardiac output in emergency resuscitation and critical illness. *Crit Care Med* 1993;**21**(2):218–23.

8. Beal AL, Cerra FB. Multiple organ failure syndrome in the 1990s. Systemic inflammatory response and organ dysfunction. *JAMA* 1994;**271**(3):226–33.

9. Kern JW, Shoemaker WC. Meta-analysis of hemodynamic optimization in high-risk patients. *Crit Care Med* 2002;**30**(8):1686–92.

10. Mythen MG, Webb AR. Perioperative plasma volume expansion reduces the incidence of gut mucosal hypoperfusion during cardiac surgery. *Arch Surg* (Chicago, Il : 1960) 1995;**130**(4):423–9.

11. Fiddian-Green RG, Baker S. Predictive value of the stomach wall pH for complications after cardiac operations: comparison with other monitoring. *Crit Care Med* 1987;**15**(2):153–6.

12. Polonen P, Ruokonen E, Hippelainen M, Poyhonen M, Takala J. A prospective, randomized study of goal-oriented hemodynamic therapy in cardiac surgical patients. *Anesth Analg* 2000;**90**(5):1052–9.

13. McKendry M. Randomised controlled trial assessing the impact of a nurse delivered, flow monitored protocol for optimisation of circulatory status after cardiac surgery. *BMJ (Clin Res Ed)* 2004;**329**(7460):258–60.

14. Kapoor PM, Kakani M, Chowdhury U, et al. Early goal-directed therapy in moderate to high-risk cardiac surgery patients. *Ann Card Anaesth* 2008;**11**(1):27–34.

15. Smetkin AA, Kirov MY, Kuzkov VV, et al. Single transpulmonary thermodilution and continuous monitoring of central venous oxygen saturation during off-pump coronary surgery. *Acta Anaesth Scand* 2009;**53**(4):505–14.

16. Reuter DA, Felbinger TW, Moerstedt K, et al. Intrathoracic blood volume index measured by thermodilution for preload monitoring after cardiac surgery. *Yjcan*, 2002;**16**(2):191–5.

17. Aya HD, Cecconi M, Hamilton M, Rhodes A. Goal-directed therapy in cardiac surgery: a systematic

review and meta-analysis. *Br J Anaesth* 2013;**110**(**4**):510–17.

18. Giglio M, Dalfino L, Puntillo F, et al. Haemodynamic goal-directed therapy in cardiac and vascular surgery. A systematic review and meta-analysis. *Interac CardioVasc Thor Surg* 2012;**15**(**5**):878–87.

19. Welsby IJ, Bennett-Guerrero E, Atwell D, et al. The association of complication type with mortality and prolonged stay after cardiac surgery with cardiopulmonary bypass. *Anesth Analg* 2002;**94**(**5**):1072–8.

20. Michalopoulos A, Tzelepis G, Pavlides G, et al. Determinants of duration of ICU stay after coronary artery bypass graft surgery. *Br J Anaesth* 1996;**77**(**2**):208–12.

21. Goepfert MSG, Reuter DA, Akyol D, et al. Goal-directed fluid management reduces vasopressor and catecholamine use in cardiac surgery patients. *Intens Care Med* 2006;**33**(**1**):96–103.

22. Katz AM. The "modern" view of heart failure: how did we get here? *Circ Heart Failure* 2008;**1**(**1**):63–71.

23. Holubarsch C, Ruf T, Goldstein DJ, et al. Existence of the Frank–Starling mechanism in the failing human heart. Investigations on the organ, tissue, and sarcomere levels. *Circulation* 1996;**94**(**4**):683–9.

24. Doherty M, Buggy DJ. Intraoperative fluids: how much is too much? *Br J Anaesth* 2012;**109**(**1**):69–79.

Chapter

28

Goal directed therapy and hemodynamic optimization in the critical care setting: practical applications and benefits

Trung Vu, Davinder Ramsingh, William Wilson, and Maxime Cannesson

Introduction

In the operating room and in the intensive care units, the optimization of a patient's hemodynamics is key to improving morbidity and mortality. Evidence suggests that either too little or too much fluid administration during the perioperative period can worsen tissue perfusion and oxygenation leading to organ dysfunction. Further, this impairment may not be reliably revealed by alterations in conventional hemodynamic indices such as heart rate, urine output, central venous pressure, or blood pressure. Numerous investigative studies in a spectrum of patient populations (sepsis, cardiovascular surgery, trauma, and other critical illnesses) have challenged the notion that these indicators accurately predict volume status.[1–7] **Goal directed therapy (GDT) is the concept of using indices of continuous blood flow and/or tissue oxygen saturation to optimize end-organ function.** By using the flow-related parameters, such as stroke volume (SV), cardiac output (CO), and markers of fluid responsiveness such as stroke volume variation (SVV), pleth variability index (PVI), and corrected aortic flow time (FTc), one is able to precisely infer where the patient is on their Frank–Starling relationship, and thus, optimize oxygen delivery. Similarly, by using markers of tissue oxygenation/extraction, such as central venous saturation (ScvO$_2$) and somatic tissue oxygenation (StO$_2$), one is able to provide GDT therapy to improve end-organ oxygenation. The body of evidence in favor of GDT continues to grow; therefore, GDT is rapidly becoming the standard of care in the ICU, emergency department, and in the operating rooms.

Goal directed therapy in the ICU and in the emergency department

Shoemaker et al. were one of the first to show that, in the critically ill patient, one should treat by physiologic criteria, and administration of therapy should be monitored to attain optimal physiologic goals.[8] These concepts have been advanced by the landmark study by Rivers et al. that showed improved patient outcome using early goal directed therapy based on a protocol maintaining ScvO$_2$ >70% during treatment of severe sepsis and septic shock.[9] Pearse et al. showed that it is possible to bridge intraoperative GDT to the ICU, and by maximizing patients' oxygen delivery index, postoperative complications and duration of postoperative hospital stay can be decreased.[10] This has been extensively discussed earlier in this book.

With regard to this, emergency physicians in the perioperative period serve a key role in recognition of early disease presentation and the implementation of GDT therapy. During the past few years, several randomized, controlled trials in patients with severe sepsis and septic shock have demonstrated significant reductions in mortality rates with the institution of GDT therapies.[9,11]

While these have shown the importance of hemodynamic flow guided indices, there are still many areas of clinical practice that need to be further developed. These include the more widespread use of SV optimization algorithms in the intensive care and emergency departments.

Perioperative Hemodynamic Monitoring and Goal Directed Therapy, ed. Maxime Cannesson and Rupert Pearse.
Published by Cambridge University Press. © Cambridge University Press 2014.

GDT in the perioperative period

The use of flow-related indices to guide intraoperative goal directed fluid therapy has appeal, since these parameters provide a numeric representation of the patient's volume status, which can frequently be difficult to ascertain using standard hemodynamic monitors, urine output, or even CVP.[12–14] Gan et al. in 2002 reported earlier return of bowel function, lower incidence of postoperative nausea and vomiting, and decrease in length of hospital stay in patients whose stroke volume was optimized using an esophageal Doppler.[15] Intraoperative GDT has also reported to improve outcomes following surgery in high-risk patients, decreasing both morbidity and length of hospital stay.[16–19] Previously published studies have shown decreased complications and hospital length of stay in high-risk patients undergoing major abdominal surgery with SVV guided GDT therapy.[20–22] In addition, similar results have been shown in non-high-risk surgical patients undergoing elective total hip arthroplasty[23] and major abdominal surgery.[22] These studies support that the use of flow-guided parameters can aid in continuous maintenance of a euvolemic state by indicating the appropriate timing of fluid administration and improve postoperative outcome.[24–26]

Fluid administration

Optimal fluid administration in the critically ill patient is important because prior reports indicate that both hypo- and hypervolemia may deleteriously affect perioperative organ function. High volume perioperative fluid therapy has been shown to have deleterious effects on cardiac and pulmonary function, recovery of gastrointestinal motility (postoperative ileus), tissue oxygenation, wound healing, and coagulation. On the other hand, one of the major concerns with intraoperative fluid restriction is unrecognized hypovolemia resulting in organ dysfunction, particularly postoperative acute renal failure. Given these considerations, the primary resuscitation goal in the critical patient is to restore tissue perfusion/cellular oxygenation, and maintain end-organ function through volume resuscitation. The optimal resuscitation fluid, however, remains a subject of debate.

The decision whether to use crystalloid versus colloid as the primary resuscitation fluid in the critically ill remains contentious. Two previous meta-analyses of the numerous prospective clinical trials

in this area suggested that colloid resuscitation may be associated with increased patient mortality. A large multicenter, randomized, double-blind trial, however, documented the safety of colloid-based resuscitation using albumin, but failed to demonstrate either an economic or survival benefit to such therapy.[27] The SAFE study authors subsequently performed a post hoc analysis of their data to confirm the suggestion that albumin is associated with a higher mortality rate in patients with traumatic brain injury (TBI).[28] These studies do not refute the fact that: (1) colloids remain intravascular longer than crystalloids, (2) colloids expand plasma volume to a greater extent, and (3) crystalloids are more likely to cause edema formation.

Protocols for goal directed therapy

Many protocols have been proposed for goal directed therapy in the critical care setting. While they are relatively clear for the management of the septic patient in the emergency department and in the intensive care unit (i.e., the Rivers protocol is the most widely accepted), the range of protocols available for the perioperative setting is much wider and depends mainly on the patient's vascular access and the availability of the monitors. Recently, the European Society of Anaesthesiology has released recommended protocols for perioperative goal directed therapy during surgery.[29] These protocols as well as others are presented below.

GDT protocols in the intensive care unit and the emergency department

In the intensive care unit and in the emergency department, the Rivers protocol for the management of the septic patient has been widely accepted. This protocol is presented here as Figure 28.1. This protocol relies on the early optimization of mean arterial pressure, central venous pressure, and ScvO$_2$. The interventions used in this protocol are volume expansion in order to keep central venous pressure between 8 and 12 mmHg, vasopressors to maintain mean arterial pressure between 65 and 90 mmHg, and transfusion and/or inotropes to keep ScvO$_2$ more than 70%. The implementation of this protocol within 6 hours following the diagnosis of sepsis has been shown to decrease mortality in this setting. (Figure 28.1)[9]

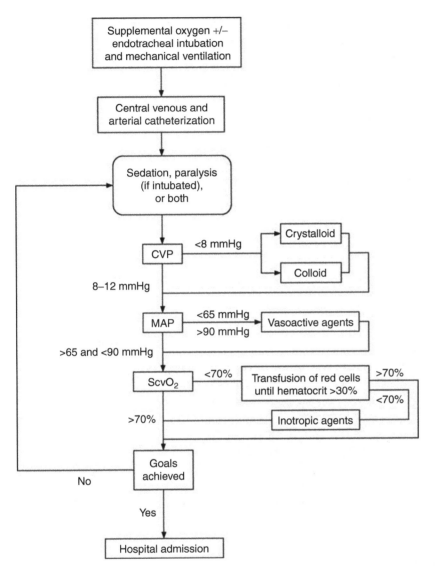

Figure 28.1. Goal directed therapy protocol developed by Emmanuel Rivers for sepsis.[9]

GDT protocol in the operating room

The first step in the operating room is to identify the patient's risk and then to define the vascular access. Then, based on the vascular access, the monitoring approach is chosen and the hemodynamic optimization protocol is applied. Figure 28.2 is a suggestion for the choice of the hemodynamic monitoring system based on patient's risk and vascular access. In all proposed GDT protocols, baseline crystalloid administration ranges from 1.5 to 5 mL/kg/h and additional fluid boluses are based on physiological endpoints and driven by the protocol.

Protocol for low-risk surgery

Patients ASA 1 or 2, with expected blood loss less than 500 mL.

Surgeries: breast, stomatology, ophthalmology, gynecology, endocrinology (except pheochromocytoma and carcinoid tumor), plastic surgery, minor orthopedic surgery, minor urology surgery.

Vascular access: one or two peripheral IV.

Monitoring: standard ASA monitors +/–respiratory variations in the plethysmographic waveform (pleth variability index) if the conditions of applications are met (sinus rhythm, general anesthesia with mechanical ventilation, tidal volume > 7 mL/kg).

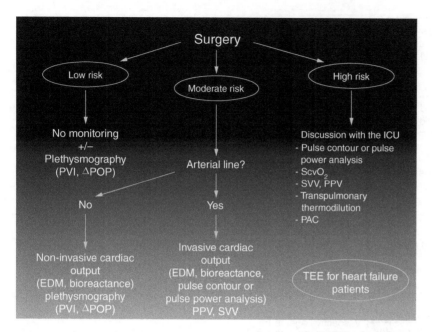

Figure 28.2. Proposed algorithm developed and implemented at the University of California Irvine for the choice of hemodynamic monitoring during sugery.
PVI: pleth variability index, ΔPOP: respiratory variations in the pulse oxymeter waveform, EDM: esophageal Doppler monitor, PPV: respiratory variations in pulse pressure, SVV: respiratory variations in stroke volume, ScvO$_2$: central venous oxygen saturation, PAC: pulmonary artery catheter, TEE: trans esophageal echocardiography.

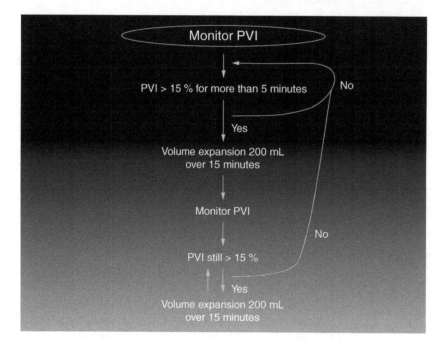

Figure 28.3. Goal directed therapy protocol based on pleth variability index. Adapted from Forget et al.[30]

The protocol for fluid administration is shown in Figure 28.3. The goal is to use a baseline crystalloid administration of 3 to 5 mL/kg/h and to titrate volume expansion based on the pleth variability index (PVI).[30]

Protocol for moderate and high-risk surgery in a patient who is not equipped with an arterial line

Patients ASA 2 or 3, with expected blood loss less than 1500 mL.

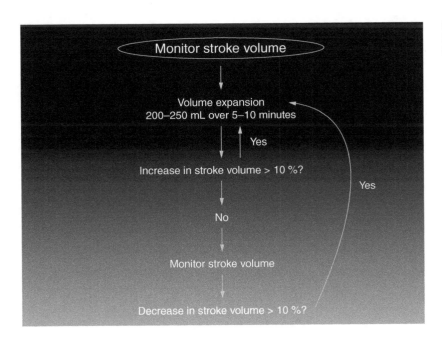

Figure 28.4. NICE Protocol.[31] Recommended by the European Society of Anaesthesiology.[29]

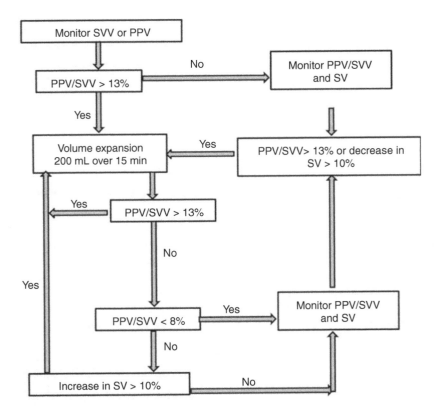

Figure 28.5. Goal directed therapy protocol based on PPV/SVV and stroke volume monitoring based on the gray zone approach.[32] Adapted from the Gan et al. protocol.[15]

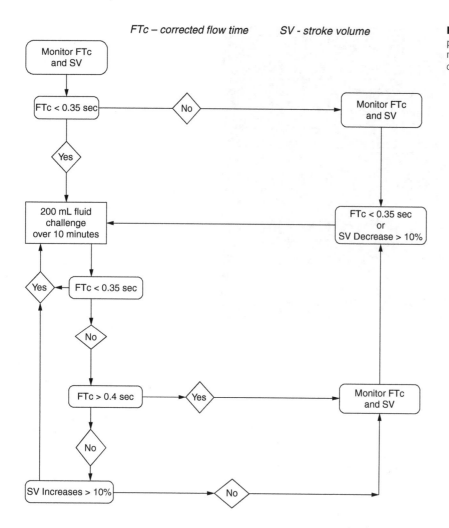

FTc – corrected flow time   *SV - stroke volume*

Figure 28.6. Goal directed therapy protocol based on esophageal Doppler monitoring using stroke volume (SV) and corrected flow time (FTc).[15]

Surgeries: vascular, abdominal, peripheral angiography, head and neck, major orthopedic and gynecology surgery, urology.

Vascular access: one or two peripheral IV ± central venous access with or without venous oxygen saturation monitoring.

Monitoring: standard ASA monitors +/–respiratory variations in the plethysmographic waveform (pleth variability index) if the conditions of applications are met (sinus rhythm, general anesthesia with mechanical ventilation, tidal volume > 6 mL/kg) and/ or non-invasive cardiac output monitoring.

If a non-invasive cardiac output monitor is used, the NICE protocol can be applied (see Figure 28.4). The goal is to titrate fluid administration in order to maximize stroke volume.

Protocol for moderate and high-risk surgery in a patient equipped with an arterial line

Monitoring: standard ASA monitors +/–stroke volume variation or pulse pressure variation (sinus rhythm, general anesthesia with mechanical ventilation, tidal volume > 6 mL/kg) and/or cardiac output monitoring based on arterial pressure waveform monitoring (pulse contour analysis or pulse power analysis) or non-invasive cardiac output monitor (esophageal Doppler or bioreactance).

In this case, stroke volume can be optimized using the NICE protocol[31] released in March 2011 by the National Health Service in the UK (see Figure 28.4), in conjunction with SVV or PPV monitoring (Figure 28.5), or following the Gan et al. algorithm (Figure 28.6).[15] If only pulse pressure variation is monitored, a PPV

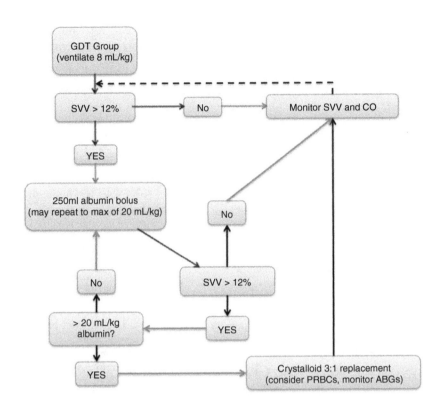

Figure 28.7. Goal directed therapy protocol based on PPV/SVV alone (adapted from Ramsingh et al.).[22] Recommended by the European Society of Anaesthesiology.[29]

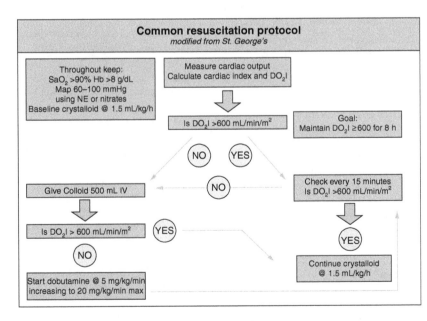

Figure 28.8. Modified version of the St. George's protocol based on oxygen delivery index.[10] Recommended by the European Society of Anaesthesiology.[29] In all cases, standard hemodynamic management for arterial pressure, urine output, and heart rate must be respected.

minimization protocol aimed at keeping PPV/SVV below 13% can be used (Figure 28.7).[22]

If oxygen delivery index is monitored, a GDT protocol including this variable has been shown to improve outcome in high-risk surgery patients (Figure 28.8).[10]

Conclusions

We believe that GDT is a powerful clinical approach for managing critically ill patients. Evidence supporting the role of GDT in improving patient outcomes is becoming well established. Further implementation of protocols of GDT will likely provide consolidation and streamlining of care for the patients by minimizing variability in clinical practice. This also has potential for improving resource utilization while implementing evidence-based medicine.

References

1. Bendjelid K, Romand JA. Fluid responsiveness in mechanically ventilated patients: a review of indices used in intensive care. *Intens Care Med* 2003;**29**(3):352–60.

2. Diebel L, Wilson RF, Heins J, et al. End-diastolic volume versus pulmonary artery wedge pressure in evaluating cardiac preload in trauma patients. *J Trauma* 1994;**37**(6):950–5.

3. Hollenberg SM, Ahrens TS, Annane D, et al. Practice parameters for hemodynamic support of sepsis in adult patients: 2004 update. *Crit Care Med* 2004;**32**(9):1928–48.

4. Kumar A, Anel R, Bunnell E, et al. Pulmonary artery occlusion pressure and central venous pressure fail to predict ventricular filling volume, cardiac performance, or the response to volume infusion in normal subjects. *Crit Care Med* 2004;**32**(3):691–9.

5. Michard F, Teboul JL. Predicting fluid responsiveness in ICU patients: a critical analysis of the evidence. *Chest* 2002;**121**(6):2000–8.

6. Osman D, Ridel C, Ray P, et al. Cardiac filling pressures are not appropriate to predict hemodynamic response to volume challenge. *Crit Care Med* 2007;**35**(1):64–8.

7. Tavernier B, Makhotine O, Lebuffe G, Dupont J, Scherpereel P. Systolic pressure variation as a guide to fluid therapy in patients with sepsis-induced hypotension. *Anesthesiology* 1998;**89**(6):1313–21.

8. Shoemaker WC, Appel P, Bland R. Use of physiologic monitoring to predict outcome and to assist in clinical decisions in critically ill postoperative patients. *Am J Surg* 1983;**146**(1):43–50.

9. Rivers E, Nguyen B, Havstad S, et al. Early goal-directed therapy in the treatment of severe sepsis and septic shock. *N Engl J Med* 2001;**345**(19):1368–77.

10. Pearse R, Dawson D, Fawcett J, et al. Early goal-directed therapy after major surgery reduces complications and duration of hospital stay. A randomised, controlled trial {ISRCTN38797445}. *Crit Care* 2005;**9**:R687–93.

11. Bernard GR, Vincent JL, Laterre PF, et al. Efficacy and safety of recombinant human activated protein C for severe sepsis. *N Engl J Med* 2001;**344**(10):699–709.

12. Gelman S. Venous function and central venous pressure: a physiologic story. *Anesthesiology* 2008;**108**(4):735–48.

13. Marik PE, Baram M, Vahid B. Does central venous pressure predict fluid responsiveness? A systematic review of the literature and the tale of seven mares. *Chest* 2008;**134**(1):172–8.

14. Howell MD, Donnino M, Clardy P, Talmor D, Shapiro NI. Occult hypoperfusion and mortality in patients with suspected infection. *Intens Care Med* 2007;**33**(11):1892–9.

15. Gan TJ, Soppitt A, Maroof M, et al. Goal-directed intraoperative fluid administration reduces length of hospital stay after major surgery. *Anesthesiology* 2002;**97**(4):820–6.

16. Abbas SM, Hill AG. Systematic review of the literature for the use of oesophageal Doppler monitor for fluid replacement in major abdominal surgery. *Anaesthesia* 2008;**63**(1):44–51.

17. Bundgaard-Nielsen M, Holte K, Secher NH, Kehlet H. Monitoring of peri-operative fluid administration by individualized goal-directed therapy. *Acta Anaesthesiol Scand* 2007;**51**(3):331–40.

18. Giglio MT, Marucci M, Testini M, Brienza N. Goal-directed haemodynamic therapy and gastrointestinal complications in major surgery: a meta-analysis of randomized controlled trials. *Br J Anaesth* 2009;**103**(5):637–46.

19. Rahbari NN, Zimmermann JB, Schmidt T, et al. Meta-analysis of standard, restrictive and supplemental fluid administration in colorectal surgery. *Br J Surg* 2009;**96**(4):331–341.

20. Lees N, Hamilton M, Rhodes A. Clinical review: Goal-directed therapy in high risk surgical patients. *Crit Care* 2009;**13**(5):231.

21. Mayer J, Boldt J, Mengistu AM, Rohm KD, Suttner S. Goal-directed intraoperative therapy based on autocalibrated arterial pressure waveform analysis reduces hospital stay in high-risk surgical patients: a randomized, controlled trial. *Crit Care* 2010;**14**(1):R18.

22. Ramsingh DS, Sanghvi C, Gamboa J, Cannesson M, Applegate RL, 2nd. Outcome impact of goal directed fluid therapy during high risk abdominal surgery in low to moderate risk patients: a randomized controlled trial. *J Clin Monit Comput* 2013;**27**(3):249–57.

23. Cecconi M, Fasano N, Langiano N, et al. Goal-directed haemodynamic therapy during elective total hip arthroplasty under regional anaesthesia. *Crit Care* 2011;**15**(3):R132.

24. Hamilton MA, Cecconi M, Rhodes A. A systematic review and meta-analysis on the use of preemptive hemodynamic intervention to improve postoperative outcomes in moderate and high-risk surgical patients. *Anesth Analg* 2011;**112** (6):1392–402.

25. Knott A, Pathak S, McGrath JS, et al. Consensus views on implementation and measurement of enhanced recovery after surgery in England: Delphi study. *BMJ Open* 2012;**2**(6): ii.

26. Moonesinghe SR, Mythen MG, Grocott MP: High-risk surgery: epidemiology and outcomes. *Anesth Analg* 2011;**112** (4):891–901.

27. Finfer S, Bellomo R, Boyce N, et al. A comparison of albumin and saline for fluid resuscitation in the intensive care unit. *N Engl J Med* 2004;**350** (22):2247–56.

28. Myburgh J, Cooper DJ, Finfer S, et al. Saline or albumin for fluid resuscitation in patients with traumatic brain injury. *N Engl J Med* 2007;**357**(9):874–84.

29. Perioperative goal directed therapy protocol summary {http://html.esahq.org/ patientsafetykit/resources/ downloads/05_Checklists/ Various_Checklists/ Perioperative_Goal_ Directed_Therapy_ Protocols.pdf}.

30. Forget P, Lois F, de Kock M. Goal-directed fluid management based on the pulse oximeter – Derived Pleth Variability Index reduces lactate levels and improves fluid management. *Anesth Analg* 2010;**111**:910–14.

31. NICE draft guidance on cardiac output monitoring device published for consultation {http://www.nice.org.uk/ newsroom/pressreleases/ DraftGuidanceOnCardiac OutputMonitoringDevice.jsp}.

32. Cannesson M, Le Manach Y, Hofer CK, et al. Assessing the diagnostic accuracy of pulse pressure variations for the prediction of fluid responsiveness: a "gray zone" approach. *Anesthesiology* 2011;**115**:896–7.

Chapter

29

Goal directed therapy at the bedside: the nurse perspective

Elizabeth J. Bridges and Debra R. Metter

The "Consensus of 16" paper outlined principles for hemodynamic monitoring, including that hemodynamic data must be relevant to the patient, sufficiently accurate to influence therapeutic decision making and that changes in care related to the data must improve patient outcomes.[1] Nurses play a role in ensuring each of these principles is met. Specifically, the nursing role in goal directed therapy requires knowledge of the pathophysiology of the process being managed and the goals for the condition, the principles underlying the goals, and strategies to achieve the goals. Nurses also have a responsibility for the correct performance of the measurements and monitoring outcomes of therapeutic interventions. This chapter addresses commonly asked questions related to the monitoring and interpretation of indicators used routinely in goal directed therapy for conditions, such as septic shock, and cardiac and general surgery.[2–4]

Blood pressure

Three aspects of blood pressure (BP) monitoring are frequent sources of questions: (1) which BP to believe, the invasive arterial pressure (IAP) or the non-invasive BP (NIBP), (2) does an increase in BP indicate an improvement in perfusion, and (3) are the forearm and upper arm BP measurements interchangeable.

Arterial blood pressure versus non-invasive blood pressure – which to believe?

The practice of using oscillometric brachial BP to determine if an arterial pressure monitoring system is accurate (i.e., the radial IAP and NIBP must be within 10 mmHg) is not evidence based.[5] Under healthy conditions, as the pulse pressure wave moves toward the periphery, the SBP increases, the diastolic

BP (DBP) decreases, and the mean arterial pressure (MAP) is relatively unchanged;[6] thus, the assumption that the radial SBP and the brachial SBP should be the same is incorrect.[7,8] In a study of 825 critically ill patients, at an SBP greater than 95 mmHg, the NIBP SBP was lower than the IAP; however, in hypotensive states, the NIBP SBP was higher than IAP, with increased bias with more severe hypotension. In contrast, the bias for the MAP was similar, despite the severity of hypotension.[8] There was wide variability in the bias for all pressures, which indicates that, for any given BP, the NIBP may underestimate, overestimate, or be the same as the IAP, negating the use of a standard correction.

Another aspect of correct BP measurement is attention to the technical details of each method.[9] For example, optimizing the dynamic response characteristics of the IAP system, through actions such as removing air bubbles and simplifying the system as appropriate,[10,11] improves the accuracy of the measurements. Correctly referencing the system to the phlebostatic axis is imperative.[11] Similarly, the NIBP measurements should be optimized through the use of a correct cuff size, placement and position, and supporting the arm at heart level.[9,12–16]

Does an increase in BP indicate an improvement in perfusion?

A vasopressor-induced increase in MAP is not always indicative of improved perfusion. In patients with septic shock, a norepinephrine-induced increase in MAP > 65 mmHg improved perfusion only in patients who also demonstrated a concurrent improvement in microcirculation.[17–19] In contrast, in patients with septic shock with normalized microcirculation after initial volume resuscitation, a further increase in MAP

Perioperative Hemodynamic Monitoring and Goal Directed Therapy, ed. Maxime Cannesson and Rupert Pearse.
Published by Cambridge University Press. © Cambridge University Press 2014.

did not improve perfusion.[20] Evaluation of microcirculatory state, for example, using tissue oxygen saturation (StO_2) response to a vascular occlusion test in conjunction with macrocirculatory indicators, may provide a bedside method to tailor therapy.[20,21]

Are the forearm and upper arm BP measurements interchangeable?

Questions arise regarding the use of forearm blood versus brachial BP under conditions where the upper arm is not available. In 51 severely obese surgical patients,[22] the forearm SBP overestimated the IAP-SBP (6 ± 16 mmHg, 95% LOA – 25 to 40 mmHg) and underestimated the DBP (2 ± 11 mmHg, 95% LOA – 10 to 18 mmHg). In the same patients, the forearm SBP overestimated the upper arm SBP (13 ± 14 mmHg, 95% LOA – 47 to 31 mmHg) and underestimated the DBP (4 ± 7 mmHg, 95% LOA – 11.5 to 29 mmHg). These results are similar to other studies conducted in acute and critically ill patients,[23,24] and demonstrate that forearm BP is not interchangeable with other sites. If forearm BP is used, the site should be documented in the record to ensure consistency of measurements. Technical aspects of forearm BP measurements include correct positioning of the arm (supported at the level of the heart), correct cuff size (guidelines for forearm BP cuff size are similar to the guidelines for upper arm circumference)[14] and cuff position (centered between the elbow and wrist).

Central venous pressure

Although CVP is not an accurate predictor of fluid responsiveness,[25] it remains a target for septic shock resuscitation and may be useful in the diagnosis of right heart failure. If a central line is not available, the question arises whether peripheral venous pressure (PVP), which is obtained from a catheter in the dorsum of the hand or forearm, is an accurate alternative. In ventilated and spontaneously breathing patients, and in a variety of surgeries (neurosurgical, laparoscopic colorectal, cardiac, renal and hepatic transplant) and positions (supine, Fowlers, prone, Trendelenburg),[26-32] the PVP-CVP bias (~2–3 mmHg) was statistically, but not clinically significant, and the PVP-CVP were highly correlated over time. If PVP is used, continuity between the peripheral catheter tip and central circulation must be ascertained by noting an increase in the PVP in response to a sustained inspiratory breath,[33] Valsalva maneuver,[34] or circumferential occlusion of the arm proximal to the catheter.[28] If continuity is present, the PVP closely approximates the CVP (bias 2 ± 1 mmHg).[35] If continuity is absent, the PVP is not an accurate indirect measurement of CVP (bias 13 ± 4 mmHg).[33] Other factors that may affect agreement include low filling pressures, severe hypotension, and non-sinus rhythms.[32] There is limited research on the PVP-CVP agreement in the ICU or postoperative setting. One study found poor PVP-CVP agreement in patients in the PACU in contrast to their OR measurements,[29] highlighting the importance of attention to the technical aspects of monitoring. Specifically, the transducer should be leveled at the phlebostatic axis and measurements obtained at end-expiration. To further optimize the PVP, the arm and shoulder should be in a neutral position, if possible.[36] No significant differences were found if the peripheral catheter was in the dorsum versus the forearm, although there was an increased bias with a smaller catheter.[30]

Use of femoral venous pressure (FVP) as an alternative for CVP has also been questioned. A systematic review[37] found that, on average, the IVC pressure is 0.5 mmHg lower than SVC. A recent postcardiac arrest study[38] found good agreement between the SVC-CVP and pressure from a femoral endovascular cooling catheter (bias −0.45 mmHg; 95% LOA −2.9 to 2.1 mmHg). Similarly, in ICU patients,[39] the bias between the FVP and CVP was small (1.1 ± 2.4 mmHg), but there was a potentially clinically significant lack of precision (95% LOA − 3.8 to 5.9 mmHg). In the latter study, intrathoracic pressure did not affect the agreement; but the FVP was directly related to intra-abdominal pressure. The FVP-CVP also varies with 30-degree head of bed elevation (bias = 0.4 mmHg; 95% LOA – 10.0 to 10.8 mmHg) compared to 0-degree elevation (bias = −1.9 mmHg; 95% LOA – 10.3 to 6.5 mmHg).[40] Based on these studies, FVP can be recommended only in supine patients without increased intra-abdominal pressure.

Another alternative if a central line is not available is to measure the CVP via a peripherally inserted central venous catheter (PICC). Only a small number of studies evaluated the agreement between the PICC-CVP and central line CVP, but all found good agreement and correlation in perioperative and ICU patients.[41-44] For example, in hepatic transplant patients there was good agreement (bias = 0.14 mmHg, 95% LOA = −1.7 to 2.0) and correlation ($r = 0.97$, $P < 0.001$) across the phases of surgery. Similarly in ICU patients,[42,43] there was good agreement (bias = 1 ± 3.2 mmHg) and correlation (r = 0.99).[43] Recently, in a study of ten critically ill patients using a Bard PowerPICC, the mean difference between the PICC and CVC was 0.17 ± 1.1 mmHg (NS).[26] This study is important, as the Power-PICC has an internal valve in contrast to all previous research, which used open-ended catheters. Technical aspects of monitoring using the PICC include correct position of the catheter tip in the SVC, use of a continuous infusion (i.e., 3 mL/hr)[42] and referencing the transducer at the phlebostatic axis.[45] There are anecdotal reports that creation of a no-flow state by turning off the stopcock eliminates any difference between the PICC-CVP and central line CVP; however, this recommendation has not been studied. A slow downslope in the pressure waveform after flushing and a damped waveform suggest PICC occlusion, which must be resolved to ensure accuracy of the PICC-CVP.

Pulmonary artery pressure monitoring

A recent meta-analysis[46] concluded that the use of a PA catheter did not affect patient outcomes. However, the debate continues regarding the interpretation of studies that solely evaluate the presence of a PA catheter versus efficacy studies involving the systematic integration of data from the PAC into care decisions.[47] The PA catheter remains an important diagnostic tool in complex cases, such as right ventricular dysfunction, fluid management and cardiac failure.[1] A challenge facing clinicians is that, with the decreased use of PA catheters, there may be a lack of familiarity with both the technical and clinical aspects of monitoring. Standardized, evidence-based protocols are available and address various factors including setting up the pressure monitoring system, referencing, zeroing, positioning the patient, measuring PA and CVP relative to the ventilatory cycle and interpretation of analog waveforms.[48]

Functional hemodynamics

There is a growing body of literature supporting the use of functional hemodynamic indicators (systolic pressure variation – SPV; pulse pressure variation – PPV; stroke volume variation – SVV; pleth variability index – PVI) to assess fluid responsiveness and guide fluid therapy.[49,50] While there are proprietary technologies available for continuous measurements, it is also possible to obtain accurate intermittent SPV and PPV measurements directly from the bedside using the stop-cursor method;[51] however, the "eyeball" technique is

not accurate.[52] Awareness of technical aspects for the correct monitoring and interpretation of these various indicators is imperative.[53]

Functional indicators (SPV, PPV, SVV, and PVI) cannot be obtained in all patients. The patient must be intubated and ventilated and the acronym SOS (**S**mall tidal volume [< 8 mL/kg]/**S**pontaneous ventilation, **O**pen chest, and **S**ustained arrhythmias) identifies the major limiting factors.[54] In these cases, a passive leg-raising maneuver may be useful in assessing the patient's fluid response status.[55–58] Other factors that affect functional hemodynamic indicators are summarized in Table 29.1.

SvO$_2$, ScvO$_2$ and SfvO$_2$ – are they interchangeable?

SvO$_2$ and ScvO$_2$ are commonly used in goal directed resuscitation,[2] but they are not interchangeable. Although the ScvO$_2$ and SvO$_2$ correlate over time,[81–84] the correlation may vary depending on the absolute ScvO$_2$.[82] On average, the ScvO$_2$ is 4%–7% higher than the SvO$_2$, meaning an ScvO$_2$ of 65% indicates a critically low SvO$_2$.[83] However, there is considerable variability in the difference between the measurements. The ScvO$_2$ value may be as much as 16% higher or 6% lower than the SvO$_2$; thus, simply correcting for the difference is not supported.[81,82,85] Similarly, femoral venous O$_2$ saturation (SfvO$_2$) is not interchangeable with ScvO$_2$ or SvO$_2$.[39,86,87] In stable patients undergoing cardiac catheterization, the bias between the SvO$_2$ and SfvO$_2$ was 2.1% ± 7.9% (95% LOA − 13.0% to 17.5%). In surgical patients the SfvO$_2$ was lower than the ScvO$_2$ (bias −1.9% ± 9.3%; 95% LOA − 20.0% to 16.3%), whereas in ICU patients with cardiogenic or septic shock, the SfvO$_2$ overestimated the ScvO$_2$ (bias 4.6% ± 14.3%; 95% LOA − 23.5% to 32.6%).

Lactate

In the setting of shock, an increase in lactate is most likely related to hypoxia or decreased clearance, although other factors causes should be considered.[88,89] A question is whether arterial and venous lactate are interchangeable. Under stable conditions, lactate obtained from peripheral, central venous, and arterial sites are interchangeable and trend over time.[90–92] However, during unstable conditions, such as acute hemorrhage[93] or septic shock,[90] there is an increased difference between the measurements. For example, in patients with septic shock,[90] there was increased bias

Table 29.1. Other factors that affect functional hemodynamic indicators

Intra-abdominal hypertension	SPV, PPV, and SVV are sensitive and specific predictors of fluid responsiveness with increased intra-abdominal pressure; however, the threshold increases.[59–62] In an animal study, the PPV threshold increased from 11.5% at baseline (IAP = 7 mmHg) to $\geq$ 20.5% (IAP = 25 mmHg). PPV remained a sensitive (75%) and specific (83%) predictor of fluid responsiveness at IAP = 25 mmHg.
Ventilator mode	There is limited research on the effect of ventilator modes on functional indicators. • *Spontaneous intermittent mandatory ventilation (SIMV):* PPV and SVV measurements obtained during SIMV were similar to those obtained during volume controlled ventilation (VCV) • *Pressure support ventilation:* SVV did not discriminate between responders and non-responders (AUC 0.56).[63,64] • *Volume controlled ventilation:* SVV threshold higher in VCV patients compared to pressure controlled ventilation.[65] • *High frequency ventilation*[66] – see respiratory rate • *Airway pressure release ventilation (APRV):* No research has been conducted; however, the short expiratory period may limit the ability to observe ventilator-induced changes in SV or BP. Additionally, spontaneous ventilations during APRV will invalidate functional indicators.
Positive end-expiratory pressure (PEEP)	PPV accurately predicts the effect of a change in PEEP on CO (i.e., a high PPV suggests that the CO will decrease with an increase in PEEP and an increase in PPV associated with an increase in PEEP suggests a decrease in CO).[67]
Respiratory rate	An increase in respiratory rate from 14–16 breaths/minute to 30–40 breaths/minute without a change in Vt decreases the PPV. A key factor may be the number of cardiac beats per respiratory cycle. When the HR/RR ratio is < 3.6 (e.g., HR 100/RR 30 = 3.3) the PPV becomes negligible due to insufficient time for the ventilator-induced change in SV to be observed.[66]
Vasoactive medications	Vasopressors have different effects on each functional indicator[68,69] and vasopressor may mask an underlying volume deficit. Vasodilator therapy[70] or a decrease in vasopressor dose[71] may unmask or create a relative hypovolemia as indicated by an increase in functional hemodynamic values.
Ventricular function	There is limited research in patients with ejection fraction (EF) < 40%. In cardiac surgery patients an SVV > 9.5% predicted fluid response status in patients with an EF < 35% (AUC 0.76) and an EF > 50% (AUC 0.88).[72] In an animal study of post-cardiac arrest where there was an acute decrease in left ventricular EF, the PPV and SVV did not predict fluid response status. However, at 4-hours post-arrest the PPV was an accurate predictor of fluid response status.[73]
Right ventricular dysfunction/*cor pulmonale*	With severe right ventricular dysfunction, the effects of ventilation are reversed, causing increased SBP during inspiration.[74] Under these conditions, the functional indicators *do not* reflect fluid responsiveness, but rather right ventricular dysfunction.[75] In cardiac and septic shock patients with elevated PA pressures, the PPV was not an accurate predictor of fluid response status (AUC 0.45).[76]
Body position (head of bed elevation and lateral position)	One study found that head of bed elevation was associated with an increase in SVV and decreased SV (suggesting position-induced decrease in preload) compared to supine measurements. Thirty degree lateral recumbent position did not affect SVV or SVI.[77]

Table 29.1. *(cont.)*

Prone position	Prone positioning effect on functional indicators and threshold values is variable. In one study of patients undergoing scoliosis surgery there was no difference in PPV in the supine versus prone position.[78] However, in another study, the PPV threshold values increased (supine 11%; prone 15%), but PPV remained an accurate predictor of fluid responsive status.[79] The increase in PPV threshold, independent of fluid response status, may be due to a decrease in compliance of the respiratory system. The prone position may also cause an increase in SV and decrease in CI, particularly in patients who are fluid responders.[77,79,80] In this case the position-induced change in hemodynamic status suggests cardiovascular compromise. Preoptimization (i.e., administering fluids to bring the functional indicator into the non-responder category – SV < 14% for 5 minutes) has been found to prevent a position-induced decrease in CI.[80]

and lack of precision between the arterial and peripheral lactate (-3.2 ± 4.5 mg/dL; 95% LOA – 12.1 to 5.4 mg/dL) compared to a non-shock state (bias -2.6 ± 3.9 mg/dL; 95% LOA – 10.2 to 5.1). However, there was no significant difference in the central venous and arterial lactate under shock (0.4 ± 2.1 mg/dL; 95% LOA – 3.8 to 4.5 mg/dL) and non-shock states (0.4 ± 2.3 mg/dL; 95% LOA – 6.2 to 5.5 mg/dL). Additionally, there was concordance in treatment decisions in 96% of the cases for the arterial and central venous specimens, but use of the peripheral lactate would have resulted in different treatment compared to the arterial lactate in ten cases (13% discordance); with the peripheral lactate overestimating the arterial lactate. These results suggest the need to obtain lactate specimens from one source (arterial or venous) only and to be aware of the potential overestimation of the lactate if a peripheral venous specimen is used.

In healthy subjects with normal venous lactate, tourniquet time, transporting the specimen on ice versus room temperature and a 15-minute delay in processing the blood sample did not significantly affect lactate level.[94] However, a second study of healthy subjects[95] found a significant increase in lactate at 10 minutes when the tube was stored at room temperature (20 °C) compared to dry or wet iced (0 °C) conditions. Given these equivocal results, if a delay in specimen processing is anticipated, there may be benefit to storing the specimen on ice.[89]

Implementing and sustaining goal directed therapy

Multidisciplinary commitment is crucial in the implementation, uptake and sustainment of goal directed therapy. One challenge is that nurses and physicians have different perceived barriers to goal directed therapy. For example, emergency department (ED) nurses identified delays in central venous catheter insertion and physician diagnosis as barriers. In contrast, ED physicians identified lack of agreement with the resuscitation protocol, lack of access to CVP and $ScvO_2$ monitoring.[96,97] These perceived differences highlight the need for multidisciplinary strategies to enhance the uptake of goal directed therapies. Lessons from other goal directed initiatives highlight the importance of multidisciplinary collaboration. For example, a before–after study evaluated the effect of nursing input into protocol compliance for tight glycemic control.[98] Initially, a physician-derived protocol was implemented. After 3 months, nursing input was sought. The nurses agreed with all aspects of the protocol, but requested additional responsibility in the initiation and maintenance of glycemic control. After implementation of these requested changes, the mean glucose and time to target decreased, although the incidence of severe hypoglycemia increased (one to five cases).

Nurses play a central role in the early identification and initiation of care for patients whose condition is deteriorating.[99,100] Strategies to facilitate early identification of patients and implementation of goal directed therapy by nurses are associated with improved outcomes.[100] Advanced practice nurses (i.e., clinical nurse specialists, educators, and nurse practitioners) play crucial roles in the implementation and sustainment of goal directed therapy, including the development of nursing specific protocols, multidisciplinary order sets, staff education, and the use of evidence-based strategies to optimize the dissemination, uptake, and institutionalization of guidelines.[101,102]

References

1. Vincent JL, Rhodes A, Perel A, et al. Clinical review: update on hemodynamic monitoring – a consensus of 16. *Crit Care* 2011;**15**:229.

2. Dellinger RP, Levy MM, Rhodes A, et al. Surviving sepsis campaign: international guidelines for management of severe sepsis and septic shock: 2012. *Crit Care Med* 2013;**41**:580–637.

3. Aya HD, Cecconi M, Hamilton M, et al. Goal-directed therapy in cardiac surgery: a systematic review and meta-analysis. *Br J Anaesth* 2013;**110**:510–17.

4. Lobo SM, de Oliveira NE. Clinical review: what are the best hemodynamic targets for noncardiac surgical patients? *Crit Care* 2013;**17**:210.

5. Bridges EJ, Bond EF, Ahrens T, et al. Direct arterial vs. oscillometric monitoring of blood pressure: stop comparing and pick one. *Crit Care Nurse* 1997;**17**: 96–7, 101–2.

6. Mignini MA, Piacentini E, Dubin A. Peripheral arterial blood pressure monitoring adequately tracks central arterial blood pressure in critically ill patients: an observational study. *Crit Care* 2006;**10**:R43.

7. Lakhal K, Macq C, Ehrmann S, et al. Noninvasive monitoring of blood pressure in the critically ill: reliability according to the cuff site (arm, thigh, or ankle). *Crit Care Med* 2012;**40**:1207–13.

8. Lehman LW, Saeed M, Talmor D, et al. Methods of blood pressure measurement in the ICU. *Crit Care Med* 2013;**41**:34–40.

9. Rauen CA, Chulay M, Bridges E, et al. Seven evidence-based practice habits: putting some sacred cows out to pasture. *Crit Care Nurse* 2008;**28**:98–124.

10. Melamed R, Johnson K, Pothen B, et al. Invasive blood pressure monitoring systems in the ICU: influence of the blood-conserving device on the dynamic response characteristics and agreement with noninvasive measurements. *Blood Press Monit*;**17**:179–83.

11. Bridges E, Evers K, Schmelz J, et al. Invasive pressure monitoring at altitude. *Crit Care Med* 2005;**33**: A13.

12. Ogedegbe G, Pickering T. Principles and techniques of blood pressure measurement. *Cardiol Clin* 2010;**28**:571–86.

13. Gore S, Middleton R, Bridges E. Analysis of an algorithm to guide decision making regarding direct and oscillometric blood pressure measurement [abstract]. *Am J Respir Crit Care Med* 1995;**151**: A331.

14. Bur A, Hirschl MM, Herkner H, et al. Accuracy of oscillometric blood pressure measurement according to the relation between cuff size and upper-arm circumference in critically ill patients. *Crit Care Med* 2000;**28**:371–6.

15. AACN Practice Alert: *Noninvasive Blood Pressure*. Aliso Viejo, CA: American Association of Critical Care Nurses; 2010 [cited 2013 25 July]; Available from: http://www.aacn.org/wd/practice/docs/practicealerts/nibp%20monitoring%2004-2010%20final.pdf.

16. Pickering TG, Hall JE, Appel LJ, et al. Recommendations for blood pressure measurement in humans and experimental animals: part 1: blood pressure measurement in humans: a statement for professionals from the Subcommittee of Professional and Public Education of the American Heart Association Council on High Blood Pressure Research. *Circulation* 2005;**111**:697–716.

17. LeDoux D, Astiz ME, Carpati CM, et al. Effects of perfusion pressure on tissue perfusion in septic shock. *Crit Care Med* 2000;**28**:2729–32.

18. Thooft A, Favory R, Salgado DR, et al. Effects of changes in arterial pressure on organ perfusion during septic shock. *Crit Care* 2011;**15**:R222.

19. Dubin A, Pozo MO, Casabella CA, et al. Increasing arterial blood pressure with norepinephrine does not improve microcirculatory blood flow: a prospective study. *Crit Care* 2009;**13**:R92.

20. Georger JF, Hamzaoui O, Chaari A, et al. Restoring arterial pressure with norepinephrine improves muscle tissue oxygenation assessed by near-infrared spectroscopy in severely hypotensive septic patients. *Intens Care Med* 2010;**36**:1882–9.

21. Teboul JL, Duranteau J. Alteration of microcirculation in sepsis: a reality but how to go further? *Crit Care Med* 2012;**40**:1653–4.

22. Leblanc ME, Croteau S, Ferland A, et al. Blood pressure assessment in severe obesity: validation of a forearm approach. *Obesity (Silver Spring)* 2013 (in press). doi: 10.1002/oby.20458.

23. Schell K, Morse K, Waterhouse JK. Forearm and upper-arm oscillometric blood pressure comparison in acutely ill adults. *West J Nurs Res* 2010;**32**:322–40.

24. Watson S, Aguas M, Bienapfl T, et al. Postanesthesia patients with large upper arm circumference: is use of an "extra-long" adult cuff or forearm cuff placement accurate? *J Perianesth Nurs* 2011;**26**:135–42.

25. Marik PE, Cavallazzi R. Does the central venous pressure predict fluid responsiveness? An updated meta-analysis and a plea for some common sense*. *Crit Care Med* 2013;**41**:1774–81.

26. Amar D, Melendez JA, Zhang H, et al. Correlation of peripheral venous pressure and central venous pressure in surgical patients. *J Cardiothorac Vasc Anesth* 2001;**15**:40–3.

27. Kim SH, Park SY, Cui J, et al. Peripheral venous pressure as an alternative to central venous pressure in patients undergoing laparoscopic colorectal surgery. *Br J Anaesth* 2011;**106**:305–11.

28. Munis JR, Bhatia S, Lozada LJ. Peripheral venous pressure as a hemodynamic variable in neurosurgical patients. *Anesth Analg* 2001;**92**:172–9.

29. Bombardieri AM, Beckman J, Shaw P, et al. Comparative utility of centrally versus peripherally transduced venous pressure monitoring in the perioperative period in spine surgery patients. *J Clin Anesth* 2012;**24**:542–8.

30. Tugrul M, Camci E, Pembeci K, et al. Relationship between peripheral and central venous pressures in different patient positions, catheter sizes, and insertion sites. *J Cardiothorac Vasc Anesth* 2004;**18**:446–50.

31. Hadimioglu N, Ertug Z, Yegin A, et al. Correlation of peripheral venous pressure and central venous pressure in kidney recipients. *Transpl Proc* 2006;**38**:440–2.

32. Hoftman N, Braunfeld M, Hoftman G, et al. Peripheral venous pressure as a predictor of central venous pressure during orthotopic liver transplantation. *J Clin Anesth* 2006;**18**:251–5.

33. Tobias JD. Measurement of central venous pressure from a peripheral intravenous catheter in the prone position during spinal surgery. *South Med J* 2009;**102**:256–9.

34. Memtsoudis SG, Jules-Elysse K, Girardi FP, et al. Correlation between centrally versus peripherally transduced venous pressure in prone patients undergoing posterior spine surgery. *Spine* 2008;**33**:E643–7.

35. Wardhan R, Shelley K. Peripheral venous pressure waveform. *Curr Opin Anaesthesiol* 2009;**22**:814–21.

36. Stoneking L, Deluca LA, Jr., Fiorello AB, et al. Alternative methods to central venous pressure for assessing volume status in critically ill patients. *J Emerg Nurs* 2012. Doi:10.1016/j.jn.2012.04.018 (Accessed July 20, 2013).

37. Desmond J, Megahed M. Is the central venous pressure reading equally reliable if the central line is inserted via the femoral vein. *Emerg Med J* 2003;**20**:467–9.

38. Lee BK, Lee HY, Jeung KW, et al. Estimation of central venous pressure using inferior vena caval pressure from a femoral endovascular cooling catheter. *Am J Emerg Med* 2013;**31**:240–3.

39. Groombridge CJ, Duplooy D, Adams BD, et al. Comparison of central venous pressure and venous oxygen saturation from venous catheters placed in the superior vena cava or via a femoral vein: the numbers are not interchangeable. *Crit Care Resusc* 2011;**13**:151–5.

40. Pacheco Sda S, Machado MN, Amorim RC, et al. Central venous pressure in femoral catheter: correlation with superior approach after heart surgery. *Rev Bras Cir Cardiovasc* 2008;**23**:488–93.

41. Yun JY, Park SH, Cho DS, et al. Comparison of the central venous pressure from internal jugular vein and the pressure measured from the peripherally inserted antecubital central catheter (PICCP) in liver transplantation recipients. *Korean J Anesthesiol* 2011;**61**:281–7.

42. Black IH, Blosser SA, Murray WB. Central venous pressure measurements: peripherally inserted catheters versus centrally inserted catheters. *Crit Care Med* 2000;**28**:3833–6.

43. Latham HE, Rawson ST, Dwyer TT, et al. Peripherally inserted central catheters are equivalent to centrally inserted catheters in intensive care unit patients for central venous pressure monitoring. *J Clin Monit Comput* 2012;**26**:85–90.

44. McLemore EC, Tessier DJ, Rady MY, et al. Intraoperative peripherally inserted central venous catheter central venous pressure monitoring in abdominal aortic aneurysm reconstruction. *Ann Vasc Surg* 2006;**20**:577–81.

45. Alansari M, Hijazi M. Central venous pressure from peripherally inserted central catheters correlates well with that of centrally inserted central catheters. *Chest* 2004;**126**:873S.

46. Rajaram SS, Desai NK, Kalra A, et al. Pulmonary artery catheters for adult patients in intensive care. *Cochrane Database Syst Rev*;**2**: CD003408. doi: 10.1002/14651858.CD003408.pub3.

47. Greenberg SB, Murphy GS, Vender JS. Current use of the pulmonary artery catheter. *Curr Opin Crit Care* 2009;**15**:249–53.

48. AACN Practice alert: pulmonary artery/central venous pressure measurement. AACN; 2009 [cited 14 Jul 2013]; Available from: http://www.aacn.org/wd/practice/docs/pap-measurement.pdf.

49. Marik PE, Monnet X, Teboul JL. Hemodynamic parameters to guide fluid therapy. *Ann Intens Care* 2011;**1**:1.

50. Perel A, Habicher M, Sander M. Bench-to-bedside review: functional hemodynamics during surgery – should it be used for all high-risk cases? *Crit Care* 2013;**17**:203.

51. Tyler L, Greco S, Bridges E, et al. Accuracy of stop-cursor method for determining systolic and pulse pressure variation. *Am J Crit Care* 2013;**22**:298–305.

52. Rinehart J, Islam T, Boud R, et al. Visual estimation of pulse pressure variation is not reliable: a randomized simulation study.

J Clin Monit Comput
2012;**26**:191–6.

53. Bridges E. Using functional hemodynamic indicators to guide fluid therapy. *Am J Nurs*;**113**:42–50.

54. Michard F. Stroke volume variation: from applied physiology to improved outcomes. *Crit Care Med* 2011;**39**:402–3.

55. Monnet X, Dres M, Ferre A, et al. Prediction of fluid responsiveness by a continuous non-invasive assessment of arterial pressure in critically ill patients: comparison with four other dynamic indices. *Br J Anaesth* 2012;**109**:330–8.

56. Cavallaro F, Sandroni C, Marano C, et al. Diagnostic accuracy of passive leg raising for prediction of fluid responsiveness in adults: systematic review and meta-analysis of clinical studies. *Intens Care Med* 2010;**36**:1475–83.

57. Michard F, Descorps-Declere A, Lopes MR. Using pulse pressure variation in patients with acute respiratory distress syndrome. *Crit Care Med* 2008;**36**:2946–8.

58. Monge Garcia MI, Gil Cano A, Gracia Romero M, et al. Non-invasive assessment of fluid responsiveness by changes in partial end-tidal CO2 pressure during a passive leg-raising maneuver. *Ann Intens Care* 2012;**2**:9.

59. Malbrain ML, de Laet I. Functional hemodynamics and increased intra-abdominal pressure: same thresholds for different conditions . . .? *Crit Care Med* 2009;**37**:781–3.

60. Renner J, Gruenewald M, Quaden R, et al. Influence of increased intra-abdominal pressure on fluid responsiveness predicted by pulse pressure variation and stroke volume variation in a porcine model. *Crit Care Med* 2009;**37**:650–8.

61. Jacques D, Bendjelid K, Duperret S, et al. Pulse pressure variation and stroke volume variation during increased intra-abdominal pressure: an experimental study. *Crit Care* 2011;**15**:R33.

62. Tavernier B, Robin E. Assessment of fluid responsiveness during increased intra-abdominal pressure: keep the indices, but change the thresholds. *Crit Care* 2011;**15**:134.

63. Perner A, Faber T. Stroke volume variation does not predict fluid responsiveness in patients with septic shock on pressure support ventilation. *Acta Anaesthesiol Scand* 2006;**50**:1068–73.

64. Heenen S, De Backer D, Vincent JL. How can the response to volume expansion in patients with spontaneous respiratory movements be predicted? *Crit Care* 2006;**10**:R102.

65. Lee JY, Park HY, Jung WS, et al. Comparative study of pressure- and volume-controlled ventilation on stroke volume variation as a predictor of fluid responsiveness in patients undergoing major abdominal surgery. *J Crit Care* 2012; **27**:531.e9–14.

66. De Backer D, Taccone FS, Holsten R, et al. Influence of respiratory rate on stroke volume variation in mechanically ventilated patients. *Anesthesiology* 2009;**110**:1092–7.

67. Michard F, Chemla D, Richard C, et al. Clinical use of respiratory changes in arterial pulse pressure to monitor the hemodynamic effects of PEEP. *Am J Respir Crit Care Med* 1999;**159**:935–9.

68. Renner J, Meybohm P, Hanss R, et al. Effects of norepinephrine on dynamic variables of fluid responsiveness during hemorrhage and after resuscitation in a pediatric porcine model. *Paediatr Anaesth* 2009;**19**:688–94.

69. Sakka SG, Becher L, Kozieras J, et al. Effects of changes in blood pressure and airway pressures on parameters of fluid

70. Hadian M, Severyn DA, Pinsky MR. The effects of vasoactive drugs on pulse pressure and stroke volume variation in postoperative ventilated patients. *J Crit Care* 2011;**26**:328.e1–8.

71. Vallet B, Tygat H, Lebuffe G. How to titrate vasopressors against fluid loading in septic shock. *Adv Sepsis* 2007;**6**:34–40.

72. Reuter DA, Kirchner A, Felbinger TW, et al. Usefulness of left ventricular stroke volume variation to assess fluid responsiveness in patients with reduced cardiac function. *Crit Care Med* 2003;**31**:1399–404.

73. Gruenewald M, Meybohm P, Koerner S, et al. Dynamic and volumetric variables of fluid responsiveness fail during immediate postresuscitation period. *Crit Care Med* 2011;**39**:1953–9.

74. Jardin F. Cyclic changes in arterial pressure during mechanical ventilation. *Intens Care Med* 2004;**30**:1047–50.

75. Mahjoub Y, Pila C, Friggeri A, et al. Assessing fluid responsiveness in critically ill patients: false-positive pulse pressure variation is detected by Doppler echocardiographic evaluation of the right ventricle. *Crit Care Med* 2009;**37**:2570–5.

76. Wyler von Ballmoos M, Takala J, Roeck M, et al. Pulse-pressure variation and hemodynamic response in patients with elevated pulmonary artery pressure: a clinical study. *Crit Care*;**14**:R111.

77. Daihua Y, Wei C, Xude S, et al. The effect of body position changes on stroke volume variation in 66 mechanically ventilated patients with sepsis. *J Crit Care* 2012;**27**:416.e7–12.

78. Marks R, Silverman R, Fernandez R, et al. Does the systolic pressure variation change in the prone

position? *J Clin Monit Comput* 2009;**23**:279–82.

79. Biais M, Bernard O, Ha JC, et al. Abilities of pulse pressure variations and stroke volume variations to predict fluid responsiveness in prone position during scoliosis surgery. *Br J Anaesth* 2010;**104**:407–13.

80. Wu CY, Lee TS, Chan KC, et al. Does targeted pre-load optimisation by stroke volume variation attenuate a reduction in cardiac output in the prone position. *Anaesthesia* 2012;**67**:760–4.

81. Chawla LS, Zia H, Gutierrez G, et al. Lack of equivalence between central and mixed venous oxygen saturation. *Chest* 2004;**126**:1891–6.

82. Varpula M, Karlsson S, Ruokonen E, et al. Mixed venous oxygen saturation cannot be estimated by central venous oxygen saturation in septic shock. *Intens Care Med* 2006;**32**:1336–43.

83. Reinhart K, Kuhn HJ, Hartog C, et al. Continuous central venous and pulmonary artery oxygen saturation monitoring in the critically ill. *Intens Care Med* 2004;**30**:1572–8.

84. Dueck MH, Klimek M, Appenrodt S, et al. Trends but not individual values of central venous oxygen saturation agree with mixed venous oxygen saturation during varying hemodynamic conditions. *Anesthesiology* 2005;**103**:249–57.

85. Kopterides P, Bonovas S, Mavrou I, et al. Venous oxygen saturation and lactate gradient from superior vena cava to pulmonary artery in patients with septic shock. *Shock* 2009;**31**:561–7.

86. van Beest PA, van der Schors A, Liefers H, et al. Femoral venous oxygen saturation is no surrogate for central venous oxygen

saturation. *Crit Care Med*;**40**:3196–201.

87. Davison DL, Chawla LS, Selassie L, et al. Femoral-based central venous oxygen saturation is not a reliable substitute for subclavian/internal jugular-based central venous oxygen saturation in patients who are critically ill. *Chest* 2010;**138**:76–83.

88. Bakker J, Nijsten MW, Jansen TC. Clinical use of lactate monitoring in critically ill patients. *Ann Intens Care* 2013;**3**:12.

89. Jansen TC, van Bommel J, Bakker J. Blood lactate monitoring in critically ill patients: a systematic health technology assessment. *Crit Care Med* 2009;**37**:2827–39.

90. Nascente AP, Assuncao M, Guedes CJ, et al. Comparison of lactate values obtained from different sites and their clinical significance in patients with severe sepsis. *Sao Paulo Med J* 2011;**129**:11–16.

91. Weil MH, Michaels S, Rackow EC. Comparison of blood lactate concentrations in central venous, pulmonary artery, and arterial blood. *Crit Care Med* 1987;**15**:489–90.

92. Middleton P, Kelly AM, Brown J, et al. Agreement between arterial and central venous values for pH, bicarbonate, base excess, and lactate. *Emerg Med J* 2006;**23**:622–4.

93. Theusinger OM, Thyes C, Frascarolo P, et al. Mismatch of arterial and central venous blood gas analysis during haemorrhage. *Eur J Anaesthesiol* 2010;**27**:890–6.

94. Jones AE, Leonard MM, Hernandez-Nino J, et al. Determination of the effect of in vitro time, temperature, and tourniquet use on whole blood venous point-of-care lactate concentrations. *Acad Emerg Med* 2007;**14**:587–91.

95. Seymour CW, Carlbom D, Cooke CR, et al. Temperature and time stability of whole blood lactate: implications for feasibility of pre-hospital measurement. *BMC Res Notes* 2011;**4**:169.

96. Carlbom DJ, Rubenfeld GD. Barriers to implementing protocol-based sepsis resuscitation in the emergency department – results of a national survey. *Crit Care Med* 2007;**35**:2525–32.

97. Burney M, Underwood J, McEvoy S, et al. Early detection and treatment of severe sepsis in the emergency department: identifying barriers to implementation of a protocol-based approach. *J Emerg Nurs* 2011;**38**:512–17.

98. DuBose JJ, Nomoto S, Higa L, et al. Nursing involvement improves compliance with tight blood glucose control in the trauma ICU: a prospective observational study. *Intensive Crit Care Nurs* 2009;**25**:101–7.

99. Aitken LM, Williams G, Harvey M, et al. Nursing considerations to complement the Surviving Sepsis Campaign guidelines. *Crit Care Med*;**39**:1800–18.

100. Tromp M, Hulscher M, Bleeker-Rovers CP, et al. The role of nurses in the recognition and treatment of patients with sepsis in the emergency department: a prospective before-and-after intervention study. *Int J Nurs Stud* 2010;**47**:1464–73.

101. Winterbottom F. Nurses' critical role in identifying sepsis and implementing early goal-directed therapy. *J Contin Educ Nurs* 2012;**43**:247–8.

102. Winterbottom F, Seoane L, Sundell E, et al. Improving sepsis outcomes for acutely ill adults using interdisciplinary order sets. *Clin Nurse Spec* 2011;**25**:180–5.

Chapter

30

A nurse anesthetist perspective: does perioperative goal directed fluid management yield better patient outcomes compared to the traditional method?

Ann B. Singleton

The primary goal of fluid administration is to restore circulating blood volume to a level that ensures adequate tissue oxygenation. The traditional method of perioperative fluid management accounts for fluid deficit, maintenance requirements, and insensible losses.[1,2,3]

Maintenance fluid guidelines were based on a landmark paper published in 1956 by Holliday and Segar. It compared patients' energy requirements from various studies and determined that 100 milliliters of water was needed for 100 calories metabolized.[3] The fluid replacement formula received criticism because it did not consider energy requirements by elderly patients, patient co-morbidities, and active infection. In the context of perioperative management, it did not take into account decreased metabolism from general anesthesia and decreased urine output from antidiuretic hormone secretion during surgery.[2,3] Conventional parameters to guide perioperative fluid management such as blood pressure (BP), heart rate, and central venous pressure (CVP) remain the standard of care for assessment of fluid requirements.

An alternative method to perioperative fluid management is a goal directed approach. Goal directed therapy (GDT) in fluid management provides hemodynamic optimization by using cardiac output parameters to measure blood flow and tissue perfusion. Cardiac monitoring includes the use of a monitor for cardiac output (CO), stroke volume (SV), and stroke volume variation (SVV) optimization. A restrictive goal directed (GD) approach usually results in the administration of less fluid. This method uses crystalloid fluid to replace extravascular losses and colloid fluid to replace intravascular losses. This review

examines the evidence using restrictive goal directed IV fluid management in the perioperative period.

History and review of the literature

History

This author's practices are at a 422-bed capacity Level 1 trauma center located in Southern California with 19 main operating rooms (OR), 4 outpatient surgery ORs, 2 gastrointestinal (GI) ORs, interventional radiology (IR), cardiac catherization, and magnetic resonance imaging (MRI) suites. The institution serves a community that consists largely of elderly, and indigent populations. In the postoperative period, there have been increases in morbidity and mortality associated with perioperative fluid overload. These complications included pulmonary edema, respiratory distress, disseminated coagulopathy, congestive heart failure, bowel obstruction, delayed wound healing, and prolonged hospital stay.

The medical practitioners in this institution rely on clinical judgment for intraoperative fluid management. Additionally, a goal directed fluid management protocol for intra-abdominal surgeries is recommended.

The PICO question

A common model used in developing a clinical question is to use the mnemonic PICO: P (patient/population), I (intervention), C (comparison), O (outcome).[4] This format is purported to aid in focusing the clinical question and to help in rapidly locating the current best evidence addressing the problem. The clinical question in the PICO format is as follows:

Perioperative Hemodynamic Monitoring and Goal Directed Therapy, ed. Maxime Cannesson and Rupert Pearse.
Published by Cambridge University Press. © Cambridge University Press 2014.

P: Adults undergoing major abdominal or gastrointestinal surgeries
I: Goal directed restrictive fluid management
C: Current practice using the traditional method of perioperative fluid management, which estimates fluid deficits, maintenance, and third space losses.
O: Patient morbidity defined by the degree of patients' deteriorating health condition.

Search strategy

The following approaches were used to gather evidence: online searches (PubMed and Cochrane Database of Systematic Reviews), ancestry approach, and informal networking. Textbooks were searched for possible evidence sources. The evidence was restricted to English language full text systematic reviews with or without meta-analysis and human clinical studies from peer-reviewed journals comparing GD restrictive fluid administration to traditional fluid administration methods in adults undergoing major abdominal or gastrointestinal surgery unrelated to trauma. Sources included in systematic reviews were not reviewed separately. Sources were noted if included in more than one systematic review. Specific keywords or word strings were, "perioperative fluid management," "abdominal surgery," "gastrointestinal surgery," "goal directed," and "restrictive fluid management." The evidence was included from 1997 to 2013. The exclusion criteria included evidence examining the incidence of the problem, trauma patients, adults undergoing surgery other than major abdominal or gastrointestinal surgery, and pediatric patients.

Critical appraisal of the literature

Five evidence sources[5–12] met the inclusion criteria. The search revealed systematic reviews with or without meta-analysis and a randomized controlled clinical trial (RCT). The evidence was appraised by the method proposed by Melnyk and Fineout-Overholt.[13]

The systematic reviews with meta-analysis[5–7] were the highest level of evidence for this review. The investigators used a defined search method. Their appraisal method included assessing sample size, allocation sequence, concealment, randomization, protocol deviations, and blinding. Trained independent researchers screened the evidence for review examined characteristics and outcomes. Measures of effect included odds ratio (OR) for dichotomous variables and weighted

mean difference (WMD) for continuous variables, both with 95% confidence intervals (95% CI). Only studies of moderate to high quality were included. Statistical heterogeneity was assessed by graphic presentations of confidence intervals on a forest plot[2] and I^2 statistics where values greater than 50% indicated high heterogeneity. A stratified analysis[5] was added to reduce heterogeneity between trials. Sensitivity analysis for bias used a funnel plot[5,6] where an inverted funnel showed no publication bias. Two RCTs[8,9] were included in three systematic reviews.[5,6,7]

The first systematic review with meta-analysis[5] included five RCTs totaling 420 patients. Two trials contributed greater than 50% of the subjects and weighted the highest in the statistical evaluation of the data. Strengths included clinical homogeneity in patient co-morbidities, mean age, and type of surgery that were measured with the American Society of Anesthesiologist physical classification, and Goldman cardiac risk score. A weakness was the absence of a cost–benefit analysis on the use of esophageal Doppler (Doppler) monitoring. Also, Doppler monitoring was only used intraoperatively. Postoperative Doppler monitoring was not applied due to its cumbersome use and patient discomfort.

The second review[6] included nine RCTs with a total of 971 patients. The authors proposed standardized definitions for the terms "standard fluid therapy," "restrictive fluid therapy," and "supplemental fluid therapy." This systematic review examined fluid therapy in the intraoperative and postoperative period. There was significant heterogeneity between the evidence sources; therefore a stratified analysis of the studies on fluid amount was carried out for timing of the intervention. A weakness was that the studies within this review had varied results in bowel preparation and epidural catheter use. The inconsistencies in these variables may have altered outcome measures. For example, some studies did not have bowel preparation, and the management of epidural catheters differed between the studies examined.

The third systematic review with meta-analysis[7] included 35 RCTs with a total of 5021 patients. This stratified meta-analysis observed two strategies of fluid management. The first group observed traditional therapy versus GD therapy. The second group observed liberal versus restrictive (LVR) fluid therapy. Twenty-three RCTs ($N = 3861$) were assigned to the GD group and 12 RCTs ($N = 1160$) were assigned to the LVR group. The analysis was restricted to high-quality studies. Secondary outcomes measured organ-specific complications unlike previous reviews[5,6] that measured composite secondary endpoints. This method avoided double counting of patients. A stratified analysis within subgroups was carried out to confirm differences in the outcomes. The weakness in this review was heterogeneity in the continuous variables that included inconsistent timing of interventions and preoperative instruction. This is due to differences in case mix, standard management of patients, and trial design. Many studies were in single center trials, and the total sample size may still have been too small to detect a clinically important difference in mortality. A sample size of 3800 patients only had a power of 72% to detect a reduction in hospital mortality from 2% to 1%.[7] Also, the types of fluids varied between the groups: one used more colloid fluid and the other crystalloid IV fluid.

The systemic review[8] without meta-analysis included seven RCTs and totaled 705 subjects. The distribution of subjects varied between the studies, and the subjects from assessor-blinded studies[9,10] weighted the most. This systematic review contained inconsistencies in outcome results and study design. The inconsistencies related to the amount of IV fluid administered between the traditional and restrictive groups, indications for additional IV fluid, perioperative care principles, and definition of the perioperative period hindered comparison and interpretation of the data. These inconsistencies revealed that evidence-based guidelines for optimal procedure-specific with fixed-volume regimen cannot be formulated. The authors[7,8] suggested heeding caution when traditional fluid therapy is used in patients with multiple co-morbidities, and individualized GD therapy was recommended to guide fluid management in this patient population.

Last, a prospective single blind RCT observed 38 patients scheduled for major abdominal non-vascular surgery. The trial observed the outcomes of goal directed fluid therapy monitoring SVV during abdominal surgery. All procedures were open laparotomy procedures. The exclusion criteria included less than 18 years old, coagulopathy, history of cerebrovascular disease, significant kidney or liver disease (creatinine >50% or liver enzymes >50% of normal values), congestive heart failure, ischemic heart disease, cardiac arrhythmias, and significant lung disease. A computerized algorithm was used to randomly assign patients to either GDT or control groups. Patients were ventilated at 8 mL/kg of ideal body weight and minute ventilation of 7–8 L/min with an I:E ratio of 1:2. Radial arterial lines were inserted

on all patients. The arterial catheters were connected to a cardiac output monitoring device and SVV data was collected throughout surgery. A fluid management protocol was used.

The limitation in this trial was its size; 38 patients compared to RCTs[9,10] that were included in the previously mentioned systematic reviews. The cardiac output device used in this trial had limitation in its accuracy when cardiac arrhythmias were detected. Intraoperative vasoactive drug boluses also altered SVV data. There was no standard of care protocol during the postoperative period, rather patient care management was left to the discretion of each surgical team.

Discussion of state of the art

The highest level of evidence reviewed favored GD restrictive fluid management compared to traditional methods.[6–10] This approach to perioperative fluid therapy relies on non-invasive monitoring of cardiac output variables such as stroke volume (SV) to determine volume responsiveness. The evidence showed that GD restrictive fluid therapy of crystalloid fluid to replace extravascular losses, and colloid fluid to replace intravascular losses improved outcomes in abdominal and colorectal surgeries. The outcomes measured patient complications, morbidity, mortality, and hospital stay. The evidence showed decreased morbidity and hospital stay when this method was used to guide fluid administration. Less cardiovascular, respiratory, and gastrointestinal complications occurred in the subjects in the GDT groups. However, patient mortality was not improved.

In the first systematic review with meta-analysis,[5] pooled analysis of the evidence showed decreased patient complications (fewer ICU admissions) when perioperative IV fluid management was guided by Doppler, compared with the traditional method in patients who had major abdominal surgeries. The evidence showed overall fewer patient complications that favored Doppler group (OR 0.28, 95% CI 0.17 to 0.46) and less ICU admissions (0.20 OR, 95% CI 0.07 to 0.57). Hospital stay favored the Doppler group (−1.60 OR, 95% CI −2.58 to −0.62). Mortality measures between the groups showed no significant difference (−0.97 WMD, 95% CI −1.31 to −0.63). The evidence showed no changes in standard monitor values (systolic blood pressure, urine output, and central venous pressure) in the presence of hypovolemia in the control groups. Signs of hypovolemia are often delayed for a significant period of time following the reduction of intravascular volume. Therefore, hypovolemia can occur without noticeable changes in these parameters. The author observed that GD therapy guided by a Doppler to measure tissue perfusion detects hypovolemia more rapidly.[5]

The second systematic review with meta-analysis[6] showed a decrease in morbidity in four trials with a sample size of 393 patients. This showed a significant reduction of postoperative morbidity in favor of restrictive fluid therapy (0.45 OR, 95% CI 0.28 to 0.72). The data showed no statistical significance on mortality (0.5 OR, 95% CI 0.09 to 2.65). Data on cardiopulmonary complications and bowel function recovery were presented as total number of events but were not summarized as pooled analysis. However, RCTs[9,10] within this review reported statistically significant faster recovery in bowel function and shorter hospital stay in favor of the restrictive group. Goal directed approach with Doppler guided the administration of colloid fluid boluses to achieve maximum stroke volume. Pooled analysis revealed significant reduction in postoperative morbidity in favor of Doppler guidance (0.43 OR, 95% CI 0.26 to 0.71), and number needed to treat (NNT) of six. This indicated that six patients would have had to receive GDT by means of Doppler in order to prevent one patient with complications.[11] There was no significant difference in mortality between the conventional and Doppler guided groups (0.32 OR, 95% CI 0.03 to 3.17).

A systematic review with stratified meta-analysis[7] hypothesized that traditional fluid therapy is not equivalent to goal directed restrictive fluid therapy. Two stratum were compared: the liberal fluid therapy (traditional) and GDT groups. The evidence favored GDT guided with Doppler over the traditional method.[6] Monitoring of cardiac output variables gave information on fluid responsiveness, therefore indicating when a fluid bolus is needed for tissue perfusion rather than risk excessive fluid administration based on traditional measures such as blood pressure and heart rate. The results showed decreased complications related to cardiac, pulmonary, renal, and gastrointestinal in the GDT group. These patients showed quicker return of bowel function, faster recovery, and shorter hospital stay. The patients assigned to the traditional group received more crystalloid fluids. Complications were greater in the traditional group, such as pneumonia (relative risk (RR) 3.0, 95% CI 1.8 to 4.8), and pulmonary edema (RR 3.8, 95% CI 1.1 to 13).[7]

The administration of crystalloid fluid for extravascular losses and colloid fluid boluses for hemodynamic stability in the GDT group reduced the incidence of pulmonary edema and pneumonia. Hospital stay was longer in the traditional group with a 4-day mean difference (95% CI 3.4 to 4.4).[7] The results must be interpreted with caution because hospital mortality did not differ between the groups. Although more colloid IV fluids were administered in the GDT group, its use should be cautioned with critically ill patients due to increased co-morbidities, and coagulopathy from synthetic colloid fluids.

A systematic review without meta-analysis[8] compared liberal versus restrictive IV fluid therapy on major abdominal surgeries experienced by patients assigned in the restrictive groups. The evidence showed decreased incidence in patient complications and shorter hospital stay. Inconsistent outcome results and study designs have been reported, which hindered direct comparison and interpretation. However, the studies suggested that excessive crystalloid fluid during the perioperative period impaired postoperative outcomes.[8–10] The authors suggested that crystalloids should be used as a maintenance fluid regimen to replace extravascular fluid losses. The evidence also suggested that GD fluid therapy guided by cardiac output monitoring optimized intravascular volume by the administration of colloid fluid IV boluses instead of by crystalloid.[6,7]

Two RCTs[9,10] were consistently included in the previously mentioned systematic reviews[6–8] and deserved separate mentioning. A randomized, multicenter trial[9] compared liberal and restrictive fluid management on 172 patients who had colorectal surgeries. The aim of the study was to compare the effect of fluid management on complication rate after colorectal surgery. The restrictive group was designed to retain preoperative weight and received a mean volume of 2.7 liters. The standard group represented traditional fluid management practice and received a mean volume of 5.4 liters. The restrictive group received more colloid fluid than the standard group, which received more normal saline solution. Postoperative patient outcomes showed significantly less complications in the restrictive group than in the traditional group with 4 NNT ($P = 0.032$).[9] Four patients died from the traditional group due to pulmonary edema, pneumonia with septicemia, and pulmonary embolism. The restrictive group resulted in less crystalloid fluid volume, less postoperative complications, and no deaths compared to the standard group. Dose–response correlation between excessive IV fluid administration and patient complications was higher in the traditional group.[9] The omission of fluid replacement for third space losses in the restrictive group reduced complications. In conclusion, perioperative fluid management, aimed to retain preoperative body weight, reduced complications after colorectal surgery.

The other RCT[10] mentioned in the previous systematic reviews[6-8] was a prospective trial that observed 152 patients who had intra-abdominal surgeries. This trial acknowledged the results from the previous trial.[9] Restrictive and traditional fluid therapy groups were randomly assigned. Outcome endpoints were patient complications, death, hospital stay, return of gastrointestinal function, and body weight. The fluid volume delivered in the restrictive group was significantly less than the liberal group. The findings favored the restrictive group with less complications ($P = 0.046$), less weight gain ($P < 0.01$), quicker return of bowel function ($P < 0.001$), and shorter hospital stay ($P = 0.01$).[10] Increased body weight observed in the traditional group was due to fluid overload and altered fluid balance, which led to gastrointestinal edema and delayed bowel function. Large fluid volume infusions exert harmful effects on cardiac and pulmonary function, tissue oxygenation, coagulation, and wound healing.[1,10]

The prospective single blind RCT[11] observed two groups. The control group was guided by conventional methods of fluid management and the anesthesiologists' clinical judgment. The GDT group was guided per fluid management protocol to maintain SVV less than 12%. There was no standard protocol for crystalloid fluid maintenance for both groups, and the transfusion of blood products was at the discretion of the anesthesiologist, as clinically indicated. Data that were nonnormally distributed used a Mann–Whitney test and normally distributed data used the Student t test. Ordinal and nominal data were compared using the chi-square (χ^2) test. A P value ≤ 0.05 was considered significant.[11]

The primary outcome measure was the return of GI function. Secondary outcomes measured length of hospital stay and recovery scores on postoperative day 2 and day 4.[11] There was no statistical difference between the groups on the amount of crystalloid, colloid, and blood product administration. It was important to note that both groups were instructed to transfuse crystalloid and blood products, based on standard practice. The difference in the GDT group was that the anesthesiologists followed the SVV guided protocol in addition to their standard practice.

This may be the reason why there was no significant difference in the total fluid administered. However, the GDT group received more frequent colloid boluses than the control group, $P = 0.003$. The average SVV in the control group was higher with readings of 12% to 20% than the GDT group. Early SVV optimization ($<12\%$) was achieved in 77% in the GDT group compared with only 19% in the control group, $P = 0.001$.[11] Interestingly, SVV optimization was achieved sooner in the GDT group (within 10 minutes) compared with the control group, which took approximately 60 minutes. The results showed that the GDT group had earlier GI recovery ($P = 0.004$) and oral intake ($P = 0.004$) than the control group. The GDT group had shorter hospital stay ($P = 0.04$) and higher quality of recovery score on postoperative day 2 ($P = 0.05$) and day 4 ($P = 0.03$) than the control group.[11] Consistent with previous evidence,[6-8] the results revealed the importance of timely administration of colloid boluses to optimize tissue perfusion and hemodynamic stability.

Summary

The primary goal of perioperative fluid management is to restore circulating blood volume, which ensures adequate perfusion to vital organs and traumatized tissues. Fluid management requires the optimization of cardiac output stroke volume. Fluid therapy includes the infusion of crystalloid and colloid IV solutions. More crystalloid fluids are necessary to equal the hemodynamic effects of colloids, but excessive infusion of crystalloids lead to pulmonary and peripheral edema which interferes with tissue perfusion.[6-10] On the other hand, colloid-accentuated fluid resuscitation would improve oxygen tissue delivery by limiting fluid shifts to the interstitial space. But, concerns of renal insufficiency and coagulopathy are associated with excessive colloid IV infusion. Other sources[1-3] recommended that crystalloid fluid is used to replace extravascular losses and that colloid fluid is used to replace plasma deficits from acute blood loss, or protein-rich pathologic shift to the interstitial space. A goal directed approach to perioperative fluid management, such as a balanced fluid replacement for extravascular losses and timely replacement of intravascular loss, were observed to maintain hemodynamic optimization.[5-8]

Current practice of perioperative fluid management assumes that a fasted patient is dry. The traditional method of fluid therapy is guided by an algorithmic approach, taking account of preoperative deficits, maintenance requirements, and third space loss.[3] This method has had a sustained influence on the clinical practice of perioperative fluid management. Based on the evidence[6-10] and other sources,[1,3] the Holliday–Segar guidelines for fluid replacement overestimates the needs of the surgical patient. The evidence showed that the groups that followed the traditional method resulted in excessive administration of fluid volume, increased patient complications and morbidities.[5-10] Also, perioperative fluid management aimed to maintain preoperative weight (a restrictive approach) yielded reduced morbidity, complications, and length of hospital stay.[9,10]

Trials that observed restrictive versus liberal perioperative fluid management showed favorable outcomes in the restrictive group.[6-10] The restrictive goups received more colloid fluid than the liberal groups. It has been demonstrated that protocol-based fluid restriction reduced the incidence of perioperative complications, GI disturbance, cardiopulmonary events, and delay in hospital stay. However, the major problem within the evidence[6-10] was the heterogeneity between the groups, and the studies within those groups. Inconsistencies were found in study design, definition of terminology, volume of fluid administered, patient population, and perioperative care principles. Lack of consistency in continuous variables required more research, emphasizing a GD approach in fluid therapy, guided by hemodynamic monitoring for volume responsiveness.

A goal directed approach to perioperative fluid management relies upon close monitoring of changes in cardiac output variables, such as SV, systolic flow times, and respiratory cyclic variations of stroke volume and pulse pressure. Reliable markers of fluid responsiveness including CO, SV, pleth variability index (PVI), and SVV optimization have been used in fluid management protocols.[13] The evidence showed that patients who received restrictive GD fluid therapy had fewer patient complications, less morbidity, faster recovery, and shorter hospital stay compared with traditional methods on surgical patients who had major abdominal and colorectal surgeries.[6-10] Despite fewer patient complications, the evidence[5-8] was not significant in reducing patient mortality. Continuous monitoring of cardiac variables for fluid responsivenes (SV, SVV, CO) provided earlier intervention of fluid boluses in the restrictive groups, which resulted in less total fluid administration than the standard groups. Also, the evidence[5-11] only observed intra-abdominal and bowel surgeries. A trial on healthy patients who had laparoscopic outpatient procedures

resulted in reduced incidence of postoperative nausea, vomiting, dizziness, and pain from liberal fluid management.[14] This suggested that liberal fluid management is acceptable in minor outpatient surgeries where major trauma and fluid shifts are unlikely.[1,14] However, careful fluid management is beneficial in patients with high co-morbidities and is scheduled for major surgeries.

GDT trials that used Doppler[5-7] and SVV[11] achieved tissue perfusion optimization sooner than the standard groups that used conventional hemodynamic monitoring. It is important to note that the total fluid administered was similar between the GDT and the standard groups.[5,11] GDT with Doppler provided early monitoring for timely colloid boluses that were found to be significant in maximizing stroke volume.[5-7] GDT guided by SVV showed statistically significant (P value ≤ 0.05) postoperative recovery outcomes on day 2 and day 4.[11] The evidence also showed significance ($P = 0.003$) in the frequency of colloid boluses, which suggested the importance of timing to achieve hemodynamic optimization. Unlike conventional monitoring, GD fluid management using cardiac output parameters (SVV, SV, CO) guided anesthesiologists to administer timely fluid boluses to optimize tissue oxygenation and organ perfusion.[6-8,11] An important note on this trial[11] was that, even though the anesthesiologists in the control group were blind to SVV data, they were able to visualize and assert clinical judgment on fluid therapy based on pulse pressure variability that was seen on the arterial waveform. However, when SVV greater than 12% was sustained, the researchers concluded that the visual inspection of the arterial waveform was not as reliable.[11]

So, how much is enough? The evidence demonstrated that the goal directed approach to fluid management guided by continuous cardiac output monitoring improved patient outcomes in abdominal and bowel surgeries.[5-11] The standard method of perioperative fluid management using conventional hemodynamic monitoring was not adequate to assess fluid responsiveness in major surgeries. Although favorable outcomes were seen in the evidence, a restrictive fluid therapy is not recommended for all surgeries. Rather, an individualized goal directed approach with a fixed fluid regimen and continuous cardiac output monitoring for major surgeries seemed reasonable. Goal directed fluid therapy using a balanced fluid regimen to replace extracellular losses, and continuous non-invasive monitoring of cardiac output variables for timely replacement of intravascular losses requires more review.

References

1. Chappell D, Jacob M, Hofmann-Kiefer K, Conzen P, Rehm M. A rational approach to perioperative fluid management. *Anesthesiology* 2008;**109**(4):723–40.

2. Ganter MT, Hofer CK, Pittet JF. Postoperative intravascular fluid therapy. In Miller RD. *Miller's Anesthesia*. 7th edn. Philadelphia, PA: Churchill Livingstone, Elsevier Inc., 2010, pp. 2796–802.

3. Barash P, Cullen B, Stoelting R, et al. *Clinical Anesthesia*. 7th edn. Philadelphia, PA: Wolters Kluwer Health/Lippincott Williams & Wilkins, 2013, pp. 333–41.

4. Cannesson M. Arterial pressure variation and goal-directed fluid therapy. *J Cardiothorac Vasc Anesth* 2010;**24**(3):487–97.

5. Abbas SM, Hill AG. Systematic review of the literature for the use of oesophageal Doppler monitor for fluid replacement in major abdominal surgery. *Anaesthesia* 2008;**63**(1):44–51.

6. Rahbari NN, Zimmermann JB, Schmidt T, et al. Meta-analysis of standard, restrictive and supplemental fluid administration in colorectal surgery. *Br J Surg* 2009;**96**(4):331–41.

7. Corcoran T, Rhodes JE, Clarke S, et al. Perioperative fluid management strategies in major surgery: a stratified meta-analysis. *Anesth Analg* 2012;**114**(3):640–51.

8. Bundgaard-Nielsen M, Secher NH, Kehlet H. Liberal vs. restrictive perioperative fluid therapy – a critical assessment of the evidence. *Acta Anaesthesiol Scand* 2009;**53**(7):843–51.

9. Brandstrup B, Tonnesen H, Beier-Holgersen R, et al. Effects of intravenous fluid restriction on postoperative complications: comparison of two perioperative fluid regimens: a randomized assessor-blinded multicenter trial. *Ann Surg* 2003;**238**(5):641–8.

10. Nisanevich V, Felsenstein I, Almogy G, et al. Effect of intraoperative fluid management on outcome after intraabdominal surgery. *Anesthesiology* 2005;**103**(1):25–32.

11. Ramsingh D, Sanghvi C, Gamboa J, et al. Outcome impact of goal directed fluid therapy during high risk abdominal surgery in low to moderate risk patients: a randomized control trial. *J Clin Monit Comput* 2013;**27**:249–57.

12. Biddle C. *Evidence Trumps Belief: Nurse Anesthetists and Evidence-Based Decision Making*. Park Ridge, IL: AANA Publishing, Inc, 2010, pp. 19–35.

13. Melnyk BM, Fineout-Overholt E. *Evidence-Based Practice in Nursing and Healthcare*. 2nd edn. Philadelphia, PA: Wolters Kluwer Health/Lippincott Williams & Wilkins, 2011, pp. 40–69.

14. Maharaj CH, Kallam SR, Malik A, et al. Preoperative intravenous fluid therapy decreases postoperative nausea and pain in high risk patient. *Anesth Analg* 2005;**100**:675–82.

Chapter

31

How to implement GDT in an institution and at the national level

Timothy E. Miller and Michael Mythen

Each year millions of pounds are spent around the world on health care research with the aim of developing interventions, practices, and guidelines that can improve human health.[1] Yet only a small proportion of these innovations are ever implemented in routine practice, and the process of change for implementation to occur can frequently take many years.[2]

The implementation of evidence-based health care is a complex process. There are many factors involved such as the innovation itself, the strength of the evidence, and the local context into which the implementation may or may not occur. There are also significant challenges in measuring implementation, which has developed into a new field of medicine known as implementation science.[3] At the nexus between research and practice, implementation science has a potential key role in measuring and defining factors that affect implementation success.

Evidence-based perioperative care is the focus of interventions aimed at improving outcomes after major surgery. Some of these interventions have been detailed in different chapters throughout this book. However, changing traditional components of perioperative care is challenging. As reported in a review of the difficulties in applying the principles of evidence-based medicine (EBM) to surgical care, "the immediate challenge to improving the quality of surgical care is not discovering new knowledge, but rather how to integrate what we already know into practice."[4]

Recent surveys in Europe, North America, and Australia have demonstrated some of these challenges and have shown the slow pace of change in perioperative practice toward evidence-based medicine.[5-7] Clinician's compliance with evidence-based guidelines is also inconsistent. The simple availability of evidence in the form of guidance is not sufficient to prompt its adoption, and it is estimated that only approximately 50% of patients receive recommended therapies.[8,9]

There are many barriers to the implementation of evidence-based medicine: these can be broadly categorized as knowledge/skills, attitude, and external factors.[10]

First, lack of awareness or familiarity of the evidence will obstruct clinicians' *knowledge*. It is obviously not possible to deliver best practice if a clinician is not familiar and up to date with current evidence and consensus guidelines. The clinician must also be familiar with the latest techniques and equipment that are recommended.

Second, clinicians must be motivated and interested in searching for the best evidence and working according to the principles of EBM. Lack of agreement with the available evidence, disbelief that the evidence will lead to the desired outcome, and inertia from established routines and habits will influence clinicians' *attitudes* about EBM.

Third, appropriate knowledge and attitudes are necessary, but not sufficient for implementation of EBM. There may still be many *external factors* that negatively impact a clinicians' ability to implement EBM. These include, but are not limited to, tension for change, funding availability, and senior clinician involvement and support.

Barriers to implementation of GDT

These barriers can play a significant role in success or failure of implementation of goal directed therapy (GDT) regimes at an institutional level. In order to eliminate barriers, and thereby overcome problems with unsuccessful implementation of GDT, it is necessary to focus on all three components.

Perioperative Hemodynamic Monitoring and Goal Directed Therapy, ed. Maxime Cannesson and Rupert Pearse.
Published by Cambridge University Press. © Cambridge University Press 2014.

Knowledge of the evidence and familiarity with the monitors

Knowledge about the evidence that supports goal directed therapy varies throughout the world. In the UK, where a significant portion of the GDT research originates, knowledge of the GDT literature is generally strong. This has been enhanced by regular seminars, workshops, and lectures at both a local and national level. Published guidelines that recommend the use of GDT in major abdominal surgery have provided further impetus.[11,12] In other parts of the world GDT has not achieved that level of prominence.[13]

Lack of familiarity with the monitors that are used to perform GDT is also common. For example, one of the main barriers for widespread adoption of esophageal Doppler monitoring (EDM) after publication of the UK's NICE guidelines[11] recommending its use for selected patients in 2007 was a lack of confidence using the new technology among anesthetists.[14] This is still a significant problem, and a recent survey showed that lack of availability of monitoring tool or a lack of experience with the monitors was the largest single barrier to conducting GDT.[13] Training in EDM is required to obtain a consistent stroke volume trace. A survey of clinicians before implementation of EDM by the UK's National Technology Adoption Centre (NTAC) showed that most accepted the benefits of EDM, but were concerned that they lacked training to use the devices confidently.[14] Indeed, even in experienced users, difficulty in obtaining an optimal signal and dislodgement of probe during the procedure can be a source of frustration.

The arterial waveform devices also need training to be used correctly. The user must be familiar with the principles and limitations of the heart–lung interaction. This is particularly the case in laparoscopic surgery when high intrathoracic pressures will increase the threshold for fluid responsiveness.

Attitude and agreement with the evidence

Lack of agreement with the available evidence is still common. The evidence base supporting GDT is fairly comprehensive, and this has led to the development of national guidelines supporting GDT.[11,12] However, some authors have expressed reservations. The criticisms come from the fact that most of the studies supporting GDT are relatively small single center studies. Most are also now 10–15 years old and were performed in the era before enhanced recovery. In a recent international survey 30% of responders felt that GDT provided no perceived benefit.[13]

There have also been some recent studies that did not show a benefit of GDT over a restrictive or zero balance approach within an enhanced recovery program.[15,16] This is perhaps not surprising, as surgery and anesthesia have improved over the last 15 years. When a relatively healthy patient undergoes laparoscopic surgery within an enhanced recovery program with minimal blood loss, it is less likely that GDT is going to show a benefit, especially if the control group is managed according to modern standards rather than using the excessive crystalloid approach that was common in the past. In patients undergoing major surgery with an estimated blood loss >500 mL the evidence base supporting GDT is still strong; however, in the enhanced recovery era it may be that the "threshold" for considering GDT has been raised, although this should still be an individualized decision.[17]

Additionally, the best monitoring system for GDT is still a matter of debate. EDM is the most commonly utilized cardiac output monitor in the UK, with significant variation in preferences in other areas of the world.[13]

External factors

The main external factor that is a barrier to the widespread uptake of GDT is cost. The cost of noninvasive cardiac output monitors typically falls on the anesthesia department, whereas the gains in terms of reduction in complications and length of stay are realized by the hospital. This silo-budgeting can limit the use of GDT.[14]

How to implement GDT at an institutional level

As detailed above, implementation of GDT is not an easy process, and can take up to a year to achieve. Before implementation occurs, there needs to be a desire for change at a clinician and management level. Implementation of GDT affects multiple departments within a hospital and requires cooperation from surgical teams, management, and procurement. The presence of an anesthesia champion to lead the process is one of the most important factors in ensuring successful implementation.[18]

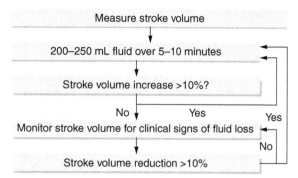

Figure 31.1. The algorithm used by the NTAC for intraoperative fluid management with EDM to optimize stroke volume.

The need for GDT is patient, surgeon, procedure, and institution specific. Each institution needs to look at its outcomes and benchmark data for the benefiting population against other institutions before making an informed decision about appropriate implementation of GDT. This data should include length of stay, readmission rate, and mortality. It is necessary to develop a strong business case and obtain managerial support at a high level to overcome silo budgetary concerns, where costs and benefits are not spread equally among departments.

Many of the cardiac output monitors used to conduct GDT are simple to use, but some training is necessary. This can be achieved through peer-led training, both in theatre and in the anesthetic department. Positioning and focusing the esophageal probes correctly can be particularly challenging. In the UK a structured and certified training program, which can include additional "doctor to doctor" support, is provided free of charge by the supplier.[14] With training, the learning curve for EDM can be overcome after approximately 12 insertions.[19]

After training, the highest success has been achieved when anesthetists are encouraged to use EDM-guided intravenous fluid in all eligible cases according to a fluid administration algorithm. A typical algorithm for EDM is shown in Figure 31.1. However, this algorithm has been criticized for oversimplification and lack of a "brake" to prevent fluid overload in healthier patients.[20] As a rule, algorithms should be developed locally to suit the needs of the institution. A tradeoff is generally needed to avoid both oversimplification and overcomplication.

After successful implementation audit and regular meetings between anesthetists and surgeons, they are encouraged to facilitate feedback and ensure

sustainability. Sustainability is as important as implementation and is not well described in the literature with regards to GDT. A recent consensus statement in implementation on enhanced recovery in the UK asked experts for proposals about sustainability, and a number of the proposals are applicable to GDT.[18]

Proposals to sustain success include:

- Clinical champion plus enthusiastic team
- Employing the GDT protocol as standard of care
- Feed back success to team
- Audit of compliance to protocol
- Continuing education of new team members
- Regular team update sessions
- Challenge of negative perspectives.

The key to sustaining success is to adopt GDT as the standard of care for appropriate cases at each institution. With the help of an enthusiastic team, this ensures that GDT will continue beyond the initial trial or implementation period.

How to implement GDT at a national level

National spread and adoption of GDT has probably been most successful in England as part of a more holistic enhanced recovery after surgery (or fast track) program.[21] Despite a strong evidence base including endorsement from the UK's National Institute for Health and Care Excellence (NICE), independent health economic analysis, and a National Technology Adoption Centre (NTAC) multicenter evaluation concluding that GDT is cost effective in the UK NHS, adoption was low.[11] Within hospitals, reasons for this included non-committal executive sponsorship, lack of endorsement from professional bodies, silo-budgeting separating "the spend" (intraop) from "the save" (postop), and weak change management capacity or tactics. Enhanced recovery pathways transpired to be a more compelling reason to effect widespread change than GDT in isolation.[22]

ER pathways are patient-centered, optimal care for patients having surgery starting prehospital and continuing to rehabilitation. Individualized goal directed fluid therapy using advanced hemodynamic monitoring was at the heart of the intraoperative pathway, combined with avoidance of excess intravenous crystalloid administration and rapid introduction of oral fluids in the immediate postoperative period. A National Consensus statement was published by the national clinical leaders and advisors appointed by the UK Department of Health to clearly define expectations for high-quality perioperative fluid management.[22] A national program to encourage the spread and adoption of ER ran over 3 years (2009–12) and delivered improved quality, patient satisfaction, and reduced LOS to predetermined targets with no increase in readmission rates. Significant increases in case load, reduced bed utilization, and financial savings were realized.[22]

Attempts to implement enhanced recovery and GDT at a national level in the NHS adopted diverse tactics, including pamphlets, toolkits, website promotion, and collaborative workshops, but probably most significantly a cadre of Department of Health appointed clinical leaders and patient representatives who got out there and drove the process supported by an expert team of "change managers."[22]

In one sector of Central London a novel three-pronged approach to spread and adoption that included a financial incentive added to the standard tariff was tested.[21] Novel approaches to spread and adoption included a commitment to upfront investment to secure buy-in and commitment of participating organizations. Key stakeholders and leaders within individual hospitals were asked to produce a signed "Demonstration of Intent". This involved assessment of each hospital's "…readiness to deliver, with acceptance in the Programme dependent on signed off dedicated clinical and project facilitator resources, either named individuals or funding to recruit."[21]

The national ER partnership program team had experience in implementation of change and clinical expertise. They focused upon securing change management capacity, with high-calibre improvement experts within the hospitals supported by external mentors to drive implementation. There was flexibility around how each hospital delivered these expectations, but commitment to appoint these internally funded lead roles was not negotiable.[21,22]

A multidisciplinary team was established in each hospital to drive the project. Collaborating hospitals were then required to form a collaborative "community of practice" that was directed using the following methods:

- Quarterly program education events. Initially, these focused on presenting examples of successful

implementation, along with support and ideas, to ensure teams returned to their trusts with all the products they needed to facilitate prompt local implementation.

- Mentoring opportunities and on-site learning from reference sites in London, to demonstrate enhanced recovery in operation.
- Explicit direction and homework requests from the program's leadership so that Trust teams knew what was required of them to prove delivery.[21]

As the program progressed, regional and national learning events focused less on external expertise and instead served as a platform for individual hospital teams to present and showcase their achievements and also to ask the community to offer solutions for issues they were facing. This generated an environment of support and recognition for the efforts of the participating teams, along with a healthy element of competition!

The final important factor was a public signing of a joint supportive statement from all the major professional bodies and clinician representatives such as the Royal College of Surgeons and Royal College of Anaesthetists in April 2012, agreeing that ER and GDT was a new standard of care and best practice.

Key success factors for implementation

- Expert clinical and managerial facilitation
- Engagement of senior representatives of key stakeholders
- Executive sponsorship of participating teams secured up front
- Aligning financial and clinical objectives
- Examples of good practice and advice on implementation strategies
- Emphasis on common sense with no overkill on particular improvement methodologies
- Participants treated as adults, with devolved responsibility to plan local implementation
- Progress driven by agreeing goals and deadlines with close monitoring of delivery
- Mandatory data collection central to driving improvement
- Regular "showcasing" by participating teams invaluable to support peer learning
- Unconditional public support from national professional bodies.

References

1. Cooksey D. *A Review of UK Healthcare Funding*. London: HM Treasury, 2006.

2. Haines A, Kuruvilla S, Borchert M. Bridging the implementation gap between knowledge and action for health. *Bull World Health Org* 2004;**82**:724–31.

3. Proctor E, Silmere H, Raghavan R, et al. Outcomes for implementation research: conceptual distinctions, measurement challenges, and research agenda. *Admin Policy Ment Health* 2011;**38**:65–76.

4. Urbach DR, Baxter NN. Reducing variation in surgical care. *BMJ* 2005;**330**:1401–2.

5. Kahokehr A, Robertson P, Sammour T, Soop M, Hill AG. Perioperative care: a survey of New Zealand and Australian colorectal surgeons. *Colorect Dis* 2011;**13**:1308–13.

6. Delaney CP, Senagore AJ, Gerkin TM, et al. Association of surgical care practices with length of stay and use of clinical protocols after elective bowel resection: results of a national survey. *Am J Surg* 2010;**199**:299–304.

7. Hasenberg T, Keese M, Langle F, et al. 'Fast-track' colonic surgery in Austria and Germany – results from the survey on patterns in current perioperative practice. *Colorect Dis* 2009;**11**(2):162–7.

8. McGlynn EA, Asch SM, Adams J, et al. The quality of health care delivered to adults in the United States. *N Engl J Med* 2003;**348**:2635–45.

9. Baker R, Camosso-Stefinovic J, Gillies C, Shaw EJ, et al. Tailored interventions to overcome identified barriers to change: effects on professional practice and health care outcomes. *Cochrane Database Syst Revs* 2010 (3):CD005470.

10. Cabana MD, Rand CS, Powe NR, et al. Why don't physicians follow clinical practice guidelines? A framework for improvement. *JAMA* 1999;**282**:1458–65.

11. MTG3 CardioQ-ODM oesophageal doppler monitor (2011) National Institute for Health and Clinical Excellence. http://guidance.nice.org.uk/MTG3.

12. Powell-Tuck J, Gosling P, Lobo DN, et al. British Consensus Guidelines on Intravenous Fluid Therapy for Adult Surgical Patients (GIFTASUP). 2011. http://www.surgicalresearch.org.uk.

13. Srinivasa S, Kahokehr A, Soop M, Taylor M, Hill AG. Goal-directed fluid therapy-a survey of anaesthetists in the UK, USA, Australia and New Zealand. *BMC Anesthesiol* 2013;**13**:5.

14. Quality, Innovation, Productivity and Prevention (QIPP) Case Series. Available from: http://www.evidence.nhs.uk/qipp.

15. Brandstrup B, Svendsen PE, Rasmussen M, et al. Which goal for fluid therapy during colorectal surgery is followed by the best outcome: near-maximal stroke volume or zero fluid balance? *Br J Anaesth* 2012;**109**:191–9.

16. Srinivasa S, Taylor MH, Singh PP, et al. Randomized clinical trial of goal-directed fluid therapy within an enhanced recovery protocol for elective colectomy. *Br J Surg* 2013;**100**:66–74.

17. Hamilton MA, Cecconi M, Rhodes A. A systematic review and meta-analysis on the use of preemptive hemodynamic intervention to improve postoperative outcomes in moderate and high-risk surgical patients. *Anesth Analg* 2011;**112**:1392–402.

18. Knott A, Pathak S, McGrath JS, et al. Consensus views on implementation and measurement of enhanced recovery after surgery in England: Delphi study. *BMJ Open* 2012;**2**.

19. Lefrant JY, Bruelle P, Aya AG, et al. Training is required to improve the reliability of esophageal Doppler to measure cardiac output in critically ill patients. *Intens Care Med* 1998;**24**:347–52.

20. Challand C, Struthers R, Sneyd JR, et al. Randomized controlled trial of intraoperative goal-directed fluid therapy in aerobically fit and unfit patients having major colorectal surgery. *Br J Anaesth* 2012;**108**:53–62.

21. Grace C, Kuper M, Weldon S, et al. Service redesign. Fitter, faster: improved pathways speed up recovery. *Health Serv J* 2011;**121**:28–30.

22. Fulfilling the potential: a better journey for patients, a better deal for the NHS. http://www.improvement.nhs.uk/documents/er_better_journey.pdf.

Chapter

32

Decision support and closed-loop systems for hemodynamic optimization and fluid management

Joseph Rinehart

Introduction

In 2001, the National Institutes of Health identified the variance in health care practices across different institutions and providers, and the inequalities this created as one of the challenges of the modern age of medicine.[1] Reducing variability in testing, treatment, and outcomes between institutions and providers will be a major focus of health care reform in the coming decades, as insurers and governments seek to obtain maximum value for cost from the health care system. Clinical decision support systems (CDSS) and closed-loop (CL) systems are two approaches to standardizing protocols and practices for clinical care.

Decision support for hemodynamic and fluid management

Clinical decision support systems come in many forms. Pop-up alerts in electronic health records, physician order-entry alerts and notices, clinical guidelines and clinical pathways, and premade order sets are all forms of decision support that are readily recognized as such. But even premade note templates and EMR patient summary pages are a form of decision support; the former because they provide a guide for the practitioner as to what information to seek and record, the latter because they present all of the relevant information in a context from which the practitioner can more readily analyze and act upon the available data.[2] In examining the modern practice environment, it becomes obvious that decision support tools are pervasive.

There are primarily two classes of decision support – active and passive. Passive decision support must be accessed by the provider in some fashion in order to "work"; document templates and medication dosing ranges in ordering forms are examples of passive decision support. Active decision support, on the other hand, may actually interrupt the provider to alert him or her of some event or otherwise present information to the provider that was not necessarily being sought. Graphical displays and alarms are an example of active decision support, as are "pop-up" alerts and direct-to-provider pages. Both types have a role in clinical care, but active CDSS is actually more difficult to implement properly because of the factors discussed below.

Decision support – design

A large determinant of the efficacy of decision support tools is the design of the tool. For applications such as document templates, design may simply mean the elements that are included or excluded from the template. For active real-time decision support systems, design refers to the entire implementation of the decision support, including graphical elements, decision trees, and user interaction. All must be carefully planned for optimal use.[2] There are entire fields of study devoted to human factors and good design principles for usability, and these principles play a very real role in how clinical decision support tools are received and actually used.[3]

One of the current challenges faced by clinical care providers is that all of the monitors and clinical systems a provider interacts with are designed by different companies. Each of these companies presents information differently; different colors mean different things on different systems, information such as patient name and ID may be located in

Perioperative Hemodynamic Monitoring and Goal Directed Therapy, ed. Maxime Cannesson and Rupert Pearse.
Published by Cambridge University Press. © Cambridge University Press 2014.

different places on displays, and even alarms and alerts are implemented uniquely. Instead of having to learn a standard convention, providers must learn the nuances of every device and this can lead to errors. Common standards and design elements (fonts, units, color schemes, lists, etc.) across an institution's systems is one factor that could substantially improve usability, but may be difficult to achieve in practice.[2] One such effort to provide standardization was undertaken, however, by the NHS in the UK and Microsoft.[4] The goal of this initiative is to provide a common appearance to similar information across health applications, allowing users to rapidly identify the information they need.

The key characteristics that make medical information useful to practitioners are relevance, validity, and accessibility.[5] Other factors which contribute, however, are clinical context of the information and acceptability.[6] Context of the information is important because, even if information is relevant, valid, and easily accessible, if it does not guide decision making in a meaningful way (whether or not to apply treatment, or the odds of developing a disease), then it is not useful. For example, a rule set that identifies a disease with 80% accuracy is not useful if the 20% of misidentified patients will have bad outcomes that could have been prevented with low-risk treatment. It makes more sense just to give everyone at risk the treatment until a better diagnostic rule set is found. Acceptability plays a role in advice that may be accurate, but will be ignored for medico-legal or financial reasons. A good example is CDSS that help triage patients in the emergency room – if the medico-legal risk of a missed diagnosis is sufficiently high, then all patients will receive treatment, despite advice that it is not indicated.

Another key element of good CDSS is providing relevant information at the time it is needed. For example, having patient allergy list and body weight visible (or readily available) when entering medication orders is obviously relevant. A pop-up alert during cardiopulmonary bypass, reminding a care provider that the current patient is due for colonoscopy screening, is obviously not relevant and may even be dangerous if it distracts the provider from essential tasks. Evidence to date shows that the more specific and appropriate the advice a diagnostic system can give, the more it will be accepted by clinicians; low specificity and relevance quickly results in system fatigue and dismissal of the advice.[7]

Improving human-user interfaces has been identified as one of the most important challenges facing CDSS development.[8,9] At the very least, interface design choices should be tested and refined by the intended users of the system. Good graphical displays can improve accuracy and reduce decision making time, while increasing adherence to established protocols. Indeed, usability testing is a requirement by the FDA for medical devices, though the rigor of testing is often left to the discretion of the device developer.

Decision support – clinical impact

Studies have examined the impact of CDSS and have found that, regardless of whether commercially developed or locally developed, they are effective in improving process measures – hospital guidelines are followed more frequently and recommended treatments are actually prescribed more often. There is very sparse evidence for clinical outcome improvements, workload benefits, economic impacts, or efficiency gains, however.[10,11] This may be due more to difficulty in designing and executing studies that focus on these factors as opposed to a lack of actual effect, but unfortunately many studies that did attempt to examine these factors were equivocal.[12–14]

For example, specific CDSS were able to show a reduction in variance in order sets in the NICU, an improvement in blood utilization based on recommended guidelines, and a reduction in length of time of ER visits.[15–18] A study designed to look at the impact on clinical outcomes in the ICU, however, did not show any significant gains.[19]

While optimal patient outcomes with the most efficient possible use of resources is the ultimate goal of process improvement in health care, the existing evidence base alone is more than enough justification for implementation of CDSS in many situations. The proven ability of CDSS to reduce variability in practice is a laudable and necessary first step in any process improvement pathway, for as long as practice is "provider dependent" there is no true underlying "process" that can improved upon. Standardization must therefore precede efforts aimed at improving patient outcomes.

Another benefit of CDSS (and CL systems) is that they enable non-expert users to achieve expert-grade clinical performance. For example, Sondergaard et al. developed a computerized clinical decision support system making recommendations to novices regarding goal directed fluid therapy, and found a high concordance between the recommendations of the system and the actions of expert anesthesiologists. As such, this study is a good example of an "exportable expert" that could be used by practitioners with minimal training to obtain near equivalent quality GDT to the experts.[20]

Decision support – challenges

Despite the safety and standardization gains that CDSS can provide, there are a variety of challenges that must be overcome. As already discussed, good design and implementation are essential for optimal impact of CDSS. There are other considerations that limit or otherwise make CDSS complicated, however. For example, hospitals and health systems require a supportive infrastructure before CDSS can be implemented.[21] Also, there is no standardization of codification of data with CDSS, making data sharing and cooperation across systems very difficult.[22]

Another non-trivial factor is that physicians may perceive that advice and guidelines coming from CDSS infringe on their professional autonomy.[22] In some regards, they are right: the CDSS are often recommending a pathway that the physician *should* follow as opposed to following his or her "gut" or personal algorithm. This is an incomplete view, however. CDSS recommend an algorithm in an effort to standardize care and reduce variability between providers and events. This does not mean the provider must *always* follow the advice of the CDSS, however, it just means that deviations from recommended care should be *justified*. As an example, a clinical pathway may recommend beta-blockers as a first-choice therapy for patients with hypertension. In a patient with severe asthma, however, a beta-blocker may not be the best first choice. If the CDSS didn't account for this, a provider would be completely justified in prescribing a different class of agents. As no CDSS can possibly account for all of the potential scenarios, clinical providers are still required to use their own judgment in application of the tool. In fact, one potential new risk introduced by CDSS is automation bias – a tendency to *over*-rely on the information provided by the system.[23] As evidence has shown that the way information is presented to the physician plays a key role in how decision support is accepted and physician attitudes toward the systems,[24] careful design and testing is warranted before clinical implementation.

As noted, timeliness of event reporting and subsequent notification to providers may be a limiting factor in CDS design.[25] In fact, interruptions and the disruption of workflow they bring are a major potential drawback of active decision support systems. Interruptions have variable influences (sometimes positive, sometimes negative) on workflow,[26] and often lead to reduction of time and attention to clinical tasks, and interrupted tasks may not be returned to a significant proportion of the time.[27]

Decision support for hemodynamic and fluid management

CDSS for hemodynamic and fluid management are still in their early stages, especially in the intraoperative and critical care environments. Perhaps the most-studied CDSS "class" in current intraoperative use are the various goal directed fluid therapy protocols, the best known of which is probably the "Rivers" protocol for sepsis.[28] Following this pathway resulted in a 30% reduction in mortality in ICU patients presenting with sepsis. Subsequently, a variety of studies looking at similar protocols in surgical and intensive care patients have shown benefits ranging from improved outcomes to lower length of stay.[29–32] Protocols like these will doubtlessly continue to be studied and improved upon in the coming years. In addition to recommendations for fluid administration, the Rivers protocol also includes inotropic and vasoactive agents. CDSS for pharmacologic agents like these are not really found outside of more comprehensive management protocols because of the risks of under-resuscitation if a vasopressor is started instead of proper volume replacement therapy.

Since the development of the Rivers sepsis protocol, CDS tools have been developed for other specific scenarios including massive transfusion[3] and battlefield trauma.[33] One study looking at fluid resuscitation following severe burns in ICU patients showed a reduction in crystalloid volumes, while simultaneously keeping patients within urinary output targets a higher percentage of the time.[34] Another study on trauma patients showed that real-time CDSS resulted in improved protocol compliance and reduced errors and morbidity when applied during the first 30 minutes of trauma resuscitation.[35] CDSS have also been shown to help providers maintain a higher MAP in an ICU setting versus a standard alarm-based monitor.[36]

It is likely that hemodynamic management will become more heavily guided by CDSS like these in the coming years, especially given the impressive results that many of these studies have reported on outcomes. From there, protocol variations can be tested and steadily improved upon for patient, surgical, or disease-based factors.

Closed-loop hemodynamic and fluid management

A control unit that measures some variable in a system and then intervenes in the same system based on the measurement is a closed-loop (Figure 32.1). Simple common examples are household air conditioners and automobile cruise control; a sophisticated example is airline autopilot. Despite their ubiquity in engineering and life in general, they have not found wide use in medical applications to date, at least not from the standpoint of the clinician. The lag between the potential applications and implementation in medicine is largely due to regulatory factors, the complicated nature of biologic systems, inaccuracies in measurement methodologies, and physician acceptance.[37] Nevertheless, the stability and consistency afforded by well-designed closed-loops makes them potentially powerful tools for improving patient care, while reducing costs,[38] and they are beginning to find use in clinical care.

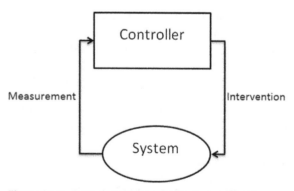

Figure 32.1. Basic closed-loop scheme. A controller takes some form of measurement from a system; it then uses that measurement to direct some form of intervention on the system. A simple example is home air conditioning: the system is the house, the measurement is the thermometer reading, and the intervention is heating or cooling by the unit.

Probably the best known medical example is the "artificial pancreas" – the idea of an automated insulin pump, which matches insulin level to glucose level and can maintain tight control with minimal patient interaction. The limiting factor in developing these systems to date has primarily been the quality of the insulin sensor, but otherwise the control algorithms themselves have been studied by a variety of groups in both simulation and clinical settings.[39–43]

Closed-loop research for hemodynamic control began in 1979 with research into heart rate control during rehabilitation[44] and computer-controlled nitroprusside infusions for hypertension.[45] Pacemakers, of course, are closed-loop devices, many of which have sophisticated respiratory rate and atrial tracking algorithms, which attempt to optimize heart rate to physiologic demand.

Closed-loop hemodynamic management

As noted above, closed-loop control of hemodynamic parameters really began in the late 1970s with work on computer-controlled nitroprusside infusions.[45] Nitroprusside has actually been the most heavily investigated vasoactive agent, probably because its short duration of action makes it easy to titrate. Additional studies were published through the 1980s and 1990s, all of which showed tighter and more consistent control with the closed-loop system.[46–50] Very little work has been published on nitroprusside in the last 15 years or so, however.

Other studies have been published, looking at blood pressure control in critical care settings, using vasopressors to support blood pressure,[51–57] treat circulatory shock[58] or in one case, study efficiency of weaning from vasopressors.[59] A recent study looking at closed-loop control of phenylephrine infusion for blood pressure support during spinal anesthesia showed tighter control of patient blood pressure in the target range.[60]

Despite more than 30 years of research into closed-loop controllers for direct management of infusion of vasoactive agents, to date, no systems have been widely accepted or commercialized. The reasons for this are probably myriad, but one of the chief difficulties is ensuring patient safety with agents that may literally be supporting life, or in the case of nitroprusside, have a very narrow safety margin with severe consequences of overdose. These features don't make closed-loop control of vasoactive

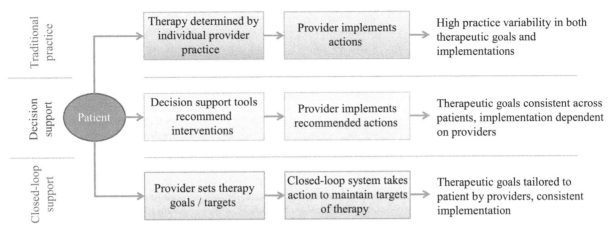

Figure 32.2. Roles of clinical decision support (CDS) and closed-loop (CL) in clinical care and comparison to traditional practice. Both CDS and CL reduce variability in practice. CDS helps with selection of appropriate interventions, thereby reducing variability, but is dependent on providers for acceptance and implementation. CL requires a deeper understanding of both the system and the therapy goals so that the providers can set appropriate targets, but once set the system will autonomously perform the interventions in a consistent manner.

agents impossible or even impractical – after all, we let computers manage commercial flights all the time and they have an incredible safety record – but the overall design, safety, and regulatory challenges have not been worth the potential commercial benefit to date. These factors may be changing, however, as cost pressure on the health care system is driving insurers and regulators to seek consistent outcomes.

Closed-loop fluid administration

Like vasoactive agents, closed-loop control of fluid administration was first reported around 1980 with a computer-controlled IV fluid infusion in burn patients directed by urine output.[61] Additional studies targeting urine output[61] and even postoperative autotransfusion followed.[62] Real work on closed-loop fluid administration has really resumed in earnest in the last decade, however. Along with closed-loop propofol infusions for anesthesia and closed-loop insulin infusion for glucose control, fluid resuscitation has been one of the major medical closed-loop research topics in the last 10 years.[38,63,64]

One of two prime areas of focus has been closed-loop control (as well as decision support) in burn and shock resuscitation.[65–67] A variety of feedback signals have been used to direct infusion rates, including blood pressure and near-infrared spectroscopy, and as with other closed-loop applications these systems show improved consistency and stability of the

controlled variable. Shock and burn resuscitation are a natural target for closed-loop control, as the fluid needs in these patients can be considerable and may vary significantly as the pathophysiology evolves. A closed-loop system can maintain constant vigilance, administering fluid when needed and backing off when patients stabilize.

The other area of active research is intraoperative fluid administration. A great deal of work has shown that various goal directed fluid therapy approaches can improve patient outcomes and reduce length of stay.[29] These protocols, however, can be time-consuming to implement and require a constant high level of vigilance by the care provider, which may distract from other essential tasks. Automation of goal directed fluid therapy with a closed-loop system can ease implementation and standardize performance on these protocols. Simulation and engineering work, as well as animal studies, suggest that this approach may be clinically effective.[64,68–70]

Conclusions

Decision support and closed-loop systems are still finding their place in hemodynamic and fluid management (Figure 32.2). Given the increasing attention being paid to disparities in outcomes and care decisions across providers and institutions, it is likely that the coming years will see an increase in development and use of tools like these to standardize health care delivery.

References

1. Medicine Io. *Crossing the Quality Chasm: A New Health System for the 21st Century*. National Academy of Sciences Washington DC, 2001.

2. Horsky J, Schiff GD, Johnston D, et al. Interface design principles for usable decision support: a targeted review of best practices for clinical prescribing interventions. *J Biomed Inform* 2012;**45**(6):1202–16.

3. Enticott JC, Jeffcott S, Ibrahim JE, et al. A review on decision support for massive transfusion: understanding human factors to support the implementation of complex interventions in trauma. *Transfusion* 2012;**52**(12):2692–705.

4. Microsoft. Microsoft Health Common User Interface. 2010; Available from: http://www.mscui.net/.

5. Shaughnessy AF, Slawson DC, Bennett JH. Becoming an information master: a guidebook to the medical information jungle. *J Fam Pract* 1994;**39**(5):489–99.

6. Ahmadian L, van Engen-Verheul M, Bakhshi-Raiez F, et al. The role of standardized data and terminological systems in computerized clinical decision support systems: literature review and survey. *Int J Med Inform* 2011;**80**(2):81–93.

7. Jaspers MW, Smeulers M, Vermeulen H, Peute LW. Effects of clinical decision-support systems on practitioner performance and patient outcomes: a synthesis of high-quality systematic review findings. *J Am Med Inform Assoc* 2011;**18**(3):327–34.

8. Sittig DF, Wright A, Osheroff JA, et al. Grand challenges in clinical decision support. *J Biomed Inform* 2008;**41**(2):387–92.

9. Kanstrup AM, Christiansen MB, Nohr C. Four principles for user interface design of computerised clinical decision support systems.

Stud Health Technol Inform 2011;**166**:65–73.

10. Bright TJ, Wong A, Dhurjati R, et al. Effect of clinical decision-support systems: a systematic review. *Ann Intern Med* 2012;**157**(1):29–43.

11. Wolfstadt JI, Gurwitz JH, Field TS, et al. The effect of computerized physician order entry with clinical decision support on the rates of adverse drug events: a systematic review. *J Gen Intern Med* 2008;**23**(4):451–8.

12. Sahota N, Lloyd R, Ramakrishna A, et al. Computerized clinical decision support systems for acute care management: a decision-maker-researcher partnership systematic review of effects on process of care and patient outcomes. *Implement Sci* 2011;**6**:91.

13. Eslami S, Abu-Hanna A, de Jonge E, de Keizer NF. Tight glycemic control and computerized decision-support systems: a systematic review. *Intens Care Med* 2009;**35**(9):1505–17.

14. Eslami S, de Keizer NF, Abu-Hanna A. The impact of computerized physician medication order entry in hospitalized patients–a systematic review. *Int J Med Inform* 2008;**77**(6):365–76.

15. Taylor JA, Loan LA, Kamara J, Blackburn S, Whitney D. Medication administration variances before and after implementation of computerized physician order entry in a neonatal intensive care unit. *Pediatrics* 2008;**121**(1):123–8.

16. Adams ES, Longhurst CA, Pageler N, et al. Computerized physician order entry with decision support decreases blood transfusions in children. *Pediatrics* 2011;**127**(5):e1112–19.

17. Spalding SC, Mayer PH, Ginde AA, Lowenstein SR, Yaron M. Impact of computerized physician

order entry on ED patient length of stay. *Am J Emerg Med* 2011;**29**(2):207–11.

18. Schneider E, Franz W, Spitznagel R, Bascom DA, Obuchowski NA. Effect of computerized physician order entry on radiologic examination order indication quality. *Arch Intern Med* 2011;**171**(11):1036–8.

19. Al-Dorzi HM, Tamim HM, Cherfan A, et al. Impact of computerized physician order entry (CPOE) system on the outcome of critically ill adult patients: a before-after study. *BMC Med Inform Decis Mak* 2011;**11**:71.

20. Sondergaard S, Wall P, Cocks K, Parkin WG, Leaning MS. High concordance between expert anaesthetists' actions and advice of decision support system in achieving oxygen delivery targets in high-risk surgery patients. *Br J Anaesth* 2012;**108**(6):966–72.

21. Gamble KH. Wired for CPOE. CIOs are finding that computerized physician order entry starts with a solid infrastructure. *Healthc Inform* 2009;**25**(13):30–2.

22. Walter Z, Lopez MS. Physician acceptance of information technologies: role of perceived threat to professional autonomy. *Decis Support Syst* 2008;**46**(1):206–15.

23. Goddard K, Roudsari A, Wyatt JC. Automation bias—a hidden issue for clinical decision support system use. *Stud Health Technol Inform* 2011;**164**:17–22.

24. Jung M, Hoerbst A, Hackl WO, et al. Attitude of physicians towards automatic alerting in computerized physician order entry systems. A comparative international survey. *Methods Inf Med* 2013;**52**(2):99–108.

25. Epstein RH, Dexter F, Ehrenfeld JM, Sandberg WS. Implications of event entry latency on anesthesia information management

decision support systems. *Anesth Analg* 2009;**108**(3):941–7.

26. Li SY, Magrabi F, Coiera E. A systematic review of the psychological literature on interruption and its patient safety implications. *J Am Med Inform Assoc* 2012;**19**(1):6–12.

27. Westbrook JI, Coiera E, Dunsmuir WT, et al. The impact of interruptions on clinical task completion. *Qual Saf Health Care* 2010;**19**(4):284–9.

28. Rivers E, Nguyen B, Havstad S, et al. Early goal-directed therapy in the treatment of severe sepsis and septic shock. *N Engl J Med* 2001;**345**(19):1368–77.

29. Hamilton MA, Cecconi M, Rhodes A. A systematic review and meta-analysis on the use of preemptive hemodynamic intervention to improve postoperative outcomes in moderate and high-risk surgical patients. *Anesth Analg* 2011;**112**(6):1392–402.

30. Lopes MR, Oliveira MA, Pereira VO, et al. Goal-directed fluid management based on pulse pressure variation monitoring during high-risk surgery: a pilot randomized controlled trial. *Crit Care* 2007;**11**(5):R100.

31. Pearse R, Dawson D, Fawcett J, et al. Early goal-directed therapy after major surgery reduces complications and duration of hospital stay. A randomised, controlled trial [ISRCTN38797445]. *Crit Care* 2005;**9**(6):R687–93.

32. Gan TJ, Soppitt A, Maroof M, et al. Goal-directed intraoperative fluid administration reduces length of hospital stay after major surgery. *Anesthesiology* 2002;**97**(4):820–6.

33. Salinas J, Nguyen R, Darrah MI, et al. Advanced monitoring and decision support for battlefield critical care environment. *US Army Med Dept J* 2011: 73–81.

34. Salinas J, Chung KK, Mann EA, et al. Computerized decision support system improves fluid resuscitation following severe burns: an original study. *Crit Care Med* 2011;**39**(9):2031–8.

35. Fitzgerald M, Cameron P, Mackenzie C, et al. Trauma resuscitation errors and computer-assisted decision support. *Arch Surg* 2011;**146**(2):218–25.

36. Giuliano KK, Jahrsdoerfer M, Case J, Drew T, Raber G. The role of clinical decision support tools to reduce blood pressure variability in critically ill patients receiving vasopressor support. *Comput Inform Nurs* 2012;**30**(4):204–9.

37. Rinehart J, Liu N, Alexander B, Cannesson M. Review article: closed-loop systems in anesthesia: is there a potential for closed-loop fluid management and hemodynamic optimization? *Anesth Analg* 2012;**114**(1):130–43.

38. Dumont GA, Ansermino JM. Closed-loop control of anesthesia: a primer for anesthesiologists. *Anesth Analg* 2013;**117**(5):1130–8.

39. Abbes IB, Richard PY, Lefebvre MA, Guilhem I, Poirier JY. A closed-loop artificial pancreas using a proportional integral derivative with double phase lead controller based on a new nonlinear model of glucose metabolism. *J Diabetes Sci Technol* 2013;**7**(3):699–707.

40. Dauber A, Corcia L, Safer J, et al. Closed-loop insulin therapy improves glycemic control in children aged <7 years: a randomized controlled trial. *Diabetes Care* 2013;**36**(2):222–7.

41. Elleri D, Allen JM, Kumareswaran K, et al. Closed-loop basal insulin delivery over 36 hours in adolescents with type 1 diabetes: randomized clinical trial. *Diabetes Care* 2013;**36**(4):838–44.

42. Kovatchev BP, Renard E, Cobelli C, et al. Feasibility of outpatient fully integrated closed-loop control: first studies of wearable artificial pancreas. *Diabetes Care* 2013;**36**(7):1851–8.

43. Hovorka R. Closed-loop insulin delivery: from bench to clinical practice. *Nat Rev Endocrinol* 2011;**7**(7):385–95.

44. Aseltine RG, Jr., Feldman CL, Paraskos JA, Moruzzi RL. A simple device for closed loop heart rate control during cardiac rehabilitation. *IEEE Trans Biomed Eng* 1979;**26**(8):456–64.

45. Hammond JJ, Kirkendall WM, Calfee RV. Hypertensive crisis managed by computer controlled infusion of sodium nitroprusside: a model for the closed loop administration of short acting vasoactive agents. *Comput Biomed Res* 1979;**12**(2):97–108.

46. Petre JH, Cosgrove DM, Estafanous FG. Closed loop computerized control of sodium nitroprusside. *Trans Am Soc Artif Intern Organs* 1983;**29**:501–5.

47. Rosenfeldt FL, Chang V, Grigg M, et al. A closed loop microprocessor controller for treatment of hypertension after cardiac surgery. *Anaesth Intens Care* 1986;**14**(2):158–62.

48. Reid JA, Kenny GN. Evaluation of closed-loop control of arterial pressure after cardiopulmonary bypass. *Br J Anaesth* 1987;**59**(2):247–55.

49. Bednarski P, Siclari F, Voigt A, Demertzis S, Lau G. Use of a computerized closed-loop sodium nitroprusside titration system for antihypertensive treatment after open heart surgery. *Crit Care Med* 1990;**18**(10):1061–5.

50. Mackenzie AF, Colvin JR, Kenny GN, Bisset WI. Closed loop control of arterial hypertension following intracranial surgery using sodium nitroprusside. A comparison of intra-operative

halothane or isoflurane. *Anaesthesia* 1993;**48**(3):202–4.

51. Mason DG, Packer JS, Cade JF, McDonald RD. Closed-loop management of blood pressure in critically ill patients. *Australas Phys Eng Sci Med* 1985;**8**(4):164–7.

52. Colvin JR, Kenny GN. Development and evaluation of a dual-pump microcomputer-based closed-loop arterial pressure control system. *Int J Clin Monit Comput* 1989;**6**(1):31–5.

53. Murchie CJ, Kenny GN. Comparison among manual, computer-assisted, and closed-loop control of blood pressure after cardiac surgery. *J Cardiothorac Anesth* 1989;**3**(1):16–19.

54. McKinley S, Cade JF, Siganporia R, et al. Clinical evaluation of closed-loop control of blood pressure in seriously ill patients. *Crit Care Med* 1991;**19**(2):166–70.

55. Martin JF. Closed-loop control of arterial pressure during cardiac surgery. *J Clin Monit* 1992;**8**(3):252–5.

56. Nafz B, Persson PB, Ehmke H, Kirchheim HR. A servo-control system for open- and closed-loop blood pressure regulation. *Am J Physiol* 1992;**262**(2 Pt 2):F320–5.

57. Potter DR, Moyle JT, Lester RJ, Ware RJ. Closed loop control of vasoactive drug infusion. A preliminary report. *Anaesthesia* 1984;**39**(7):670–7.

58. Mason DG, Packer JS, Cade JF, Siganporia RJ. Closed-loop management of circulatory shock. *Australas Phys Eng Sci Med* 1988;**11**(4):133–42.

59. Merouani M, Guignard B, Vincent F, et al. Norepinephrine weaning in septic shock patients by closed loop control based on fuzzy logic. *Crit Care* 2008;**12**(6):R155.

60. Luginbuhl M, Bieniok C, Leibundgut D, et al. Closed-loop control of mean arterial blood pressure during surgery with alfentanil: clinical evaluation of a novel model-based predictive controller. *Anesthesiology* 2006;**105**(3):462–70.

61. Bowman RJ, Westenskow DR. A microcomputer-based fluid infusion system for the resuscitation of burn patients. *IEEE Trans Biomed Eng* 1981;**28**(6):475–9.

62. Blankenship HB, Wallace FD, Pacifico AD. Clinical application of closed-loop postoperative autotransfusion. *Med Prog Technol* 1990;**16**(1–2):89–93.

63. Hovorka R. The future of continuous glucose monitoring: closed loop. *Curr Diabetes Rev* 2008;**4**(3):269–79.

64. Rinehart J, Alexander B, Le Manach Y, et al. Evaluation of a novel closed-loop fluid-administration system based on dynamic predictors of fluid responsiveness: an in silico simulation study. *Crit Care* 2011;**15**(6):R278.

65. Chaisson NF, Kirschner RA, Deyo DJ, et al. Near-infrared spectroscopy-guided closed-loop resuscitation of hemorrhage. *J Trauma* 2003;**54**(5 Suppl): S183–92.

66. Hoskins SL, Elgjo GI, Lu J, et al. Closed-loop resuscitation of burn shock. *J Burn Care Res* 2006;**27**(3):377–85.

67. Salinas J, Drew G, Gallagher J, et al. Closed-loop and decision-assist resuscitation of burn patients. *J Trauma* 2008;**64**(4 Suppl):S321–32.

68. Rinehart J, Lee C, Cannesson M, Dumont G. Closed-loop fluid resuscitation: robustness against weight and cardiac contractility variations. *Anesth Analg* 2013;**117**(5):1110–18.

69. Rinehart J, Lee C, Canales C, et al. Closed-loop fluid administration compared to anesthesiologist management for hemodynamic optimization and resuscitation during surgery: an in vivo study. *Anesth Analg* 2013;**117**(5):1119–29.

70. Rinehart J, Chung E, Canales C, Cannesson M. Intraoperative stroke volume optimization using stroke volume, arterial pressure, and heart rate: closed-loop (learning intravenous resuscitator) versus anesthesiologists. *J Cardiothorac Vasc Anesth* 2012; **26**(5):933–9.

Index

13% difference, 9
30% percentage error, 123, 125, 134
95% limit of agreement, 9–11, 122–4, 174

AAP Patient Centered Medical Home, 25
abdominal surgery, 238, 257–60
absolute hypovolemia, 213
ACC/AHA guidelines, 5, 15, 39, 137
accuracy of individual readings, 121, 123
active decision support, 267
acute heart failure, 29
acute kidney injury (AKI), 191, 204
acute renal failure, 76, 110
acute respiratory distress syndrome (ARDS), 140, 163, 165, 168
adenylate cyclase (AC), 85
adrenergic agonists, 192
advanced monitoring, 107, 114–17
advanced practice nurses, 250
aerobic exercise, 37, 51
Affordable Care Act, 25
afterload, 101
    static heart–lung interactions, 102
    stroke volume and, 102
airway pressure release ventilation (APRV), 249
albumin, 78, 80, 238
alpha-adrenergic agonists, 52, 87
alpha-adrenergic receptors, 42, 85
American College of Surgeons (ACS), 1
anaerobic metabolism, 113
anaerobic threshold (AT), 5
anemia, 62, 67, 193
    hospital-acquired, 70
    patient blood management, 66–8
    physiologic adaptation to, 65–6
anesthesia
    CNAP study, 177
    management, 231
    mortality rates, 14
    safety record, 25
anesthesia led integrated team, 26, 263

anesthetic depth, 225
    electroencephalography and, 226–7
    hypotension and mortality, 224
    neuro-cardiovascular control, 224–5
anesthetists
    PAC knowledge deficits, 136
    perioperative physician, 14–15
angina pectoris, 42
angiogenesis, 66
angiotensin converting enzyme inhibitors, 52
animal models, 130
Anrep effect, 30
antibiotics, 194
antidiuretic hormone (ADH), 86
aortic aneurysm repair, 20, 138
aortic root, 41
APACHE II score, 4, 193
APACHE scores, 4
area under the curve (AUC), 11
arginine vasopressin (AVP), 86
arm equilibrium pressure (Parm), 161
Arozullah model, 4
arterial blood gas analysis (aBGA), 113
arterial oxygen delivery. See oxygen delivery
arterial pressure, 34–5, 47–8, 246. See also invasive arterial blood pressure (IBP). See also mean arterial pressure (MAP)
    critical closing, 53–4
    determinants of, 49
    limits of the system, 54
    measurement, 48
    responses to decreased, 52
    responses to increased, 51–2
arterial pressure regulation, 47. See also pulmonary artery catheter
    cardiac output, 50–1
    continuous non-invasive, 173–7
    drawbacks to, 171
    high values of, 48–9
    schema, 49
    vascular resistance, 49–50
arterial pulsatility, 148
arterial resistance, 52
arterial tone, 35

arterial tonometry, 172
arterial waveform analysis, 44, 263
artificial hypervolemia, 77
artificial oxygen carriers, 68
artificial pancreas, 270
ASA classification, 4
ASA Physical Status Score (ASA-PSS), 15
ASA Task Force on Pulmonary Artery Catheterization (2003), 137
at risk patient, 112–13
atherosclerosis, 42
ATP content, 57
atrial contraction, 41
atrial natriuretic peptide (ANP), 78
atrioventricular (AV) node, 39
attitude barriers, 262–3
audit data
    cardiac surgery, 2
    importance of, 1
    peer review, 1
Australian and New Zealand Audit of Surgical Mortality (ANZASM), 1
automation bias, 269
autoregulation of coronary flow, 41

bacterial peritonitis, 56
barbiturates, 187
Bard PowerPICC, 248
baroreceptor regulation, 49, 51–2
base deficit, 205, 207
base excess, 113
baseline cardiac output, 10
baseline LV reserve, 160
BASES trial, 82
Bennett, Dr David, xii
benzodiazepines, 187
best practice, 21
beta-adrenergic receptors, 42, 85
beta-blockers, 21, 39, 225, 269
bias, 9, 123–5, 200
    automation, 269
bicarbonate, 113
bioimpedance, 112, 114, 120, 147, 150
    thoracic, 150, 206
biomarkers, 4–5
    gray zone, 12
bioreactance, 112, 114, 134, 147, 150
BioZ, 147, 150

bispectral index, 224, 226
　mortality and, 227
　postoperative recovery, 227
　readings, 227–8
Bland–Altman plot, 9–11, 122–3, 125
　CO device comparison, 134
　interpreting results, 129
　modifications, 123
　parameters presented, 124
　validation studies, 174
bleeding patient model, 77
blinding in RCTs, 200, 233
blood gas analysis, 113, 188
blood loss, 62
blood oxygen content, 67
blood pressure, 171–2, 246–7.
　　　See also arterial pressure
blood transfusions, 62, 193–4
　anemia, 67, 193
　patient blood management, 68–9
blood volume, 35–7
Bohr effect, 63
BoMed, 120
brain tissue oxygen monitoring, 69
broad spectrum antibiotics, 194

calcium channel blockers, 52
calibration, imprecise, 122
capacitance, 51
capnography, 111
carbon dioxide rebreathing system,
　115, 147, 149
cardiac arrhythmia, 116, 165, 167
cardiac cycle, 40–1
　pressure and volume in, 40
cardiac events, major, 226
cardiac function, 39, 50–1, 107
　and hypotension, 53
　evaluation, 110
　increase in, 52
cardiac function curve.
　　　See Frank–Starling curve
cardiac function index, 139–40, 214
cardiac output, 97, 107
　arterial pressure, 49
　continuous assessment, 117
　decrease in, 52
　delta, 123, 125, 127–8
　dopamine effect on, 88
　oxygen delivery/consumption, 37–8
　PAC measurements, 134–5
　partial CO_2-rebreathing technique,
　　115
　perioperative optimization, 151, 197
　regulation, 50–1
　right atrial pressure, 36
　$ScvO_2$ and, 186
　systemic vascular resistance and, 110
　vasopressin effect on, 87

cardiac output measurement, 8, 123
　Bland–Altman plot, 9
　correlation, 8
　inaccuracy of, 135
　methodology concerns, 10
　trend analysis, 10
cardiac output monitors, 124, 128
　adaptation to patient, 152
　clinical safety, 121
　cost and availability, 121
　data source combination, 121
　ease of use, 120
　GDT endpoints, 204–6
　graphical presentation and analysis,
　　123–5
　institutional decisions, 152
　intended use, 120
　lack of familiarity with, 263
　non-invasive monitoring
　　ultrasound, 146–8
　overview, 147
　reliability and clinical validation,
　　121–2
　reliable trending, 125–7
　statistical approaches, 122–3
　study outcomes, 127–30
　training, 264
cardiac physiology, 39–41
cardiac surgery
　audit data, 2
　blood transfusions, 69, 193
　GDT, 231–5
　GDT endpoints, 206–8
　mortality rates, 233
　non-invasive monitoring, 175–7
　PAC in, 137
　TPTD in, 140
cardiogenic shock, 188, 192
cardiopulmonary bypass (CPB), 88,
　175, 234
cardiopulmonary exercise testing
　(CPET), 5, 16
CardioQ, 122, 146–7
cardio-renal syndrome, 98
cardiorespiratory disease, 110
cardiovascular disease, 29, 44–5,
　213
carotid artery stenting, 20
carotid sinus nerve, 51–2
carotid sinus pressure (CSP), 50, 53
carotid sinus receptors, 49
case-based analysis, 227
ccNexfin device, 116
CDSS. See clinical decision support
　systems
cellular injury, 56
cellular membrane, 75
central aortic absolute pressures, 171
central command, 51

central exclusion zone, 126–7, 129
central venous blood gas analysis
　(cvBGA), 113
central venous lines, 79, 116
　dedicated, 113
　standard, 112
　vs. PAC, 137
central venous oxygen saturation
　($ScvO_2$), 113, 116, 186, 192
　factors affecting, 189
　GDT endpoint, 205, 208
　limitations, 189
　measurement, 187–8, 248
　physiology, 186–7
　validation, 188–9
central venous pressure (CVP), 42, 79,
　107, 112, 117, 192
　fluid challenge, 213–14, 219
　GDT endpoint, 204–5
　measurement, 247–8
cerebral hypoperfusion, 228
cerebrovascular disease, 109
cesarean section, 177
Charlson Age-co-morbidity index
　(CACI), 15
CHEST trial, 21, 81–2
chloride-restrictive resuscitation, 191
citrate synthase, 57–8
Clark-type electrodes, 182
Clavien's model, 3
clinical decision support systems, 267–71
　challenges, 269
　clinical impact, 268
　design, 267
　hemodynamic and fluid
　　management, 269
clinical examination, 108–9
clinical trials, large scale, 20
clinical validation, 121–2
closed-loop control, 270–1
　fluid management, 271
　hemodynamic management, 270
CNAP technique, 112, 116, 151, 174,
　176–7
CO. See cardiac output
coagulation abnormalities, 62
coagulation tests, 69
Codman, Ernest, 1
Colin tonometer, 173
colloids, 74. See also hydroxyethyl
　starch (HES)
　complications from, 259
　fluid challenge, 214, 218
　ICU patients, 80–1, 238
　iso-oncotic, 77–8, 80
　patient outcome, 79
　volume effects, 77–8
colorectal surgery, 18, 257–8, 260
community of practice, 265

co-morbidities, 108
  hemodynamic instability and, 107
compliance, 30, 47, 53
complication rates, 3, 197–8.
    See also post operative
complications
    fluid rates and, 258
    reporting and collating, 198
concordance analysis, 126–7
  interpreting results, 129
concordance limits, 128
confidence interval, 12–13
congestive heart failure, 109
Consensus of 16 paper, 246
continuous CO (CCO), 117
continuous end-diastolic volume
    (CEDV), 117
continuous non-invasive monitoring,
    174
    arterial pressure, 173–7
    measurement techniques, 172–3
    validation, 172
continuous-wave Doppler, 44
contractility, 100–1
co-oximetry, 113, 188
coronary arteries, 41
coronary artery bypass, 137, 232–4
coronary circulation, 41–2
coronary sinus, 41
correlation, 8–9, 130
correlation coefficient, 130
cost analysis, 199
costs, 25, 234, 263–4
CQUIN payment framework, 18–19
CREST trial, 20
CRISTAL trial, 81–2
critical care, 3. *See also* emergency
    department. *See also* ICU patient
critical care nurses, 136
critical closing pressure, 53–4
crystalloids, 74
    complications from, 259
    fluid challenge, 218
    fluid losses, 76
    ICU patients, 81
    patient outcome, 79, 258
    volume effects, 77–8
    volume losses, 76
c-statistic, 11
cutoffs
    gray zone approach, 12–13
    parameter discrimination, 13
    population characteristics, 13
    rules determining, 11–12
cyclic AMP (cAMP), 85
cytochrome complexes, 57–8

day of surgery admission, 19
DDG-330®, 147, 150

DECREASE trials, 21
dedicated central venous lines, 113
delirium, 195
delta cardiac output (ΔCO), 123, 125,
    127–8
delta-POP, 45
Demonstration of Intent, 265
dextrans, 80
diastole, 40
    early, 41
    final phase, 40
    rapid filling phase, 40–1
diastolic BP, 31, 246–7
diastolic compliance, 30
diastolic function, 44
diastolic relaxation (lusitropy), 32
dilution techniques, 43
diphosphoglycerate (2,3-DPG),
    63
direct (pericardial) interaction, 41
discrimination, 11
DO_2. *See* oxygen delivery (DO_2)
dobutamine, 58, 87, 89, 136, 193,
    232
dopamine, 86, 192–3
    physiologic effects, 88
dopamine receptors, 85
dopexamine, 45
Doppler devices, 44, 147, 181.
    See also esophageal Doppler
    ease of use, 120
    echocardiography, 136
    tissue perfusion, 260
double-blinding, 233
double-label blood volume, 75, 78
double-low hypothesis, 228
downstream pressure, 97, 99
driving pressure, 41, 97

echocardiography, 43
    diastology, 44
    Doppler, 136
    GDT endpoints, 206
    limited value of, 16
    transesophageal, 117, 138, 206
ECOM, 147, 150
ejection fraction (EF), 43, 249
ejection phase, 40
elastance, 47–8. *See also* time-varying
electrocardiography (ECG), 107,
    110
electroencephalography, 226–7
emergency department
    GDT, 237
    GDT protocols, 238
    hemodynamic monitoring, 192
    nurses, 250
    older patients, 2
    physicians, 237, 250

end-diastolic volume (EDV), 29–31, 40
    continuous, 117
    global, 116, 140
    left ventricular, 33
    right ventricular, 34
end-expiratory CO_2 levels, 111
end-expiratory occlusion test, 167–8
end-hole measurement, 48
end-systole, 40
end-systolic elastance (E_{es}), 32
end-systolic pressure–volume
    relationship (ESPVR), 32–3
end-systolic volume (ESV), 40
end-tidal anesthetic concentration
    (ETAC), 226–7
endarterectomy, 20
end-expiratory occlusion test, 164
endocardium, 41
endothelial glycocalyx, 80
endothelial surface layer (ESL), 75
endothelial vasoreactivity, 182
endotoxin, 56, 158–9
endpoints
    GDT, 204–8
    hemodynamic and tissue variables,
        205
    optimal, 203
enhanced recovery (ER), 18–19, 27,
    263–5
epicardium, 41
epinene, 86
epinephrine, 86, 89, 193
equilibrium point, 36
equipoise decision, 12
errors
    PACs, 134
    percentage, 122, 125
    precision, 122
    presenting, 122
    understanding, 122
erythropoiesis-stimulating agents
    [ESAs], 67–8
erythropoietin, 66
ESCAPE trial, 133
esCCO™, 147, 150
ESL, 77
esophageal Doppler, 79, 115, 121–2,
    146–7, 151
    algorithm, 264
    GDT endpoint, 205–6, 208
    GDT protocol, 242
    lack of familiarity with, 263
    patient complications, 257–8
    perioperative monitoring, 152
    trials, 256
estrogen, 68
European Society of Anaesthesiology
    (ESA)
    protocols, 238, 241

European Society of Cardiology (ESC) guidelines, 5, 15, 137
European Surgical Outcomes Study, 2
EuroSCORE, 4
euvolemia, 45, 67
EV1000, 116
EV1000 VolumeView, 138
EVAR II trial, 20
evidence-based perioperative care, 262
EVLW, 116
exclusion zone, 127
expanded monitoring, 107, 112–14
exponential decay time, 139
external factors barriers, 262–3
extravascular lung water (EVLW), 116, 139–40
eyeball technique, 248

Fast Fourier transformation, 173
fasting, preoperative, 76
femoral artery catheterization, 138
femoral venous oxygen saturation (SfvO$_2$), 248
femoral venous pressure (FVP), 247
fiberoptic catheters, 188
Fick equation, 186
Fick method, 139
  accuracy of, 134
Fick's principle, 43, 115, 134
financial penalties, 5
Finapres, 173, 175–6
finger cuff, 175–6
finger cuff technology, 149, 151
fixed bias, 9
FloTrac, 147, 151, 232
FloTrac/Vigileo, 116, 121, 148
flow mediated dilatation, 50
flow probes, 130
fluid administration
  goal of, 255
  ICU patient, 238
  intraoperative, 271
  protocol, 240
fluid challenge, 132, 168, 218
  definition, 213
  historic review, 213–14
  literature reports, 215
  physiological rationale, 214–18
  safety, 219
  target and time, 219
  type of fluid, 218
  volume and infusion rate, 218–19
fluid compartments, 75
Fluid Expansion As Supportive Therapy, 191
fluid losses, 76
  crystalloids, 76

fluid management
  CDSS, 269
  clinical practice, 78–82
  closed-loop control, 271
  goals of, 255–61
  guidelines, 255
  outcome-based evidence, 74–5
  protocol, 257, 259
  trials, 256–7
fluid overload, 80, 213, 219, 234
  complications from, 255, 259
fluid replacement formula, 255
fluid repletion, 213
fluid responsiveness, 163
  CVP readings and, 204
  hemodynamic effects, 164–5
  passive leg raising and, 166
  predictors in practice, 168
fluid restriction, 234, 238, 258
fluid resuscitation, 157, 191
  CDSS, 269
  closed-loop control, 271
  under- and over-, 203
fluid shifting types, 78
fluid therapy review, 256
FOCUS trial, 193
forearm BP measurements, 247
four quadrant plot, 125, 127, 129
fragmented perioperative care, 24
Frank–Starling curve, 42, 114, 164
  fluid challenge, 214, 218
  fluid overload and, 234
Frank–Starling relationship, 29–30, 36, 50, 98, 163
functional capacity, 5, 108–9
functional hemodynamics, 112, 248
  assessment, 114
  factors affecting, 249
  monitoring, 151
  parameters, 152

G protein-coupled receptor, 85–6
gastric bypass surgery, 226
gastric tonometry, 183, 205, 208
gastrointestinal surgery, 18, 203
gelatins, 80
global end-diastolic volume (GEDV), 116, 139–40
glycemic control, 194, 250
goal directed fluid management, 18, 255–61
  protocols, 269
goal directed fluid restriction, 234
goal directed therapy (GDT)
  algorithms, 85
  available endpoints, 204–8
  cardiac surgery, 231–5
  cardiovascular disease, 44–5
  criticism of, xi

definition, 237
evidence for benefit of, 197–200
fluid management, 79
goals, 203
heterogeneity, 200
ICU and emergency department, 237
ideal endpoint, 203
implementation, 262–6
implementing and sustaining, 250
improved outcomes, xi
nurse's role in, 246–50
patient blood management, 62
perioperative period, 238
postoperative period, 232
protocols, 238–43
quality of evidence, 200
ScvO$_2$ and, 189
gold standard, 8, 122, 134, 171
Goldman and Lee scores, 4
gravitational energy, 48
gray zone approach, 12–13
guiding fluid therapy, 78–9
gut mucosal hypoperfusion, 232
gut mucosal pH, 231
Guyton's venous return analysis, 50

half-moon plot, 127–8
Holliday–Segar guidelines, 260
head of bed elevation, 249
health care improvement science. See quality improvement
heart failure, 29, 109
heart function curve, 99, 101
heart–lung interactions, 102–4
heart rate (HR)
  anemia, 65
  GDT endpoint, 204–5, 208
hematocrit dilution, 76–7
hematopoiesis, 66–7
hemodynamic monitoring, 29, 42–4. See also cardiac output monitors
  advanced, 114–17
  clinical examination and observation, 108–9
  closed-loop control, 270
  expanded, 112–14
  ICU and ED patients, 192
  indications for, 107–8
  integrative approach, 107–18
  optimization protocol, 239–40
  routine, 110–12
  TPTD, 139
  treatment protocols and, 151–2
  working principle and invasiveness, 115
hemodynamic signals, 164–5
hemodynamically unstable patient, 107–8, 110, 112–13, 213

hemodynamics. *See also* functional hemodynamics
  driving pressure, 98
  mechanical ventilation and, 102–4
  oxygenation and, 95–8
hemoglobin bound oxygen, 63–4
hemoglobin levels, 64, 68
hemoglobin molecule, 63
hemoglobin monitoring, 68, 112
hemoglobin saturation curve, 187
Hemosonics, 146–7
Henderson–Hasselbalch equation, 113
Henry's law, 63
HES. *See* hydroxyethyl starch (HES)
heterogeneity in perfusion, 180
high risk patients, 108, 110
  definition, 199
  mortality rates, 2–3, 14
  short-term mortality, 198–9
  supranormal hemodynamics, 231
  tissue hypoxia, 231
high-risk surgery, 109
  GDT protocols, 240, 242
  microcirculation/mitochondria dysfunction, 58
  patient outcome, 1–6
  ScvO₂ limitations, 189
high-sensitivity C-reactive protein (hs CRP), 4
Hip Fracture Perioperative Network, 15, 18
hip surgery, 193, 238
His–Purkinje system, 40
homeostasis, normal, 37
hospital length of stay, 197–8, 233–4
hospital-acquired anemia (HAA), 70
human-user interfaces, 268
hydralazine, 52
hydrostatic gradient, 48
hydroxyethyl starch (HES), 21, 78–82
hyperchloremia, 191
hyperlactemia, 194
hypertension
  and vascular resistance, 51
  intra-abdominal, 167, 249
hypervolemia, 77
hypoglycemia, 194
hypoperfusion, 109, 113, 234
  cerebral, 228
  gut mucosal, 232
hypotension, 34. *See also* intraoperative hypotension
  anesthetic depth and, 224
  oscillometry measurements, 172
  PACs and, 137
  pathological causes, 53
  systemic, 37

hypovolemia, 30, 36, 67, 213
  cardiac patients and, 234
  detection, 258
  fluid responsivess, 168
  fluid restriction and, 238
  vena cava and, 165
hypoxemia, 110
hypoxia. *See* tissue hypoxia
hypoxia inducible factors (HIFs), 66

ICU patient, 237
  blood transfusions, 193
  fluid administration, 238
  fluid management, 78–82
  GDT, 237
  GDT endpoints, 204, 208
  GDT protocols, 238
  hemodynamic monitoring, 192
  intravenous fluid therapy, 191
  length of stay, 234
  PACs, 132–3, 136
  sedation, 195
implementation of GDT, 262–5
  barriers to, 262–3
  institutional level, 263–4
  key success factors, 265
  national level, 264–6
implementation science, 262
indocyanine green, 150
infusion rate, 214, 219
inoconstrictors, 86, 88–9
inodilators, 87, 89
inotropy, 100–1, 233
inspiratory hold maneuver, 158–61
insulin, 109
integrated care pathway, 26
integrated hemodynamic monitoring, 107–17
interchangeability, 8
interclass correlation coefficient (ICC), 130
intra-abdominal hypertension, 167, 249
intra-abdominal pressure, 117
intra-abdominal surgery, 259
intraoperative fluid administration, 271
intraoperative hypotension, 224–5
  defining, 225
  mortality and, 225
  myocardial and cerebrovascular injury, 226
  perioperative complications, 226
intrathoracic blood volume (ITBV), 139
intrathoracic blood volume index (ITBVI), 233
intrathoracic pressure (PEEP), 102, 117, 167

intrathoracic thermal volume (ITTV), 140
intravascular fluid resuscitation, 191
intravenous fluid therapy, 191
invasive arterial blood pressure (IBP), 107, 112, 246
invasive devices, 117
ischemia, 66, 68, 109
isoproterenol, 87, 89
isovolumic relaxation, 40

Jadad score, 200
joint surgery, 27

kinetic energy, 47–8
knowledge deficits, 135–6, 262–3

lactate, 56, 58, 77
  clearance, 194
  GDT, 205, 207, 232
  levels, 113
  measurement, 248
  microcirculation assessment, 180
LACTATE trial, 20
Laplace relationship, 42, 47
laser Doppler, 181
Lee risk-index, 16, 108
left coronary artery, 41
left ventricular (LV)
  afterload, 31
  compliance, 99
  contractions, 41
  ejection pressure, 31–2
  filling pressures, 35
  function, 29–33
  function curve, 158
  pressure–volume loop, 30–2
  wall stress, 31
length of hospital stay, 197–8, 233–4
liberal versus restrictive (LVR) fluid therapy, 256, 258–60
LiDCO, 116, 121, 206
LiDCOplus, 116, 149, 151
LiDCOrapid, 116, 147, 149
limits of agreement, 125, 127
lithium dilution, 116
long term mortality, 199
low cardiac output syndrome, 234
low-risk surgery protocol, 239
lung auscultation, 109
lung edema, 116

macrocirculation, 95, 104
macro-microcirculatory decoupling, 95, 98
major surgery. *See* high-risk surgery

mean arterial pressure (MAP), 34–5, 37, 110, 112, 171
GDT endpoint, 204–5, 208
mean circulatory pressure (Pmsa), 161–2
fluid challenge, 219
mean difference, 9
mean polar angle, 127
mean systemic filling pressure (Pmsf), 99, 218–19
mean systemic pressure (Pms), 35–7, 157
monitoring, 157–62
stop-flow measures, 157
vascular peripheral stop-flow, 161–2
mechanical ventilation, 102–4
metabolic acidosis, 113
metabolic equivalents, 5, 108
methoxamine, 87
microcirculation, 95, 103, 181
microcirculation changes, 180
clinical examination and biomarkers, 180
consequences of, 56–7
high risk surgery, 58
occlusion tests, 182
relevance of, 58
sepsis, 56–7
sublingual, 57
techniques evaluating, 180–1
videomicroscopy, 181–2
microvascular perfusion, 57–8
mini-fluid challenge, 168
minimally invasive monitoring, 113, 117, 151
missing data, 11
mitochondrial dysfunction
evidence for, 57–8
high risk surgery, 58
relevance of, 58
mitochondrial oxidative phosphorylation, 66
mitral regurgitation, 44
moderate risk surgery protocols, 240, 242
modified risk index, 109
morbidity. See patient complications. See complication rates
mortality benefit, 198
mortality rates, 2–3
anesthesia, 14
bispectral index and, 227
cardiac surgery, 233
high-risk patients, 14
hypotension and, 224–5
intravenous fluid therapy and, 191
long term, 199
microcirculation alterations, 57
postoperative care, 3

postoperative complications, 25
pulmonary artery catheters, 133
short-term, 198–9
subgroup analyses, 199
triple low state and, 228
MostCare, 147–8
mucosal imaging, 181
multidisciplinary teams, 250, 265
muscarinic acetylcholine receptors, 42
muscular activity. See aerobic exercise
myocardial infarction, 42
myocardial injury, perioperative, 226
myocardial ischemia, 226
earliest signs, 40
myocardial oxygen consumption (MVO$_2$), 31, 42
myocardial performance index (MPI), 44
myocardial wall tension, 42
myogenic mechanism, 50

NADH, 57
National Confidential Enquiry into Patient Outcome and Death (NCEPOD), 1, 15
National Consensus statement, 265
National Emergency Laparotomy Audit (NELA), 15, 17
national registries, 1
National Technology Adoption Centre (NTAC), 264
natriuretic peptides (NP), 4, 16
near-infrared spectroscopy (NIRS), 182
neuro-cardiovascular control, 224–5
neuromuscular blockade, 67, 224
Nexfin, 112, 147, 149, 151, 174–6, 206
GDT endpoint, 205, 208
NIBP, 177
NICE protocol, 241–2, 263
NICE-SUGAR trial, 20, 194
NiCO, 147, 149
NICOM, 121, 134, 147, 150
GDT endpoint, 205–6, 208
Nidorf normogram, 122
Nightingale, Florence, 1–2
nitric oxide, 42, 50
nitroprusside, 270
nomograms, 149
non-cardiac surgery
beta-blockers, 21, 39, 225
critical care, 3
mortality rates, 2–3
ScvO$_2$ measures, 188
triple low hypothesis, 227
non-invasive advanced monitoring, 112, 117
non-invasive blood pressure (NIBP), 107, 110, 112, 246

non-invasive monitoring, 116–17, 151. See also NICOM. See also continuous non-invasive monitoring
finger cuffs, 149
pulse wave analysis, 112
non-invasive ultrasound, 146–8
non-splanchnic circulation, 52
norepinephrine, 34, 53, 86, 88, 159–60, 176, 192
first-line vasopressor, 193
normograms, 146
normovolemia, 75, 78
normovolemic hemodilution, 77
NSQIP data, 3, 6, 25
N-terminal pro-B-type natriuretic peptide (NT pro-BNP), 4
nurses
advanced practice, 250
emergency department, 250
knowledge deficits, 136
role in GDT, 246–50

observation step, 108
occlusion testing, 182
odds ratio, 197–8, 256
older patients, 2, 110
oliguria, 204
open loop analysis, 53
operating room (OR), 237
GDT endpoints, 204, 208
GDT protocols, 239–43
organ blood flow, 34–5
organ perfusion. See organ blood flow
orthogonal polarization spectral (OPS) imaging, 181
orthopedic surgery, 177
oscillometry, 110, 171
outcome-based evidence
fluid handling, 74–5
outpatient surgeries, 260
overtreatment, 136
oxygen consumption (VO$_2$), 37–8, 50, 65–6, 96
DO$_2$/VO$_2$ balance, 96
increase in, 187
peak, 5
oxygen content of blood, 64, 67
oxygen debt, xi, 197
oxygen delivery (DO$_2$), 37–8, 63–5, 96
determination, 112
DO$_2$/VO$_2$ balance, 96
perioperative optimization, 197, 231
oxygen delivery index (DO$_2$I), 45
oxygen demand. See oxygen consumption (VO$_2$)
oxygen extraction (EO$_2$), 65
oxygen hemoglobin dissociation curve, 66

oxygen partial pressure (PO$_2$), 63–4, 67

oxygen saturation, 37, 58, 110, 113. *See also* venous oxygen saturation (SvO$_2$). *See also* central venous oxygen saturation (ScvO$_2$)
  tissue, 182

oxygenation. *See also* tissue oxygenation
  adequate, xi
  hemodynamics and, 95–8

PAC. *See* pulmonary artery catheter

pacemaker cells, 39

pacemakers, 270

PAC-Man trial, 133

partial CO$_2$ rebreathing technique, 115, 147, 149

passive decision support, 267

passive leg raising (PLR), 164, 166–7
  GDT endpoint, 205, 207

patient age, 2, 108, 110

patient assessment, improvements in, 15–16

patient at risk, 107

patient bleeding model, 78

Patient Blood Management (PBM), 62–3
  anemia, 66–8
  new standard of care, 69–70
  transfusions and, 68–9

patient complications
  goal directed fluid therapy, 258

patient outcome
  crystalloids, 258
  data in surgery, 79–80
  GDT, xi
  goal directed fluid therapy, 257–8
  major surgery, 1–6
  PACs and, 133, 136
  septic shock, 80–1
  system wide strategies, 5–6

peak oxygen consumption (VO$_2$ peak), 5

peer review, 1

Peňáz principle, 175–6

percentage error, 122, 125, 134, 174

perfect correlation, 8

perfluorocarbons, 68

perfusion improvement, 246

perfusion pressure, 48–9, 97, 107

perioperative health care
  CO optimization, 151
  CO/DO$_2$ optimization, 197
  evidence-based, 262
  new trends, 14

perioperative period, 201, 238

perioperative physician, 14–15

Perioperative Surgical Home (PSH), 15, 22, 24–8
  definition, 25

peripheral edema, 35, 176

peripheral pulse amplification, 171

peripheral venous pressure (PVP), 247

peripherally inserted central venous catheter (PICC), 247

perspiration, 76

pH, 113
  gut mucosal, 231

Pharmacovigilance Risk Assessment Committee (PRAC), 82

phenylephrine, 53, 86–7, 193

photoplethysmography, 173

Physiocal algorithm, 175

PiCCO, 116, 121–2, 138, 151, 206

PiCCOplus, 116

PICO format, 256

PIVOT trial, 20

plasma volume, 77

pleth variability index (PVI), 45, 114, 151
  GDT endpoint, 205, 207–8
  GDT protocol, 240

plethysmogram waveform analysis, 45

plethysmography signal, 165

pleural pressure, 52

pneumonia, 194

PO$_2$. *See* oxygen partial pressure (PO$_2$)

POISE trial, 21, 225

Poiseuille relationship, 47, 49

polar concordance rate, 127

polar plots, 10, 126, 128–9

pop-up alert, 267–8

positive end-expiratory pressure (PEEP), 249

positive pressure ventilation, 103

positive response, fluid challenge, 219

POSSUM score, 4, 15

postoperative complications, 199. *See also* complication rates
  cardiac surgery, 233
  costs, 200, 234
  financial implications, 25
  mortality rates, 25
  prevention of, 25

postoperative morbidity survey, 3, 198

postoperative period
  cardiac surgery, 232
  mortality rates, 3

PPV. *See* pulse pressure variation (PPV)

PRAM, 121

preassessment clinic (PAC), 15

precision error, 122

preload, 51, 107
  heart contraction and, 234
  inotropy and, 100–1
  responsiveness, 163
  static heart-lung interactions, 102
  static indices, 163–4
  stroke volume and, 99
  venous return and, 98–100

preload increase, 43

preload responsive, 30

preload state, 42

preoperative C-reactive protein (CRP), 16

PreSep, 232

Pressure Record Analytic Method (PRAM), 148

pressure support ventilation, 249

prone position, 250

propofol, 187

proportional bias, 9

prostatectomy, 20

protocols
  GDT, 238–43
  hemodynamic monitoring and, 151–2
  perioperative care, 18–21

pseudonormalization, 44

pulmonary arterial hypertension (PAH), 137

pulmonary artery catheter, xi, 76, 79, 114–17, 132–4, 248
  benefits of, 136–7
  clinical safety, 121
  GDT endpoint, 204
  knowledge deficit, 135–6
  overtreatment with, 136
  perioperative indications for, 137–8
  risks from, 134–6, 186

pulmonary artery occlusion pressure (PAOP), 204–5, 214

pulmonary artery pressure (PAP), 117, 248

pulmonary artery systolic pressure (sPAP), 136

pulmonary capillary wedge pressure, 42, 117, 135

pulmonary edema, 35, 103, 139

pulmonary embolism, 36

pulmonary thermal volume (PTV), 140

pulmonary vascular permeability index (PVPI), 139

pulse contour analysis, 138–40, 147–9, 151
  GDT endpoint, 205–6, 208

pulse contour systems, 120

pulse oximetry, 107, 110, 112, 150, 207

pulse pressure variation (PPV), 11, 42, 44–5, 103–4, 112, 114
automated algorithms, 151
GDT endpoint, 205, 207
stroke volume and, 35, 164–5
pulse wave analysis, 113, 115–17
pulse wave transit time, 147, 150
PulseCO™, 149
pulsed dye densitometry, 147, 150
Pulsioflex, 116, 147–8
PVPI, 139

quality improvement, 6, 17–18
quality management, 27
Quality, Productivity and Prevention in Practice (QIPP), 18

radial limits of agreement, 127
radial vectors, 10
RaFTinG trial, 80–2
random errors, 122
randomization, 200
randomized controlled trials (RCTs), 21, 133, 256–9
quality of, 200
rapid filling phase of diastole, 40–1
RCRI risk score, 16
readmissions, costs, 25
receiver operator characteristic (ROC) curve analysis, 126
red blood cell transfusion, 193
reference methods, 11, 122–5
regression analysis, 124, 130
relative hypovolemia, 213
reliability, cardiac monitors, 121–2
renal replacement therapy (RRT), 191
resistance, 47–8
respiratory cost of breathing, 96
respiratory rate, 249
respiratory variation
hemodynamic signals, 164–5
vena cava, 165
return function, 49–50, 52
right atrial pressure (RAP), 33–4, 36, 50, 99, 159
venous return and, 99, 158
right coronary artery, 41
right ventricular
dysfunction, 249
right ventricular (RV)
contractions, 41
filling pressure, 33
function, 29, 33–4
specificity, 101
stroke volume, 158–9
right ventricular (RV) function, 31
risk assessment, 4–5
risk scores, 4

risk stratification, 39
Rivers protocol, 238–9, 269
ROC curves, 11–13
routine monitoring, 107, 110–12
rule set, 268

SAFE study, 238
saline versus albumin fluid evaluation (SAFE), 191
sample size, 129, 233
SaO_2. See total oxygen content of blood (SaO_2)
Scandinavian Starch for Severe Sepsis/Septic Shock (6S) trial, 20, 80–2
scatter plot, 8, 123–4, 127
Scottish Audit of Surgical Mortality (SASM), 1, 17
Scottish Patient Safety Programme (SPSP), 17
$ScvO_2$. See central venous oxygen saturation ($ScvO_2$)
sedation, ICU patient, 195
semi-invasive techniques.
See minimally-invasive monitoring
sensitivity analysis, 197–8, 200
septic shock
antibiotic administration, 194
blood pressure measurements, 246
cardiac output, 37
fluid responsiveness, 163, 168
GDT and, 237, 239
glycocalyx degradation, 80
hemodynamic monitoring, 29
intravenous fluid therapy, 191
lactate measurement, 248
microcirculation in, 56–7
microvascular perfusion, 57
mitochondrial dysfunction, 57–8
outcome data, 80–2
resuscitation, 191
Rivers protocol, 238
$ScvO_2$ monitoring, 188
sublingual microcirculation, 181
vascular tone, 53
vasopressor treatment, 192–3
serial cardiac output readings, 121, 125
series interaction, 41
serum creatinine, 109
shared decision making (SDM), 16–17, 26
short-term mortality, 198–9
shunt, 56
side-hole measurement, 48
sidestream dark field (SDF) imaging, 57, 181
sinoatrial (SA) node, 39
skin perfusion, 180

Snow, John, 1
SOFA score, 58
SOS acronym, 248
speckle laser Doppler, 181
speckle tracking, 44
spinal blockade, 224
splanchnic circulation, 37, 50, 52
spontaneous intermittent mandatory ventilation (SIMV), 249
spread and adoption, 265
SPV. See systolic pressure variation (SPV)
St. George's protocol, 243
stair climbing, 108
stakeholders, 265
standard central venous lines, 112
standard deviation, 122, 124, 129
Starling's law of the heart, 99
statistical analysis, 8–13
comparisons against reference method, 122
differences in, 130
precision error, 122
study design, 123
stop-cursor method, 248
stop-flow measures, Pms, 157
stop-flow vascular pressure, 161–2
strain analysis, 44
stressed volume, 49–50, 99, 218
stroke volume, 29–31
afterload and, 102
anemia, 65
effects on, 97
increase in, 43
inotropy and, 100
main determinants of, 97
optimization, 238
preload and, 99
pulse pressure variation and, 35, 164–5
right ventricular, 158–9
stroke volume index (SVI), 232
stroke volume variation (SVV), 42–3, 114
fluid management protocol, 259
fluid management trials, 259
GDT endpoint, 205, 207
tissue perfusion, 260
stroke work, 30
ST-segment changes, 110
study design, 123, 129
study size, 129
subarachnoid hemorrhage (SAH), 140
subgroup analyses, 198–9
sublingual microcirculation, 57, 181
sublingual PCO_2, 183
superior vena cava (SVC), 187

super-optimization, 203–4
supine position, 249
supranormal hemodynamics, 231
supranormal resuscitation, 199
Surgical Safety Checklist, 20
survival benefit, 199, 203
survival, factors predicting, 45
Surviving Sepsis Campaign, 79, 188, 193, 203
sustainability, 264
sympathetic tone increase, 51
systematic errors, 122
systemic circulation
    two compartment model, 52–3
systemic vascular resistance (SVR), 35, 43, 110
    equation, 43
    FloTrac measurement of, 148
systole, 40
    early, 41
    start of, 40
    time-varying elastance, 32–3
systolic BP, 31, 246–7
    overestimation, 172
systolic function assessment and monitoring, 43–4
systolic pressure variation (SPV), 42, 104

Tei index, 44
terlipressin, 86
test methods, 123–5
therapeutic trial, 29
thermal bolus technique, 116
thermodilution, 9, 121
    accuracy of, 134
    inaccuracy of, 135
    precision errors, 122
    reference method, 122
    transpulmonary, 116, 138–40
thoracic bioimpedance, 150, 206
three-element-Windkessel model, 115
thresholds definition, 11–13
thresholds determination, 13
time plot, 126
time-based analysis, 228
time-dependent analysis, 198
time-varying elastance, 30, 32–3
tissue CO_2 measurements, 183
tissue compartment pressure, 98
tissue dysoxia, 207
tissue hypoperfusion, 234
tissue hypoxia, xi, 56, 64, 66, 231
tissue oxygenation, 97, 107.
    See also oxygenation
tissue perfusion, 260
tissue perfusion imaging, 181, 183

tissue PO_2 and oxygen saturation, 182
TL-200 device, 174
TL-200pro device, 174–5
T-Line, 173–5
total body blood volume, 75
total body water, 75
total hemoglobinHb (SpHb), 68
total oxygen content of arterial blood (CaO_2), 64, 66, 97
total oxygen content of blood (SaO_2), 64, 67, 96
TRACS trial, 193
training program, 264
tranexamic acid, 68
transesophageal echocardiography (TEE), 117, 138, 206
Transfusion Requirements in Critical Care (TRICC) trial, 68, 193
transmural pressure, 47, 98
transplant surgery, 138
transpulmonary thermodilution (TPTD), 116, 138–40
transthoracic Doppler, 115
trauma patients, 188, 269
trend analysis, 10, 121–3, 126–7
tricuspid regurgitation, 135
triple low hypothesis, 224, 227–8
troponins (Tn), 4, 16, 226
two compartment model of systemic circulation, 52–3
two methods measurement, 8–11
    Bland–Altman plot, 9–11
    correlations, 8–9
    methodology concerns, 10
    planning the study, 11
    reporting the results, 11
    trend analysis, 10

UK's National Technology Adoption Center (NTAC), 263
uncalibrated devices, 116
uncalibrated pulse contour analysis, 147
uncalibrated pulse wave analysis, 113, 117
United Kingdom, mortality rates, 14
United States
    mortality rates, 14
    surgical statistics, 24
unstressed blood volume, 99, 218
upper arm BP measurements, 247
upper gastrointestinal (UGI) bleeding, 194
upstream pressure, 97, 99
urine output, 76, 204–5, 208
USCOM, 120–2, 147–8

validation studies, 129
Valsalva maneuver, 52
value in health care, 24
vascular barrier, 75
vascular endothelial growth factor (VEGF), 66
vascular occlusion testing, 182
vascular peripheral stop-flow, 161–2
vascular resistance, 50
    aerobic exercise, 51
    arterial pressure, 49
    distribution of, 54
    hypertension, 51
    regulation, 49–50
vascular surgery, 138
vascular tone loss, 53
vascular unloading method, 173
vascular waterfall effect, 52
vasoconstriction, 87
vasoconstrictors, 34, 86–8
vasodilation, 51, 87
vasodilators, 31, 42, 249
vasopressin, 86, 193
    levels, 192
    physiologic effects, 87–8
vasopressin receptors, 86
vasopressors, 34, 36–7, 192–3, 249.
    See also norepinephrine
    closed-loop control, 270
    exogenous, 54
vena cava, respiratory variation, 165
venous CO_2 measurements, 183
venous communications (Thebesian veins), 41
venous compliance, 51
venous inflow, 214
venous oxygen saturation (SvO_2), 37–8, 113, 186
    GDT endpoint, 205, 207
    GDT parameter, 232
    measurement, 248
    vs. $ScvO_2$, 187
venous pressure, 214
venous resistance, 51–2, 100
venous return, 33, 36, 49, 218
    preload and, 98–100
    resistance to, 36
    right atrial pressure and, 99
venous return curve, 36, 158
    inspiratory hold maneuver, 158–61
ventricular filling, 40–1
ventricular function, 249
ventricular interdependence, 31, 33, 41
ventricular pump function, 29–34
VERIFI algorithm, 176–7

videomicroscopy, 181–3
Vigileo, 206
viscoelastic hemostatic assays (VHAs),
    69
VISEP trial, 80, 82
VO$_2$. *See* oxygen consumption (VO$_2$)
volume clamp method, 173
volume controlled ventilation, 249
volume deficits, 76

volume effects
    crystalloids and colloids, 77–8
    iso-oncotic colloids, 78
volume responsiveness, 42, 132
volume status, 135
volumetric parameters, 116

wall stress, 47
weekend vs. weekday care, 18

weighted mean difference (WMD),
    256
Wesseling approach, 115

Youden index, 12

zero cardiac output–mean arterial
    pressure intercept, 35
zero flow pressure, 35

CPSIA information can be obtained
at www.ICGtesting.com
Printed in the USA
LVHW02*2033191217
560258LV00009B/220/P